Transcription Factors
and Human Disease

OXFORD MONOGRAPHS ON MEDICAL GENETICS

General Editors

Arno G. Motulsky   Martin Bobrow   Peter S. Harper   Charles Scriver

Former Editors

J. A. Fraser Roberts   C. O. Carter

Transcription Factors and Human Disease

Gregg L. Semenza, M.D., Ph.D.

Institute of Genetic Medicine
Johns Hopkins University
School of Medicine

New York   Oxford
Oxford University Press
1998

Oxford University Press

Oxford   New York
Athens   Auckland   Bangkok   Bogota   Buenos Aires   Calcutta
Cape Town   Chennai   Dar es Salaam   Delhi   Florence   Hong Kong   Istanbul
Karachi   Kuala Lumpur   Madrid   Melbourne   Mexico City   Mumbai
Nairobi   Paris   São Paulo   Singapore   Taipei   Tokyo   Toronto   Warsaw

and associated companies in
Berlin   Ibadan

Library of Congress Cataloging-in-Publication Data
Semenza, Gregg L.
Transcription factors and human disease / Gregg L. Semenza.
p.   cm. — (Oxford monographs on medical genetics ; no. 37)
Includes bibliographical references and index.
ISBN 0-19-511239-3
1. Transcription factors—Pathophysiology.
2. Genetic disorders—Pathophysiology.
3. Carcinogenesis.   4. Oncogenes.   I. Series.
[DNLM: 1. Hereditary Diseases—genetics.   2. Transcription Factors.
3. Neoplasms—genetics.   4. Mutation—genetics.
5. Transcription, Genetic.   QZ 50 S471t 1999]
RB155.5.S44   1999
616'.042—dc21
DNLM/DLC
for Library of Congress   97-47791

9 8 7 6 5 4 3 2 1

Printed in the United States of America
on acid-free paper

For Allison, Evan, and Laura

Preface

The Big Picture

During the past two decades, many human diseases have been explained at the molecular level by demonstrating that mutations within specific genes are responsible for, or contribute significantly to, the pathogenesis of particular clinical phenotypes. The elucidation of these molecular pathologies represents a giant step toward a more complete understanding of these disorders. In general, however, these investigations have provided little insight into one of the central questions of biology: how can a single cell, the zygote, give rise to a multicellular, multisystem organism, consisting of approximately 10^{14} cells in the case of the human body, each with its own unique biochemical, anatomical, and functional identity?

Major advances in our ability to address this fascinating issue of our own ontogeny have occurred in the past decade. Cellular identities are established through temporal and quantitative differences in the expression of each of the approximately 50,000 to 100,000 genes present within the 3 billion base pairs of DNA that compose the haploid human genome. Although gene expression can be (and is) regulated at many steps from the synthesis of a primary RNA transcript to the formation of a biologically active protein, the most efficient and most commonly utilized means of gene regulation occur at the first step of gene expression, transcription. To modulate this process, the genome encodes hundreds and perhaps thousands of transcription factors, proteins that control the quality and quantity of gene transcription within the cell.

Several important general principles have already emerged from the still nascent study of transcription factors. First, germline mutations in genes encoding transcription factors often result in malformation syndromes that affect the development of multiple body structures. These varied phenotypic consequences result from the fact that a single transcription factor may contribute to the regulation of scores of genes within dozens of different cell types. Therefore, if the identity of a cell is established by virtue of the genes expressed within it, then the loss of a single transcription factor may have a profound effect on the identity of a large number of cells. Molecular characterization of these mutations has provided insight into the mechanisms that determine whether a given mutant allele will result in a phenotype that is inherited in a dominant or recessive manner.

Second, whereas germline mutations within transcription factors can produce malformation syndromes, somatic mutations involving the same genes may contribute to the development of cancer. Transcription factors play important roles in determining the proliferative capacity of cells and the developmental transition from cellular proliferation to differentiation, a process that is at least in part reversed during oncogenesis. Thus, these discoveries have established a connection between the study of development and malformations, by embryologists and dysmorphologists, and the study of cancer by oncologists.

Third, research into the molecular basis of normal development and of malformation syndromes has revealed remarkable evolutionary conservation of transcriptional regulatory mechanisms. This research has provided further evidence of the critical importance of these pathways in mammals as well as invertebrates separated by over 500 million years of evolution and characterized by seemingly unrelated body forms. An important consequence of these relationships has been the dramatic synergy of research efforts in a variety of organisms, which is accelerating the pace of discovery within the field of human genetics. This chain reaction has been further catalyzed by nucleotide sequence data generated as part of the Human Genome Project and similar projects in model organisms and by the continued refinement of tools for sequence analysis. Conversely, changes in transcription factor structure and/or function may also represent an important driving force in evolution and speciation.

Fourth, another major connection has been established between prenatal development and postnatal physiology. When transcription factors responsible for the expression of certain cell-type-specific gene products were identified, it was found that mutations in genes encoding these transcription factors (e.g., PIT-1) resulted in the loss of expression of the target gene product (e.g., growth hormone) in the adult organism. Subsequent studies revealed that these transcription factor mutations also resulted in the loss during development of the cell type (e.g., pituitary somatotropes) that would ultimately synthesize the gene product. Thus, a single transcription factor can control both the proliferation of specific cell types during development and the ultimate expression within the differentiated cell of gene products that participate in specific physiologic responses. Another link between physiology and development has been the demonstration that in certain cases the same transcription factors are utilized to respond to both developmental signals (e.g., growth factors) and physiological signals (e.g., heat, osmotic stress, oxidative stress) and that related pathways are utilized to transduce the signal from the cell membrane, where the stimulus is received, to the nucleus, where changes in gene expression can be effected by transcription factor activity. Remarkably, in many cases, both the signal transduction pathways and transcription factors appear to have been conserved throughout the evolutionary history of the animal kingdom.

This book attempts to communicate the excitement experienced by one investigator of transcriptional regulation, who views this field as a vital center linking basic embryologic, evolutionary, and physiologic studies with clinically oriented investigations into the molecular bases for a wide variety of human diseases, regardless of whether they are due to germline or somatic mutations or are monogenic or multifactorial in their inheritance, and even whether they are considered inherited or environmental in their etiology. This book is an illustrative survey rather than an encyclopedic catalogue since, given the pace of research, no published text in this area could possibly be considered complete and up-to-date. Rather, I hope the book will provide a set of general principles that will remain applicable as this field continues to grow and as new data continue to increase our understanding of the elegant molecular mechanisms underlying human development, homeostasis, and disease.

Molecular, cellular, and developmental biologists who are interested in learning more about human disorders that are relevant to their own work and medical geneticists and other clinicians who are interested in understanding pathogenesis at the molecular level should find this text useful. It is organized according to the classical model of medical education, in which basic science precedes clinical study. In Part I, (Chapters 1 through 3), general concepts of transcriptional regulation are introduced, beginning with a simplified overview and progressing to the current understanding of transcriptional mechanisms. In Part II, (Chapters 4 through 16), disease processes are interpreted at the molecular level, starting with germline mutations in *cis*-acting DNA regulatory elements (Chapter 4) and *trans*-acting factors, including sequence-specific DNA-binding proteins (Chapters 5 through 12), coactivators (Chapter 13), and general transcription factors (Chapter 14). A summary of the inherited human disorders due to transcription factor defects that are described in Chapters 5 through 15 is provided in the accompanying table. Finally, Chapters 15 and 16 describe the involvement of transcription factors in somatic genetic disease (cancer) and epigenetic disease (teratogenesis), respectively.

Inherited human disorders due to mutations in genes encoding transcription factors

A. Nuclear Receptors (Chapter 5)
- 1. AR: androgen insensitivity syndromes; spinal/bulbar muscular atrophy
- 2. ER: estrogen resistance
- 3. GR: glucocorticoid resistance
- 4. TRβ: thyroid hormone resistance
- 5. VDR: hereditary vitamin D resistant rickets type II
- 6. DAX1: X-linked adrenal hypoplasia congenita; dosage-sensitive sex reversal

B. Other Zinc Finger (Chapter 6)
- 7. WT1: WAGR syndrome; Denys-Drash syndrome
- 8. GLI3: Greig cephalopolysyndactyly syndrome; Pallister-Hall syndrome

C. PAX (Chapter 7)
- 9. PAX2: optic nerve coloboma and renal hypoplasia
- 10. PAX3: Waardenburg syndrome types I and III; craniofacial-deafness-hand syndrome
- 11. PAX6: aniridia; Peter's anomaly; isolated foveal hypoplasia; autosomal dom. keratitis

D. bHLH (Chapter 8)
- 12. MITF: Waardenburg syndrome type II
- 13. TWIST: Saethre-Chotzen syndrome

E. Homeodomain (Chapter 9)
- 14. MSX1: autosomal dominant tooth agenesis
- 15. MSX2: Boston-type craniosynostosis
- 16. HOXD13: synpolydactyly
- 17. HOXA13: hand-foot-genital syndrome
- 18. RIEG: Rieger syndrome
- 19. SHOX: short stature
- 20. IPF1: pancreatic agenesis

F: HMG (Chapter 10)
- 21. SRY: sex reversal
- 22. SOX9: camptomelic dysplasia; sex reversal

G. POU (Chapter 11)
- 23. POU1F1 (PIT1): hypopituitary dwarfism
- 24. POU3F4 (BRN4): X-linked deafness type 3

H. Other (Chapter 12)
- 25. TBX5: Holt-Oram syndrome
- 26. TBX3: ulnar-mammary syndrome
- 27. RFX5: bare lymphocyte syndrome
- 28. RFXAP: bare lymphocyte syndrome
- 29. CIITA: bare lymphocyte syndrome
- 30. OSF2 (CBFA1): cleidocranial dysplasia
- 31. HNF1α: maturity-onset diabetes of the young
- 32. HNF4α: maturity-onset diabetes of the young

I. Coactivators (Chapter 13)
- 33. ATRX: X-linked α-thalassemia and mental retardation
- 34. CBP: Rubenstein-Taybi syndrome

J. General Transcription Factors (Chapter 14)
- 35. ERCC3 (XPB): xeroderma pigmentosa
- 36. ERCC2 (XPD): xeroderma pigmentosa
- 37. ERCC6 (CSB): Cockayne syndrome
- 38. CSA: Cockayne syndrome
- 39. P44T: Werdnig-Hoffman spinal muscular atrophy

K. Tumor Suppressors (Chapter 15)
- 40. RB: retinoblastoma
- 41. P53: Li-Fraumeni syndrome

Each chapter contains an extensive but selective list of references, including both review articles and primary literature, which allow the reader to explore areas of interest in greater detail. An additional important cited reference source is Online Mendelian Inheritance in Man (OMIM), a database catalogue of human genes and genetic disorders established and directed by Dr. Victor A. McKusick of The Johns Hopkins University School of Medicine, which is available via the Internet through the World Wide Web site of the National Center for Biotechnology Information at the National Library of Medicine (http://www.ncbi.nlm.nih.gov). Readers are encouraged to access this site for updated information on any of the diseases presented in the following chapters.

The Disclaimers

Ultimately, the pathophysiology of all human disease processes must be understood in terms of changes in gene expression within relevant cell types of the body. There is increasing evidence that genetic variation in transcription factors and/or their binding site sequences contribute to common multifactorial disorders including cancer, diabetes, and ischemic heart disease. Even in "nongenetic" infectious diseases, alterations of host cell transcriptional regulation play an important role in pathogenesis, as recent investigations of human immunodeficiency virus–related disease have demonstrated. Although brief discussions of multifactorial, somatic genetic, and epigenetic diseases are presented, the focus of this book is on disease processes that demonstrate mendelian inheritance, a decision that was no doubt influenced by the author's training and experience as a medical geneticist. This focus on mendelian disorders is not intended to minimize the important role of somatic genetic and epigenetic alterations of transcriptional regulation in disease states. Indeed, all of the major research projects in the author's own laboratory are focused on these issues.

Just as every disease will one day be understood at the level of gene expression, so too will developmental processes be interpreted as a cascade of transcription factors, each of which is responsible for the expression of a defined battery of genes. Unfortunately, there is no developmental process in mammals in which a complete molecular pathway has been delineated. Similarly, mapping the pathway from mutations in a given transcription factor to pathology will require identifying of all the genes normally regulated by that transcription factor. Thus far, there are very few points on these maps. New molecular methods of genetic analysis may allow the gaps to be filled in the near future. If this text proves useful enough to warrant a second edition, it will be possible to present a much more complete picture of development, homeostasis, and pathophysiology at the molecular level.

Acknowledgments

This work was inspired by my participation in the Short Course in Medical and Experimental Mammalian Genetics, which has been given at the Jackson Laboratory in Bar Harbor, Maine every summer since 1960. Dr. McKusick, who has co-directed this course since its inception, has kindly invited me to lecture on transcriptional regulation for each of the last nine years, thus providing an annual opportunity to present this material to a diverse group of scientists and clinicians. I am grateful to Dr. Charles Scriver and the other members of the editorial board of the *Oxford Monographs on Medical Genetics* series for their support of this project, and Jeffrey W. House, of Oxford University Press, for his forebearance.

Baltimore   G.L.S.
October 1997

Contents

Transcriptional Regulation

Part **I**

Gene Expression and 1
Transcriptional Regulation

To ensure that the subsequent discussions of transcriptional regulation and molecular pathophysiology will be accessible to those not well-versed in this literature, a brief overview will be presented first. Whereas molecular geneticists may wish to forgo this introductory course and proceed directly to the second half of the chapter (beginning with "The Transcription Initiation Complex"), the uninitiated should not do so until the definitions and organizing principles in the first three sections have been thoroughly digested. If additional introductory material is needed, a basic textbook in molecular biology should be consulted (e.g., Lewin, 1997).

Definitions

The most basic (and most misused) terminology in molecular genetics relates to gene structure (Fig. 1.1). For the purposes of this text a gene will be defined as a continuous, uninterrupted, chromosomal (genomic) DNA sequence that constitutes one (or more) transcription unit(s) from the (5'-most) transcription initiation site to the sequence corresponding to the (3'-most) polyadenylation site found in the transcribed messenger RNA(s) (mRNA). This somewhat cumbersome definition takes into account genes with multiple transcription initiation and polyadenylation sites. Sequences flanking the transcription unit(s) are referred to as 5'- and 3'-flanking sequences (5'-FS and 3'-FS). Because many *cis*-acting transcriptional regulatory elements are located within flanking sequences, they are not formally considered part of the gene proper. The rationale for this exclusion is that within some multigene clusters such as the εγδβ-globin gene family, a single *cis*-acting element may control the expression

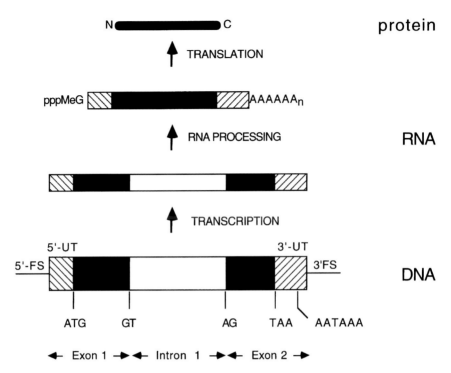

FIGURE 1-1. Gene structure and expression. A hypothetical gene consisting of two exons and one intron is depicted on the line marked DNA as follows: thin line, flanking (nontranscribed) sequences (5'-FS, 3'-FS); box, transcribed sequences; striped box, untranslated sequences (5'-UT, 3'-UT); filled box, amino acid coding sequences; open box, intervening sequences (intron). Important regulatory signals shown are ATG, translation initiation codon; GT and AG, invariant dinucleotides at 5' and 3' ends of intron, respectively; TAA, translation termination codon; AATAAA, polyadenylation signal; pppMeG, 5' cap; AAAAAA$_n$, polyadenylyl tail. Above the gene are depicted (in ascending order) the primary RNA transcript, processed mRNA, and translated protein. Ribosomal translation of mRNA coding sequences in a 5'-to-3' direction results in the synthesis of a polypeptide sequence from amino (N) to carboxyl (C) terminus.

of several contiguous genes and therefore cannot be classified as being part of any single gene.

The transcription unit or gene encodes a primary RNA transcript that is processed to a mature mRNA by modification of the 5' end (addition of a 5-methylguanine cap), splicing of intervening sequences (introns), cleavage at the 3' end, and addition of a polyadenylyl tail. The mature mRNA contains an open reading frame (ORF) that encodes a polypeptide. The ORF begins with an initiator methionine codon (which is almost always encoded by ATG in genomic DNA) and ends with a translation termination codon (TAA, TAG, or TGA). mRNA sequences 5' and 3' to the ORF are referred to as 5'- and 3'-untranslated sequences (5'-UT and 3'-UT). Frequently encountered errors in terminology include referring to cDNA sequences as a gene, referring to any sequences 5' or 3' to the coding sequences (including untranslated sequences) as flanking sequences, and referring to 5'-flanking sequences as the promoter, which must be defined by functional assays as described in Chapter 2.

Gene Expression Is Regulated at Multiple Levels

The processes of cellular proliferation and differentiation that underlie human development are controlled by programs of regulated gene expression within the embryo. Cells establish their ultimate structural and functional identities by activating unique combinations of genes. Failure to successfully execute these developmental programs of gene expression, either due to genetic defects (mutations) or environmental insults (teratogens), can result in a wide spectrum of clinical phenotypes ranging from severe malformation syndromes to more common and less debilitating birth defects. After birth, humans must respond to a variety of endogenous and exogenous stimuli in order to maintain cellular and systemic homeostasis. The ability to maintain homeostasis in the face of a physiologic challenge is a function of the genetic background and the magnitude of the challenge. Thus, the likelihood of developing atherosclerotic coronary vascular disease depends upon the presence of predisposing mutations that might, for example, affect the levels of plasma apolipoproteins as well as on environmental (behavioral) factors such as diet, exercise, and use of cigarettes. As in the case of development, postnatal structure and function are maintained by signal transduction pathways through which physiologic stimuli induce specific adaptive responses that involve quantitative or qualitative changes in gene expression.

Of the 50,000 to 100,000 genes estimated to be present in human genomic DNA, the majority encode proteins and are transcribed by RNA polymerase II (Pol II) into mRNA. Genes encoding the 5.8S, 18S, and 28S ribosomal RNA (rRNA) are transcribed by RNA polymerase I (Pol I) and genes encoding transfer RNAs, 5S rRNA, and most small nuclear RNAs (snRNAs) are transcribed by RNA polymerase III (Pol III). The scope of this book is limited to mRNA transcription by Pol II.

The steps involved in the expression of protein-coding genes are outlined in Figure 1.1 and Table 1.1. Regulation of these steps can affect both the nature (structure and function) of the final gene product and

TABLE 1.1. The regulation of gene expression

---

1. Transcription
     a. Initiation
     b. Elongation
     c. Termination
2. Posttranscriptional processing
     a. Polyadenylation
     b. Splicing
     c. Editing
     d. Transport/Localization
3. Translation
     a. Initiation
     b. Termination
4. Posttranslational processing
     a. Proteolytic cleavage
     b. Phosphorylation
     c. Glycosylation
     d. ADP-ribosylation
     e. Myristoylation
     f. Ligand/Cofactor binding
     g. Oligomerization
     h. Subcellular localization
     i. Oxidation/Reduction
     j. Degradation

---

its steady-state level. A wide variety of regulatory strategies are employed and, for any given gene, regulation at one or more steps may be of paramount importance in determining expression. In general terms, however, the most efficient and most commonly utilized mechanisms for the regulation of gene expression are exercised at the first step in the process, the transcription of DNA sequences into RNA. This process is regulated by transcription factors, which are the protein products of genes that are in turn subjected to regulation at many posttranscriptional levels, as will be described in detail below; thus the question of whether transcription can claim primacy over other regulatory events becomes something of a chicken-and-egg debate that illustrates the complex interconnectedness of biological processes.

Basic Principles of Transcriptional Regulation

The principles presented in this section represent the foundation on which this work will be constructed. The basic principles are as follows: (1) The specificity of transcription depends on the binding of *trans*-acting factors to *cis*-acting regulatory elements. (2) The quality of transcriptional regulation depends on both DNA-protein interactions and protein-protein interactions. (3) These interactions affect DNA conformation, co-valent modification of chromatin protein structure, and formation of the transcription initiation complex. (4) Combinatorial control allows several thousand transcription factors to differentially alter in every cell type the expression of each gene in response to every potential developmental or physiologic stimulus that is transmitted to the nucleus. These four principles are described in greater detail below.

Cis-trans *Interactions*

As illustrated in Figure 1.2, the molecular basis for the transcriptional regulation of gene expression is the binding of *trans*-acting proteins (transcription factors) to *cis*-acting DNA sequence elements. The transcription factor is a *trans*-acting regulator because it is the product of a gene distinct from the gene it regulates, whereas the transcription factor–binding site is a *cis*-acting regulatory element because it is present on the same strand of DNA as the gene that it regulates. The presence of *cis*-acting DNA sequences establishes the binding of transcription factors at locations from which they can interact with the transcription initiation complex, a macromolecular assembly of RNA polymerase II and associated protein cofactors. There are two general classes of proteins that participate in transcriptional regulation. The general or basal transcription factors form the transcription initiation complex that is required for the

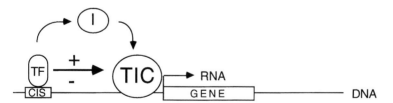

FIGURE 1-2. Principles of transcriptional regulation. A *trans*-acting factor (TF) binds to its cognate *cis*-acting DNA sequence (CIS) and interacts with the transcription initiation complex (TIC). Interaction of the TF with the TIC, either directly or indirectly via intermediate cofactors (I) may have a positive or negative effect on the rate of transcription by stabilizing or destabilizing formation of the TIC, respectively. Thus, DNA-binding activators interact with coactivators whereas DNA-binding repressors interact with corepressors to increase or decrease the rate of transcription initiation, respectively. Note that the TF is involved in protein-DNA interactions (with CIS) and protein-protein interactions (with I and TIC). (Adapted from Semenza, 1994.)

transcription of protein-encoding genes. In contrast, the transcriptional regulatory proteins either bind to specific *cis*-acting DNA sequences present within the regulatory regions of a restricted number of genes (activators, repressors) or interact with sequence-specific DNA-binding proteins (coactivators, corepressors). The binding of sequence-specific transcriptional activators is believed to recruit the general transcription factors to a specific DNA sequence. These sequence-specific transcriptional activators therefore determine the location and rate at which Pol II will initiate transcription of DNA into mRNA.

DNA-Protein and Protein-Protein Interactions

The assembly of the transcription initiation complex is believed to be the rate-limiting step in the transcription of most genes. Transcription factors affect the stability of the transcription initiation complex by direct interactions with one or more proteins within the complex or indirectly by interactions with intermediary proteins that can interact with the transcription initiation complex. These interactions may have positive or negative effects on the rate of transcription by stabilizing or destabilizing formation of the transcription initiation complex. Transcription factors thus participate in two types of molecular interactions: DNA-protein interactions that establish sequence-specific binding and protein-protein interactions that affect the rate of transcription initiation (Fig. 1.2).

Chromatin Remodeling and Formation of the Transcription Initiation Complex

Transcription in vivo occurs in the context of chromatin, a nucleoprotein complex, rather than on naked DNA. An essential aspect of transcription is the remodeling of chromatin structure, which requires conformational changes of DNA structure and enzymatic alteration of chromatin proteins. DNA conformational changes are effected in part by DNA-binding proteins whereas enzymatic modifications are effected by coactivators and corepressors that interact with the DNA-binding proteins. The coactivators thus provide two essential functions: they tether the transcription initiation complex to the transcription initiation site via interactions with sequence-specific transcriptional activators and they enzymatically alter chromatin structure to allow binding of other sequence-specific transcription factors and, subsequently, to allow transcriptional elongation to occur.

Combinatorial Control

The final principle is that transcription is subject to multiple levels of combinatorial control as follows: (1) a single gene contains binding sites for multiple positive- and negative-acting transcription factors; (2) the combination of binding sites that are present determines a gene's transcriptional potential; (3) for each developmental and physiologic state, qualitative and/or quantitative differences in the expression of factors, their DNA binding, and their interactions with other transcription factors define the transcriptional activity of the gene. Thus, within each cell, the net effect of specific positive and negative transcription factors that are present in the cell, and for which the gene possesses binding sites, will determine the level of transcription. (4) Many transcription factors function as dimeric proteins. Families of dimeric transcription factors exist, resulting in multiple homodimer and heterodimer combinations, each of which possesses differing affinity for target site binding and transcriptional activation or repression. (5) Transcription factor activity may also be modified by posttranslational covalent modifications or by binding of small molecules (ligands) or other proteins (cofactors).

The Transcription Initiation Complex

Basal (General) Transcription Factors and Pol II

The transcription initiation complex is a macromolecular assembly of approximately 50 different proteins that is required for RNA polymerase II (Pol II) transcription (reviewed by Zawel and Reinberg, 1993). The biochemical characterization of the transcription initiation complex was made possible by the establishment of conditions for promoter-dependent transcription initiation by Pol II in vitro (Weil et al., 1979). In addition to Pol II, which in yeast and mammals consists of 10 to 14 subunits with a combined mass of approximately 600 kDa (reviewed by Halle and Meisterernst, 1996; Young, 1991; Zawel and Reinberg, 1993), components of the transcription initiation complex include TFIIA, TFIIB, TFIID, TFIIE, TFIIF, and TFIIH (Table 1.2), all of which are conserved from yeast to humans (reviewed by Carey, 1995; Nikolov and Burley, 1997). These basal or general transcription factors were originally identified by fractionation of nuclear extracts by ion exchange chromatography (Dignam et al., 1983a; reviewed by Zawel and Reinberg, 1993).

TFIID. Based on electrophoretic mobility-shift assays using DNA templates and purified general transcription factors (Buratowski et al., 1989),

Table 1.2. General transcription factors of the Pol II transcription initiation complex

Factor	Number of Subunits	Subunit Sizes (kDa)	Function
Pol II	12–14	10–220	Synthesizes RNA
TFIID			
TBP	1	38	Binds DNA; interacts with TFIIB
TAFs	≥12	15–250	Interact with activators; remodel chromatin
TFIIB	1	35	Interacts with TBP, TFIIF, and Pol II
TFIIA	2	14, 32	Interacts with TBP and activators
TFIIF	2	30, 74	Interacts with TFIIB and Pol II
TFIIE	2	34, 57	Stimulates TFIIH kinase/ATPase activities
TFIIH	9	35–89	ATPase, helicase, and CTD kinase activities

Adapted from Nikolov and Burley, 1997.

the formation of the transcription initiation complex has been proposed to occur as a multistep assembly process that begins with the binding of TFIID to DNA sequences immediately 5' to the transcription initiation site (reviewed by Zawel and Reinberg, 1993). TFIID is the only general transcription factor with sequence-specific DNA-binding activity, and its binding to DNA is required for the subsequent recruitment of Pol II and the other general transcription factors (Fig. 1.3). The binding of TFIID to a specific DNA sequence, the TATA box (see Chapter 2) determines the site of transcription initiation and the direction in which transcription will proceed.

TFIID is itself a multiprotein complex consisting of the TATA-binding protein (TBP) and multiple TBP-associated factors (TAFs) ranging from 15 to 250 kd in size, many of which have been conserved throughout eukaryotic evolution from yeast to humans (Dynlacht et al., 1991; reviewed by Nikolov and Burley, 1997). The TAFs can be considered either as general components of the transcription initiation complex (with which they were isolated) or as coactivators because these proteins are required for transcriptional activators to have a stimulatory effect on transcription, as will be described in Chapter 3. In *Drosophila melanogaster*, purified TFIID has been shown to consist of TBP and eight TAFs with apparent molecular masses ranging from 30 to 250 kDa (reviewed by Goodrich and Tjian, 1994). In human cells, TFIID contains at least 13 TAFs ranging from 17 to 250 kDa in size (Chiang et al., 1993; Jacq et al., 1994; Mengus et al., 1996; Zhou et al., 1992). The 250-kDa TAF of *Drosophila* (dTAF$_{II}$250) functions as a scaffold protein that binds to TBP as well as the other TAFs to create the TFIID complex (Chen et al., 1994; Ruppert et al., 1993; Weinzierl et al., 1993). The TAF complex may play

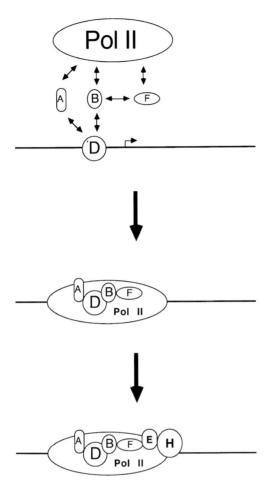

FIGURE 1-3. Formation of the transcription initiation complex. A stepwise model is presented as follows: double-headed arrows, protein-protein interaction; DNA, thin line; transcription initiation site, bent arrow; large oval, RNA polymerase II; small ovals, basal transcription factors TFIIA, TFIIB, TFIID, TFIIE, TFIIF, and TFIIH. (Adapted from Buratowski, 1994.)

an important role in integrating signals received from activators and other coactivators, as described in Chapter 3.

The structures of the amino terminal regions of dTAF$_{II}$42, dTAF$_{II}$62, and dTAF$_{II}$30 show remarkable similarity to the structures of histones H3, H4, and H2B, respectively (reviewed by Travers, 1996). Furthermore, dTAF$_{II}$42 and dTAF$_{II}$62 form heterotetramers that are strikingly similar in structure to the (H3-H4)$_2$ heterotetramer that forms the histone core

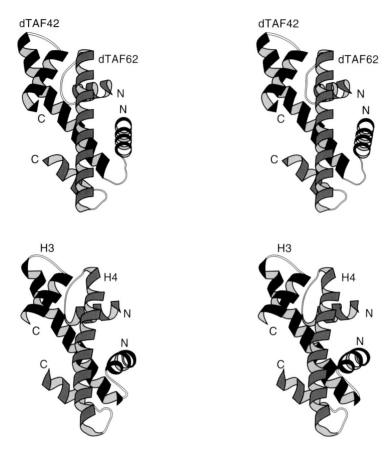

FIGURE 1-4. Structural similarity between TPB-associated factors (TAFs) and histones. The three-dimensional structures of dTAF$_{II}$42 (amino acid residues 17–86) and dTAF$_{II}$62 (amino acid residues 1–70) are compared with the structures of histones H3 and H4 as heterodimers. (Reproduced with permission from Xie et al., 1996. Copyright © 1996 by Macmillan Magazines Limited.)

of nucleosomes (Xie et al., 1996) (Fig. 1.4). Remarkably, hTAF$_{II}$20, h-TAF$_{II}$31, and hTAF$_{II}$80, which are the human homologues of dTAF$_{II}$30α, dTAF$_{II}$42, and dTAF$_{II}$62 (Table 1.3), interact with H2A, H3, and H4, respectively (Hoffmann et al., 1996). No TAF homologous to H2A has been identified, but hTAF$_{II}$20, the H2B homologue, is capable of self-association, suggesting that TAFs may form a [(hTAF$_{II}$20)$_2$-(hTAF$_{II}$31-hTAF$_{II}$80)]$_2$ octamer-like complex.

These results suggest that TFIID may form a multiprotein complex similar to the histone octamer that may function in DNA binding and

TABLE 1.3. Structurally similar histones
and TAFs

Histone	*Drosophila*	Human
H2B	dTAF$_{II}$30α	hTAF$_{II}$20
H3	TAF$_{II}$42	hTAF$_{II}$31
H4	dTAF$_{II}$62	hTAF$_{II}$80

perhaps nucleosome displacement during transcription initiation and/or elongation. The interaction of histone-like TAF domains with DNA may depend on conformational changes induced by interactions with activators or other coactivators. Alternatively, the histone-like domains may be involved only in protein-protein interactions between TAFs (Xie et al., 1996). However, it is notable that binding of DNA by TFIID and core histones is mutually exclusive (reviewed by Nikolov and Burley, 1997).

The homologous structural and functional relationships between histones and transcription factors also extends to sequence-specific transcriptional activators: the DNA-binding domain of hepatocyte nuclear factor 3 (HNF-3) closely resembles the structure of histone H5, a variant of the linker histone H1 (Clark et al., 1993). Taken together with other data presented later in this chapter and in Chapter 3, these results indicate that an important function of transcriptional activators and coactivators is to modify chromatin structure.

TBP is required for recognition of the TATA box, a canonical *cis*-acting element with a consensus sequence of 5'-TATAAA-3' that is usually located 25 to 30 base pairs (bp) 5' to the transcription initiation site. TBP alone is sufficient for basal transcription in vitro, whereas TAFs are required to mediate the effects of sequence-specific transcriptional activators on the transcription initiation complex. TAFs interact with one another (as described above), with other proteins in the initiation complex (such as TBP, TFIIB, TFIIE, and TFIIF), and with sequence-specific transcription factors, all of which suggests that they may play important roles in transcriptional regulation (Dikstein et al., 1996; Goodrich et al., 1993; Hisatake et al., 1995; Ruppert and Tjian, 1995). In genes that do not contain a TATA box, TBP is still required for transcription. In this case, however, the transcription initiation site may be determined by protein-DNA interactions involving other components of the transcription initiation complex such as TFIIA, TFIIB, and/or TAFs (Hansen and Tjian, 1995; Verrijzer et al., 1994, 1995). TBP binds to the minor groove of the DNA helix and induces a bend in the region of the TATA box that may alter the nucleosome structure at the promoter and bring the transcription initiation complex in close proximity to transcriptional activators (Guzikevich-Guerstein and Shakked, 1996; Kim et al., 1993a, b; reviewed by Travers, 1996).

Remarkably, TBP is a universal factor that is required for transcription by Pol I, Pol II, and Pol III (reviewed by Hernandez, 1993; Struhl, 1994), which probably accounts for the fact that it is one of the most highly conserved proteins in eukaryotes from yeast to humans (reviewed by Buratowski, 1994; Hernandez, 1993). The last 180 amino acids of human TBP are 88% identical to TBP from *Drosophila melanogaster* and 80% to 81% identical to TBP from the yeast species *Saccharomyces cerevisiae* and *Schizosaccharomyces pombe* (Zawel and Reinberg, 1993). Different combinations of TBP and TAFs have been shown to form: SL1, which is required for Pol I transcription of rRNAs (Comai et al., 1992); TFIID, which is required for Pol II transcription of protein-encoding genes (Dynlacht et al., 1991); SNAP$_c$, which is required for Pol II transcription of some snRNAs (Sadowski et al., 1993); and TFIIIB, which is required for Pol III transcription (Lobo et al., 1992; Taggart et al., 1992). Thus, promoter recognition by specific TBP-TAF complexes is an essential prerequisite for transcription by Pol I, II, and III.

The crystal structure of the conserved carboxyl-terminal domain of TBP revealed a saddle-like appearance in which DNA binding in the minor groove of the double helix occurs via the concave underside, and protein-protein interactions with other components of the transcription initiation complex occur on the convex upper surface (reviewed by Nikolov and Burley, 1997). A remarkable aspect of TBP is that despite its small size (38 kDa) it has a large surface area containing distinct domains that allow interaction with DNA, basal transcription factors, and transcriptional activators and coactivators (reviewed by Hansen, 1996). Among the other basal transcription factors, both TFIIA and TFIIB have been shown to bind to the TFIID-DNA complex.

TFIIA, TFIIB, and TFIIF. TFIIB, a single 35-kDa polypeptide of 316 amino acids (Ha et al., 1991), enters the transcription initiation complex after binding of TFIID to the TATA box. The crystal structure of the TBP–TATA box–TFIIB ternary complex revealed interactions of TFIIB with both TBP and the DNA along one side of the TBP-induced bend (Nikolov et al., 1995). As in the case of TFIID, TFIIA and TFIIB may also interact with sequence-specific transcription factors (reviewed by Zawel and Reinberg, 1993). For example, TFIIB interacts with the transactivation domain of the activator VP16 (Roberts et al., 1993) and with the coactivator TAF$_{II}$40 subunit of TFIID (Hori et al., 1995). TFIIB has also been shown to recruit Pol II into the transcription initiation complex in asso-

474

Customer:

Miss AS Ingraha

I

Transcription Factors and Human Disease (Oxford Monographs on Medical

Gregg L. Semenza

W1-N020-O3
RB-879-654

9780195112399

Used - Good

Picker Notes:

QA Notes:

9385312

I

10018113

ciation with the 30-kDa subunit of TFIIF (RAP30) (Buratowski et al, 1989; Flores et al., 1991). Remarkably, RAP30 contains a region of approximately 70 amino acids with sequence similarity to domains within the *E. coli* σ^{70} factor that make contact with the bacterial core RNA polymerase (reviewed by Zawel and Reinberg, 1993), which is consistent with the proposed role of TFIIF in recruiting Pol II to the transcription initiation complex. These observations also provide additional evidence that the basic transcriptional machinery has been highly conserved throughout the evolution of all living organisms.

TFIIE and TFIIH. The multimeric protein complexes TFIIE (two subunits with apparent molecular masses of 34 and 56 kDa) and TFIIH (eight subunits) are required for the conversion of the initiation complex into an elongation complex (promoter clearance), which involves phosphorylation of the carboxyl terminal domain (CTD) of the largest (240-kDa) subunit of Pol II by TFIIH (reviewed by Buratowski, 1994; Conaway and Conaway, 1993; Drapkin et al., 1994). The Pol II CTD contains the heptapeptide sequence TSPTSPS, which is repeated 26 times in yeast Pol II and 52 times in human and mouse Pol II (reviewed by Carey, 1995; Zawel and Reinberg, 1993). The CTD must be hypophosphorylated in order for Pol II to participate in formation of the transcription initiation complex (reviewed by Hansen, 1996). Reversible phosphorylation of the Pol II CTD by cyclin dependent kinases (which include one of the TFIIH subunits) appears to play an essential role in both transcription initiation and elongation (reviewed by McKnight, 1996). A TAF (TAF$_{II}$250) has also been shown to specifically phosphorylate the 74-kDa subunit of TFIIF (RAP74) (Dikstein et al., 1996). These results provide further evidence that phosphorylation events may regulate critical protein-protein interactions required for the formation of the transcription initiation complex and the transition from initiation to elongation. In addition to kinase activity, TFIIH also copurifies with DNA-dependent ATPase and DNA helicase activities that may be required for melting of the DNA at the initiation site (open complex formation) that occurs prior to promoter clearance (Drapkin et al., 1994). DNA-dependent protein kinase activity of TFIIH has also been implicated in the phosphorylation of the Pol II CTD, a process that may be stimulated by transcriptional activators such as heat shock factor (reviewed by Hansen, 1996). During the transition from initiation to elongation, Pol II begins to move in a 5'-to-3' direction along the coding strand. Some of the general transcription factors, including TFIID, may remain at the initiation site, where they may initiate another round of transcription (Zawel et al., 1995), whereas other factors (e.g., TFIIH) that are required for elongation remain bound to Pol II.

RNA transcription, splicing, and polyadenylation all occur as a continuous process that is coordinated by the interaction of the required processing factors with the Pol II CTD (McCracken et al., 1997).

The 'Transcriptosome'

In contrast to the multistep model for initiation complex formation presented above, which is based on in vitro transcription assays using purified proteins and naked DNA templates, more recent data suggest that a holoenzyme complex exists in vivo and is recruited to the transcription initiation site in a single step (Kim et al., 1994; Koleske and Young, 1994, 1995; reviewed by Carey, 1995). In yeast, the holoenzyme has been shown to consist of Pol II, TFIIB, TFIIE, TFIIF, TFIIH, and nine SRB (suppressor of RNA polymerase B) proteins (Koleske and Young, 1994), which may interact both with components of the transcription initiation complex and with transcriptional activators, similar to the proposed function of TAFs described above. In the holoenzyme model, the two key events in formation of the transcription initiation complex appear to be, first, binding of the TATA box region of the promoter by TFIID and, second, binding of the holoenzyme to the TFIID-promoter complex.

The SRB complex appears to bind to a hypophosphorylated form of the Pol II CTD, and phosphorylation of the CTD, by an SRB-associated cyclin-dependent kinase may release the SRB complex during the transition from transcription initiation to elongation (reviewed by McKnight, 1996), which is similar to the function proposed for TFIIH described above. A human holoenzyme complex containing TFIIE, TFIIH, and SRB proteins has also been isolated recently (Chao et al., 1996), again suggesting evolutionary conservation of the basic transcriptional machinery from yeast to humans.

In addition to the basal/general transcription factors and SRB complex, a third multiprotein complex associated with Pol II that is greater than one million daltons (1 MDa) in size consists of SWI/SNF proteins that play a role in chromatin remodeling (Wilson et al., 1996), as described in Chapter 3. Finally, Pol II also interacts with proteins required for nucleotide excision and double-stranded-break DNA repair (reviewed by Halle and Meisterernst, 1996). Taken together, the Pol II transcription complex contains at least 60 protein subunits with a total molecular mass of greater than 3 MDa, rivaling the ribosome in size and leading to the speculative but not unreasonable proposal that this complex represents an immobile transcriptosome through which DNA templates are threaded during the process of RNA polymerization (Halle and Meisterernst, 1996).

DNA Methylation

In mammals and other vertebrates, genomic DNA is selectively modified by methylation of cytosine residues located 5' to guanine residues (5'-CG-3') through the activity of the enzyme DNA cytosine-5-methyltransferase, which is required for normal embryonic development (Li et al., 1992). As a general rule, so-called housekeeping genes, which are expressed in a wide variety of cell types, usually contain CpG islands, or large stretches of DNA in which the sequence 5'-CG-3' is over-represented relative to the genome as a whole. These CpG islands usually extend over the 5'-flanking region and first exon and are constitutively unmethylated (Bird, 1986). In contrast, cell-type-specific genes are methylated in all cells except those in which they are transcribed (Yeivin and Razin, 1993). In vivo, the loss of cytosine methylation in promoter regions is associated with transcriptional activation (reviewed by Cedar, 1988). In cultured cells, methylated and transcriptionally inactive genes can be activated by treatment with the cytosine methylase-inhibitor 5-azacytidine (reviewed by Jones, 1985). Comparison of methylation patterns in female cells revealed methylation of promoter sequences on the inactive, but not the active, X chromosome (reviewed by Grant and Chapman, 1988). For imprinted genes, expressed alleles also appear to be hypomethylated relative to the unexpressed allele (Reik et al., 1987; Sapienza et al., 1987; Sasaki et al., 1991).

Methylation of genomic DNA is a dynamic process. After formation of the zygote, genomic DNA from the egg and sperm is demethylated and remains so throughout the blastula stage (Kafri et al., 1992; Monk et al., 1987). At the time of implantation, genomic DNA is remethylated (Jahner and Jaenisch, 1984). Embryos deficient for 5-methyltransferase activity die shortly after implantation (Li et al., 1992). Throughout development, additional demethylation events occur as transcription of individual genes is activated in a cell-type-specific manner. The *cis*-acting sequences (other than 5'-CG-3') and *trans*-acting factors (other than cytosine methyltransferase) that regulate methylation and demethylation are not well understood at the present time. However, methylation appears to be one mechanism by which the activity of a gene can be fixed in the "on" or "off" position and maintained as such as cells undergo successive rounds of DNA replication and cell division.

Chromatin

Gene transcription within the nuclei of cells does not occur on naked DNA. Instead, genomic DNA is organized by several levels of coiling and compaction that is mediated by proteins that associate with DNA to form chromatin. The binding of histones to DNA generates the primary level of chromatin organization, the nucleosome. Approximately 200 bp of DNA is packaged in each nucleosome, with 146 bp wound around a histone octamer core consisting of two molecules each of H2A, H2B, H3, and H4, and the remaining DNA present as a linker of variable length between cores to which H1 binds (reviewed by Krude and Elgin, 1996). Nucleosomes are further compacted by coiling with six nucleosomes per turn to form a 30-nm chromatin fiber (Felsenfeld, 1992). Higher-order structures have been identified in which nucleosomes are further compacted, with the highest levels of compaction seen in metaphase chromosomes of dividing cells. In vitro chromatin reconstitution experiments have provided evidence that, compared to naked DNA templates, the presence of nucleosomes inhibits each step of transcription: binding by sequence-specific transcriptional activators, formation of the transcription initiation complex, transcription initiation, and elongation (reviewed by Adams and Workman, 1993; Felsenfeld, 1992; Kingston et al., 1996).

Posttranslational modification of histones, such as acetylation (reviewed by Wolffe and Pruss, 1996), and/or the expression of nonhistone proteins may be involved in regulating the degree of chromatin compaction. Although the core histones are modified by acetylation, ADP-ribosylation, methylation, phosphorylation, and ubiquitination, reversible acetylation of the ε-amino groups of lysine residues is most strongly associated with transcriptionally active chromatin (reviewed by Vettese-Dadey et al., 1996). Mutations in yeast that inactivate histone H4 or alter the amino terminal domain result in derepression of gene expression (reviewed by Felsenfeld, 1992). In addition, the transcriptionally inactive X chromosome in female mammals is highly deficient in histone H4 acetylation in comparison to all other chromosomes (Jeppesen and Turner, 1993). Recent studies indicate that nucleosomes containing acetylated H4 are preferentially bound by the mammalian basic helix-loop-helix factor USF and the yeast zinc finger factor GAL4 (Vettese-Dadey et al., 1996). These results suggest that hypoacetylated histone H4 is involved in chromatin compaction that represses transcription and that hyperacetylation of H4 facilitates transcription factor binding and transcription initiation. As described in Chapter 3, these hypotheses have been strengthened by the recent demonstration that several transcriptional coactivators possess histone acetyltransferase activity and that several transcriptional corepressors possess histone deacetylase activity.

Because it is unlikely that transcription factors can efficiently access their cognate DNA binding sites in highly compacted chromatin, it is likely that a necessary prerequisite for gene transcription is the conversion of the chromatin to a noncompacted, "open" configuration (reviewed by van Holde, 1989). It is not unreasonable to speculate that this process also results from the binding of *trans*-acting factors to *cis*-acting elements, and evidence in support of this hypothesis will be presented in Chapters 2 and 3. Discontinuities in the nucleosomal packaging of genomic DNA in mammalian cells was first suggested by the identification of DNase I hypersensitive sites in chromatin (reviewed by Krude and Elgin, 1996). When nuclei are isolated from a mammalian tissue and exposed to DNase I, specific DNA sequences are much more sensitive to digestion than bulk chromatin. These sequences, which are usually several hundred base pairs in length, are located within promoter or enhancer elements of genes that are expressed within the tissue analyzed. DNase I hypersensitive sites are also accessible to restriction endonucleases and other nucleases and have been recovered as histone-free DNA fragments, suggesting a local absence of nucleosomes in these regions (Elgin, 1988; Krude and Elgin, 1996). However, DNase hypersensitivity may represent unfolding, sliding, or complete dissociation of the histone octamer from DNA (Felsenfeld, 1992). In the case of both developmentally regulated and physiologically inducible genes, the presence of a hypersensitive site may precede the onset of transcription, indicating that the establishment of an open chromatin configuration is a necessary prerequisite for gene expression. Specific factors involved in chromatin remodeling have recently been characterized and will be described in Chapter 3.

Conclusion

Transcription is a complex biochemical process that requires a multitude of protein components and occurs in multiple, highly regulated steps including binding of transcription factors, formation of the transcription initiation complex, chromatin remodeling by nucleosome disruption, DNA melting at the initiation site, promoter clearance, and transcript elongation (Fig. 1.5). However, transcriptional regulation cannot be understood as a simple linear process. For example, binding of a transcription factor may be crucial to reorganizing chromatin at the promoter, which in turn may allow binding of additional sequence-specific and general transcription factors, which may result in further changes in the topology of the chromatin template that are necessary for transcription initiation.

Taken together, investigations into the biochemical nature of the transcription initiation complex have revealed a tremendous degree of molecular complexity, which is necessary in order that the transcription

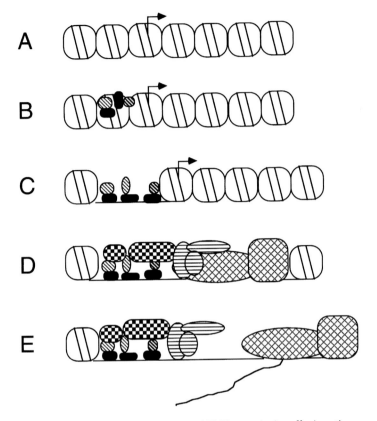

FIGURE 1-5. Steps in transcription. (A) Transcriptionally inactive gene in a closed chromatin configuration. (B) Initial binding of sequence-specific transcription factors (solid, DNA binding domain; diagonal stripes, transcriptional activation domain) to cognate sites on nucleosomal DNA upstream of the transcription initiation site (bent arrow). (C) Binding of transcription factors that disrupt nucleosomes. (D) Binding of coactivators (checkerboard) and formation of transcription initiation complex. (E) Promoter clearance and transcript elongation. Components of the transcription initiation complex (horizontal stripes) that interact with activators and coactivators remain at the initiation site where they can participate in the formation of another transcription initiation complex. Although depicted as a linear sequence of events, steps B, C, and D are interrelated and occur concomitantly as discussed in the text. (Adapted from Kingston et al., 1996.)

of thousands of different genes can each be modulated uniquely through the individual interactions of a large array of transcription factors with different components of the complex. Therefore, regardless of whether the complex is assembled in one or more steps, the stable formation of the complex at the transcription initiation site occurs as a result of multiple DNA-protein and protein-protein interactions involving sequence-specific transcription factors and components of the basal complex. The rate of transcription initiation for a gene will thus depend on the transcription factors present within the cell for which the gene contains binding sites and the strength of the interactions between those DNA-bound factors and basal factors within the transcription initiation complex. Additional regulation may occur at the level of transcription elongation, and a recent study of transcriptional activators has revealed that some stimulate transcription initiation, others affect transcription elongation, and a third group has effects on both initiation and elongation (Yankulov et al., 1994). In each case, the sequence-specific transcription factors function by specific interactions with DNA and with components of the Pol II complex. Thus, despite the biochemical complexity of the transcription reaction, the simple model presented at the beginning of this chapter (Fig. 1.2) remains a valid framework for the present efforts to understand the detailed and varied mechanisms of transcriptional regulation.

References

Adams, C. C., and J. L. Workman. Nucleosome displacement in transcription. *Cell* 72:305–308, 1993.

Bird, A. P. CpG-rich islands and the function of DNA methylation. *Nature* 321: 209–213, 1986.

Buratowski, S. The basics of basal transcription by RNA polymerase II. *Cell* 77: 1–3, 1994.

Buratowski, S., S. Hahn, L. Guarente, and P. A. Sharp. Five intermediate complexes in transcription initiation by RNA polymerase II. *Cell* 56:549–561, 1989.

Carey, M. F. A holistic view of the complex. *Curr. Biol.* 5:1003–1005, 1995.

Cedar, H. DNA methylation and gene activity. *Cell* 53:3–4, 1988.

Chao, D. M., E. L. Gadbois, P. J. Murray, S. F. Anderson, M. S. Sonu, J. D. Parvin, and R. A. Young. A mammalian SRB protein associated with an RNA polymerase II holoenzyme. *Nature* 380:82–85, 1996.

Chen, J. L., L. D. Attardi, C. P. Verrijzer, K. Yokomori, and R. Tjian. Assembly of recombinant TFIID reveals differential coactivator requirements for distinct transcriptional activators. *Cell* 79:93–105, 1994.

Chiang, C. M., H. Ge, Z. Wang, A. Hoffmann, and R. G. Roeder. Unique TATA-binding protein-containing complexes and co-factors involved in transcription by RNA polymerases II and III. *EMBO J.* 12:2749–2762, 1993.

Clark, K. L., E. D. Halay, E. Lai, and S. K. Burley. Co-crystal structure of the HNF-3/fork head DNA-recognition motif resembles histone H5. *Nature* 364: 412–420, 1993.

Comai, L., N. Tanese, and R. Tjian. The TATA-binding protein and associated factors are integral components of the RNA polymerase I transcription factor SL1. *Cell* 68:965–976, 1992.

Conaway, R. C., and J. W. Conaway. General initiation factors for RNA polymerase II. *Annu. Rev. Biochem.* 62:161–190, 1993.

Dignam, J. D., R. M. Lebovitz, and R. G. Roeder. Accurate transcription initiation by RNA polymerase II in a soluble extract from isolated mammalian nuclei. *Nucleic Acids Res.* 11:1475–1489, 1983a.

Dignam, J. D., P. L. Martin, B. S. Shastry, and R. G. Roeder. Eukaryotic gene transcription with purified components. *Methods Enzymol.* 101:582–598, 1983b.

Dikstein, R., S. Ruppert, and R. Tjian. TAF$_{II}$250 is a bipartite protein kinase that phosphorylates the basal transcription factor RAP74. *Cell* 84:781–790, 1996.

Drapkin, R., A. Sancar, and D. Reinberg. Where transcription meets repair. *Cell* 77:9–12, 1994.

Dynlacht, B. D., T. Hoey, and R. Tjian. Isolation of coactivators associated with the TATA-binding protein that mediate transcriptional activation. *Cell* 66: 563–576, 1991.

Elgin, S. C. R. The formation and function of DNAase I hypersensitive sites in the process of gene activation. *J. Biol. Chem.* 263:19259–19262, 1988.

Felsenfeld, G. Chromatin as an essential part of the transcription mechanism. *Nature* 355:219–224, 1992.

Flores, O., H. Lu, M. Killeen, J. Greenblatt, Z.F. Burton, and D. Reinberg. The small subunit of transcription factor IIF recruits RNA polymerase II into the preinitiation complex. *Proc. Natl. Acad. Sci. U.S.A.* 88:9999–10003, 1991

Goodrich, J. A., T. Hoey, C. J. Thut, A. Admon, and R. Tjian. Drosophila TAF$_{II}$40 interacts with both a VP16 activation domain and the basal transcription factor TFIIB. *Cell* 75:519–530, 1993.

Goodrich, J. A., and R. Tjian. TBP-TAF complexes: selectivity factors for eukaryotic transcription. *Curr. Opin. Cell. Biol.* 6:403–409, 1994.

Grant, S. G., and V. M. Chapman. Mechanisms of X-chromosome regulation. *Annu. Rev. Genet.* 22:199–233, 1988.

Guzikevich-Guerstein, G., and Z. Shakked. A novel form of the DNA double helix imposed on the TATA-box by the TATA-binding protein. *Nat. Struct. Biol.* 3:32–37, 1996.

Ha, I., W. S. Lane, and D. Reinberg. Cloning of a human gene encoding the general transcription initiation factor IIB. *Nature* 352:689–695, 1991.

Halle, J.-P., and M. Meisterernst. Gene expression: increasing evidence for a transcriptosome. *Trends Genet.* 12:161–163, 1996.

Hansen, S. K., and R. Tjian. TAFs and TFIIA mediate differential utilization of the tandem Adh promoters. *Cell* 82:565–575, 1995.

Hansen, U. Mechanisms of eukaryotic transcription: surfaces, complexes, and contexts. *Biochim. Biophys. Acta* 1287:59–62, 1996.

Hernandez, N. TBP, a universal eukaryotic transcription factor? *Genes Dev.* 7: 1291–1308, 1993.

Hisatake, K., T. Ohta, R. Takada, M. Guermah, M. Horikoshi, Y. Nakatani, and R. G. Roeder. Evolutionary conservation of human TATA-binding-polypeptide-associated factors TAF$_{II}$31 and TAF$_{II}$80 and interactions of TAF$_{II}$80 with other TAFs and with general transcription factors. *Proc. Natl. Acad. Sci. U. S. A.* 92:8195–8199, 1995.

Hoffmann, A., C.-M. Chiang, T. Oelgeschlager, X. Xie, S. K. Burley, Y. Nakatani, and R .G. Roeder. A histone octamer-like structure within TFIID. *Nature* 380: 356–359, 1996.

Hori, R., S. Pyo, and M. Carey. Protease footprinting reveals a surface on transcription factor TFIIB that serves as an interface for activators and coactivators. *Proc. Natl. Acad. Sci. U.S.A.* 92:6047–6051, 1995.

Jacq, X., C. Brou, Y. Lutz, I. Davidson, P. Chambon, and L. Tora. Human TAF$_{II}$30 is present in a distinct TFIID complex and is required for transcriptional activation by the estrogen receptor. *Cell* 79:107–117, 1994.

Jahner, D., and R. Jaenisch. DNA methylation in early mammalian development. In *DNA Methylation: Biochemistry and Biological Significance*, A. Razin, H. Cedar, and A. D. Riggs, eds. New York: Springer-Verlag, pp. 189–220, 1984.

Jeppesen, P., and B. M. Turner. The inactive X chromosome in female mammals is distinguished by a lack of histone H4 acetylation, a cytogenic marker for gene expression. *Cell* 74:281–289, 1993.

Jones, P. A. Altering gene expression with 5-azacytidine. *Cell* 40:485–486, 1985.

Kafri, T., M. Ariel, M. Brandeis, R. Shemer, L. Urven, J. McCarrey, H. Cedar, and A. Razin. Developmental pattern of gene specific DNA methylation of the mouse embryo and germ line. *Genes Dev.* 6:705–714, 1992.

Kim, J. L., D. B. Nikolov, and S. K. Burley. Co-crystal structure of tBP recognising the minor groove of a TATA element. *Nature* 365:520–527, 1993a.

Kim, Y., J. H. Geiger, S. Hahn, P. B. Sigler. Crystal structure of a yeast TBP/TATA-box complex. *Nature* 365:512–520, 1993b.

Kim, Y. J., S. Bjorklund, Y. Li, M. H. Sayre, and R. D. Kornberg. A multiprotein mediator of transcriptional activation and its interaction with the C-terminal domain of RNA polymerase II. *Cell* 77:599–608, 1994.

Kingston, R. E., C. A. Bunker, and A. N. Imbalzano. Repression and activation by multiprotein complexes that alter chromatin structure. *Genes Dev.* 10:905–920, 1996.

Koleske, A. J., and R. A. Young. An RNA polymerase II holoenzyme responsive to activators. *Nature* 368:466–469, 1994.

Koleske, A. J., and R. A. Young. The RNA polymerase II holoenzyme and its implications for gene regulation. *Trends Biochem. Sci.* 20:113–116, 1995.

Krude, T., and S. C. R. Elgin. Chromatin: pushing nucleosomes around. *Curr. Biol.* 6:511–515, 1996.

Lewin, B. *Genes VI*. Oxford: Oxford University Press, 1997.

Li, E., T. H. Bestor, and R. Jaenisch. Targeted mutation of the DNA methyltransferase gene results in embryonic lethality. *Cell* 69:915–926, 1992.

Lobo, S. M., M. Tanaka, M. L. Sullivan, and N. Hernandez. A TBP complex essential for transcription from TATA-less but not TATA-containing RNA polymerase III promoters is part of the TFIIIB fraction. *Cell* 71:1029–1040, 1992.

McCracken, S., N. Fong, K. Yankulov, S. Ballantyne, G. Pan, J. Greenblatt, S. D. Patterson, M. Wickens, and D. L. Bentley. The C-terminal domain of RNA polymerase II couples mRNA processing to transcription. *Nature* 385:357–361, 1997.

McKnight, S. L. Transcription revisited: a commentary on the 1995 Cold Spring Harbor Laboratory meeting "Mechanisms of Eukaryotic Transcription." *Genes Dev.* 10:367–381, 1996.

Mengus, G., M. May, X. Jacq, A. Staub, L. Tora, P. Chambon, and I. Davidson. Cloning and characterisation of hTAF$_{II}$18, hTAF$_{II}$20 and hTAF$_{II}$28: three subunits of the human transcription factor TFIID. *EMBO J.* 14:1520–1531, 1996.

Monk, M., M. Boubelik, and S. Lehnert. Temporal and regional changes in DNA methylation in the embryonic, extraembryonic and germ cell lineages during mouse embryo development. *Development* 99:371–382, 1987.

Nikolov, D. B., and S. K. Burley. RNA polymerase II transcription initiation: a structural view. *Proc. Natl. Acad. Sci. U.S.A.* 94:15–22, 1997.

Nikolov, D. B., H. Chen, E. D. Halay, A. A. Usheva, K. Hisatake, D. K. Lee, R. G. Roeder, and S. K. Burley. Crystal structure of a TFIIB-TBP-TATA-element ternary complex. *Nature* 377:119–128, 1995.

Reik, W., A. Collick, M. Norris, S Barton, and M. A. Surani. Genomic imprinting determines the methylation of parental alleles in transgenic mice. *Nature* 328: 248–251, 1987.

Roberts, S. G. E., I. Ha, E. Maldonado, and D. Reinberg, and M. R. Green. Interaction between an acidic activator and transcription factor IIB is required for transcriptional activation. *Nature* 363:741–744, 1993.

Ruppert, S., and R. Tjian. Human $TAF_{II}250$ interacts with RAP74: implications for RNA polymerase II initiation. *Genes Dev.* 9:2747–2755, 1995.

Ruppert, S., E. Wang, and R. Tjian. Cloning and expression of human $TAF_{II}250$: a TBP-associated factor implicated in cell-cycle regulation. *Nature* 362:175–179, 1993.

Sadowski, C. L., R. W. Henry, S. M. Lobo, and N. Hernandez. A TBP-containing complex activates transcription from snRNA promoters through the PSE. *Genes Dev.* 7:1535–1548, 1993.

Sapienza, C., A. C. Peterson, J. Rossant, and R. Balling. Degree of methylation of transgenes is dependent on origin of gametes. *Nature* 328:251–254, 1987.

Sasaki, H., T. Hamada, T. Ueda, R. Seki, T. Higashinakagawa, and Y. Sakaki. Inherited type of allelic methylation variations in a mouse chromosome region where an integrated transgene shows methylation imprinting. *Development* 111:573–581, 1991.

Semenza, G. L. Transcriptional regulation of gene expression: mechanisms and pathophysiology. *Hum. Mutat.* 3:180–199, 1994.

Struhl, K. Duality of TBP, the universal transcription factor. *Science* 263:1103–1104, 1994.

Taggart, A. K. P., T. S. Fisher, and B. F. Pugh. The TATA-binding protein and associated factors are components of Pol III transcription factor TFIIIB. *Cell* 71:1015–1028, 1992.

Travers, A. Transcription: building an initiation machine. *Curr. Biol.* 6:401–403, 1996.

van Holde, K. E. Chromatin structure and transcription. In *Chromatin*, K. E. van Holde, ed. New York: Springer-Verlag, pp. 355–408, 1989.

Verrijzer, P., J.-L. Chen, K. Yokomori, and R. Tjian. Binding of TAFs to core elements directs promoter selectivity by RNA polymerase II. *Cell* 81:1115–1125, 1995.

Verrijzer, C. P., K. Yokomori, J.-L. Chen, and R. Tjian. Drosophila $TAF_{II}150$: similarity to yeast gene TSM-1 and specific binding to the core promoter DNA. *Science* 264:933–941, 1994.

Vettese-Dadey, M., P. A. Grant, T. R. Hebbes, C. Crane-Robinson, C. D. Allis, and J. L. Workman. Acetylation of histone H4 plays a primary role in enhancing transcription factor binding to nucleosomal DNA in vitro. *EMBO J.* 15:2508–2518, 1996.

Weil, P. A., D. S. Luse, J. Segall, and R. G. Roeder. Selective and accurate initiation of transcription at the AD2 major late promoter in a soluble system dependent on purified RNA polymerase II and DNA. *Cell* 18:469–484, 1979.

Weinzierl, R. O. J., B. D. Dynlacht, and R. Tjian. Largest subunit of Drosophila transcription factor IID directs assembly of a complex containing TBP and a coactivator. *Nature* 362:511–517, 1993.

Wilson, C. J., D. M. Chao, A. N. Imbalzano, G. R. Schnitzler, R. E. Kingston, and R. A. Young. RNA polymerase II holoenzyme contains SWI/SNF regulators involved in chromatin remodeling. *Cell* 84:235–244, 1996.

Wolffe, A. P., and D. Pruss. Targeting chromatin disruption: transcription regulators that acetylate histones. *Cell* 84:817–819, 1996.

Xie, X., T. Kokubo, S. L. Cohen, U. A. Mirza, A. Hoffman, B. T. Chait, R. G. Roeder, Y. Nakatani, and S. K. Burley. Structural similarity between TAFs and the heterotetrameric core of the histone octamer. *Nature* 380:316–322, 1996.

Yankulov, K., J. Blau, T. Purton, S. Roberts, and D. L. Bentley. Transcriptional elongation by RNA polymerase II is stimulated by transactivators. *Cell* 77: 749–759, 1994.

Yeivin, A., and A. Razin. Gene methylation patterns and expression. In *DNA Methylation: Molecular Biology and Biological Significance*, J. P. Jost and H. P. Saluz, eds. Basel: Birkhauser-Verlag, pp. 523–568, 1993.

Young, R. A. RNA polymerase II. *Annu. Rev. Biochem.* 60:689–715, 1991.

Zawel, L., K. Kumar, and D. Reinberg. Recycling of the general transcription factors during RNA polymerase II transcription. *Genes Dev.* 9:1479–1490, 1995.

Zawel, L., and D. Reinberg. Initiation of transcription by RNA polymerase II: a multistep process. *Prog. Nucl. Acids Res. Mol. Biol.* 44:67–108, 1993.

Zhou, Q., P. M. Lieberman, T. G. Boyer, and A. J. Berk. Holo-TFIID supports transcriptional stimulation by diverse activators and from a TATA-less promoter. *Genes Dev.* 6: 1964-1974, 1992.

2 Cis-Acting Transcriptional Regulatory Elements

Although it is impossible to discuss the *cis*-acting DNA sequence elements without reference to the *trans*-acting factors that bind to these sequences, this chapter will primarily focus on defining the different types of positive and negative *cis*-acting transcriptional regulatory elements. The *trans*-acting factors will be described in considerable detail in Chapter 3.

Introductory Definitions

All the *cis*-acting elements that affect transcription are defined on the basis of functional criteria. Therefore, none of these elements can be definitively identified solely by the examination of nucleotide sequence data. In general *cis*-acting elements are DNA sequences containing binding sites for several different transcription factors that are required *en bloc* for the element to function fully. The first defining criterion is whether the putative element has a positive or negative effect on transcription. In general, positive *cis*-acting elements contain binding sites for positive *trans*-acting factors (transcriptional activators) and negative *cis*-acting elements contain binding sites for negative *trans*-acting factors (transcriptional repressors). Examples of positive *cis*-regulatory elements include promoters and enhancers, whereas silencers and transcription-arrest sites represent examples of negative regulatory elements.

Effects on transcription mediated by these elements may be, and often are, limited to a specific cell type, developmental stage, or physiologic condition. Classification in this respect can be somewhat arbitrary because a given element may contain sequences that have a positive effect on transcription in one developmental or physiologic context and a negative effect on transcription in a different context. Such elements can be classified as cell-type-restricted, inducible, or repressible positive regulatory elements. For example, a promoter may allow transcription of a gene only in a limited number of cell types. This restricted expression may be achieved by the presence of binding sites for cell-type-restricted activators and repressors. To illustrate this concept, consider a hypothetical *cis*-acting transcriptional regulatory element (for example, a promoter or enhancer) that contains binding sites for five different *trans*-acting factors (A, B, C, D, and E). The level of transcription mediated by this regulatory element in any given cell type would represent the net effect of activators and repressors that are present within the cell and for which binding sites are present within the promoter. Thus, the five different transcription factors, three of which are activators (A, B, and D) and two of which are repressors (C and E), can mediate various levels of transcription specifically within five different tissues (Fig. 2.1). This example illustrates an important principle of transcriptional regulation: *specificity is achieved by combinatorial means,* which allows the largest number of different states to be defined by the smallest number of regulators.

The second defining criterion is whether proper function of the pu-

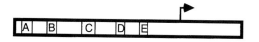

Factor	_____ Site of Expression and Effect on Transcription _____									
	Br	He	In	Ki	Li	Lu	Ov	Sp	Te	Th
A	++	++	0	0	+	+++	0	0	+	0
B	+	++	0	+	+	+	+++	+++	+++	++
C	++	0	--	--	--	0	0	0	--	--
D	+	0	+	0	+	+	0	0	0	0
E	0	0	--	--	-	-	---	-	0	0
NET	+++	++	0	0	0	++	0	+	+	0

FIGURE 2-1. Combinatorial control of transcription. A hypothetical *cis*-acting transcriptional regulatory element contains binding sites for five different *trans*-acting factors (A, B, C, D, and E) is shown. The effect of each individual factor on transcription is indicated as is the net transcription in each organ. Br, brain; He, heart; In, intestine; Ki, kidney; Li, liver; Lu, lung; Ov, ovary; Sp, spleen; Te, testis; Th, thymus.

tative element is dependent or independent of its position. The positional point of reference may be local (for example, the transcription initiation site of the gene under regulation) or it may be with respect to a more global context (for example, location within the genome). Thus, the promoter and enhancer are position-dependent and -independent positive regulatory elements with respect to the transcription initiation site, but the function of both elements is affected by genomic location, whereas a chromatin domain element, by definition, functions independently of genomic location. The classical *cis*-acting positive and negative regulatory elements will be described below, followed by a description of the more recently characterized chromatin domain elements.

Positive *Cis*-acting Regulatory Elements

Positive *cis*-acting elements are DNA sequences whose presence increases the transcriptional activity of a gene. These elements bind sequence-specific transcriptional activators. The two major types of positive *cis*-acting elements are the promoter and enhancer.

Promoter Elements

Promoter sequences encompass the transcription initiation site. The function of this element is position- and orientation-dependent, as the promoter establishes the site of transcription initiation and the direction in which transcription will proceed. The promoter can be dissected into the proximal promoter, which determines the initiation site and direction in which transcription will proceed, and the distal promoter, which determines the rate of transcription, usually by determining the frequency of transcription initiation. It should be noted that the terms promoter and 5'-flanking sequence are not synonymous. The limits of the distal promoter are defined functionally by determining the DNA sequences that are required for maximal rates of transcription. Given that transcriptional regulation often distinguishes between different cell types and physiological conditions, it should be recognized that this functional definition of the promoter prevents any absolute statements about the limits of the promoter except with respect to the particular conditions under which promoter function has been assayed.

The proximal promoter element, at a minimum, includes the DNA sequences that determine the transcription initiation site, and contains binding sites for Pol II and other components of the transcription initiation complex. Two sequence motifs that are present within the proximal promoter elements of many, but not all, genes are the TATA box and

Inr (initiator) elements. The TATA box is located 25 to 30 bp 5' to the transcription initiation site and has the consensus sequence 5'-TATAAA-3' (Breathnach and Chambon, 1981) and is recognized by the TBP (TATA binding protein) subunit of TFIID as described in Chapter 1. A generalization (with so many known exceptions as to be of limited utility) is that tissue-specific genes, the expression of which is restricted to a limited number of cell types, usually contain a TATA box whereas so-called housekeeping genes that are ubiquitously expressed often lack TATA boxes and instead contain highly GC-rich sequences in the vicinity of the transcription initiation site. A more useful generalization is that genes containing a TATA box usually initiate transcription from a single downstream site, whereas genes lacking a TATA box often initiate transcription from multiple sites that may be spread over a distance of up to several hundred nucleotides. In general, TATA-containing promoters appear to support a higher rate of transcription relative to TATA-less promoters when assayed in vitro (Zawel and Reinberg, 1993).

An obvious question arose as to the mechanism of transcription initiation site selection in TATA-less promoters. Analysis of the terminal deoxynucleotidyl transferase gene identified a novel *cis*-acting element, the initiator (Inr), a short pyrimidine-rich sequence (5-GCCCTCATTCT-3') that encompassed the transcription initiation site (the A residue) and was required for accurate and efficient transcription (Smale and Baltimore, 1989). Comparison of initiator elements from a variety of genes revealed a consensus sequence $Y_{4-5}CANTY_{4-5}$ (N, any nucleotide; Y, pyrimidine) (reviewed by Smale, 1994). Remarkably, TFIID binds to the initiator element (Kauffman and Smale, 1994), demonstrating the importance of this component of the transcription initiation complex for determining the transcription initiation site of all genes transcribed by Pol II. However, in contrast to the TATA box, which is recognized by TBP, the initiator is recognized by one of the TAFs (TBP associated factors). In addition, several sequence-specific transcription factors, including USF (Roy et al., 1991) and YY1 (Seto et al., 1991), have been shown to bind to initiator elements, but the functional significance of such binding has not been conclusively established. Although many proximal promoter elements contain either a TATA box or initiator element or both, several genes have been described that apparently lack both of these elements (Emami et al., 1995), suggesting that a third proximal promoter element motif may await discovery.

Additional transcription factor binding sites may be located either 5' or 3' to the proximal promoter. In some cases, the proximity of these sites is necessary for function, suggesting that factors binding at these sites make direct contact with components of the transcription initiation complex and are unable to do so when the site is moved to a more distal location. At present, it is not clear how factors binding at remote locations are able to interact (directly or indirectly) with the transcription initiation complex, nor is it clear why the function of some binding sites (and thus of their cognate factors) appears to be sensitive to location. Although the properties of individual transcription factors may play a role in this process, it is equally likely that each promoter has a unique architecture in which the binding of factors at proximal and distal sites allows the formation of a three-dimensional protein-DNA complex that results in a frequency of transcription initiation that is appropriate for that particular gene.

In Figure 2.2, the general promoter structure of members of the human alcohol dehydrogenase (ADH) gene family is shown with transcription factor binding sites indicated relative to the transcription initiation site. Binding sites for tissue-specific (oval), ubiquitous (rectangle), and ligand-regulated (triangle) transcription factors have been identified (van Ooij et al., 1992). Liver-specific transcription of these genes is activated by binding of the transcriptional activators C/EBP (CCAAT/enhancer-binding protein) and HNF-1 (hepatocyte nuclear factor 1), which are present at high levels in liver nuclei (see Chapter 12). RAR (retinoic acid receptor) is a transcription factor that must bind retinoic acid in order to function as a transcriptional activator (see Chapter 5). This is highly relevant to the physiologic function of ADH, which catalyzes the oxidation of vitamin A (retinol), the rate-limiting step in the metabolism of retinol to retinoic acid. Because retinoic acid then activates RAR function, this example provides an excellent illustration of the complex interactions that can exist between transcription factors, the genes they regulate, the protein products of regulated genes, and their respective enzymatic substrates and products.

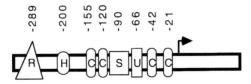

FIGURE 2-2. A prototypical *ADH* gene promoter. The coordinates of transcription factor binding sites are given relative to the transcription initiation site (bent arrow). The transcription factors are indicated as follows: C, C/EBP (CCAAT/ enhancer-binding protein); H, HNF-1 (hepatocyte nuclear factor 1); R, RAR (retinoic acid receptor); S, Sp1; U, USF (upstream stimulatory factor). (Adapted from van Ooij et al., 1992.)

Enhancer Elements

Enhancers are *cis*-acting DNA sequences that may be located 5' or 3' to the gene or within an exon or intron of the gene. In contrast to the promoter, enhancer function is by definition position- and orientation-independent (reviewed by Thompson and McKnight, 1992). Enhancers have a modular structure with each module representing a transcription factor binding site. Enhancer function is based on synergism, as individual modules may have little or no enhancing activity. Rather, it is the juxtaposition of binding sites for multiple factors in close proximity to one another that is the basis for enhancer function. This requirement for proximity suggests cooperativity of function, at the level of DNA binding and/or transactivation. Enhancer sequences often demonstrate a hypersensitivity to digestion by DNase I within nuclei isolated from cells that express the gene regulated in *cis* by the enhancer. This experimental finding indicates that these DNA sequences are less protected by histones and other chromosomal proteins. The existence of nucleosome-free DNA allows greater accessibility to DNase I in vitro and to transcription factors in vivo.

Enhancers are able to function at distances of 10 kb or more from the transcription initiation site. How can factors binding at such remote locations interact with components of the transcription initiation complex? The model that is currently favored to explain this paradox involves DNA looping (Ptashne, 1988), as illustrated in Figure 2.3. In this illustration, exon 1 of a hypothetical gene is depicted by the box. The TATA box and other sequences required for the formation of the transcription initiation complex are present in the proximal 5'-flanking region of the gene. In addition, binding sites are present in the 5'-flanking region

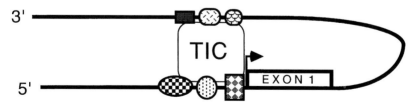

FIGURE 2-3. Chromatin looping. The 5' end of a hypothetical gene is shown with binding sites for three transcription factors in the 5'-flanking sequence and binding sites for three additional factors within the intervening sequence 3' to exon 1. The formation of a DNA loop allows the general transcription factors of the transcription initiation complex (TIC) to interact with factors bound both 5' and 3' to the transcription initiation site.

for sequence-specific transcriptional activators that interact with components of the transcription initiation complex. An enhancer, located several kilobases 3' to the hypothetical gene, contains binding sites for several additional transcriptional activators. Despite their distance from the promoter, these proteins are also able to interact with components of the transcription initiation complex by a looping out of DNA sequences between the enhancer and the gene.

Evidence in support of this model was provided by the following experiment (Li et al., 1991). A DNA fragment was constructed that contained four binding sites for the sequence-specific transcriptional activator Sp1 at one end and five binding sites for the factor E2 at the other end (Fig. 2.4). The DNA was incubated with Sp1 and E2 and the resulting complexes were examined by electron microscopy. The two factors could be distinguished by electron density because the Sp1 signal appeared lighter than the E2 signal, and their binding sites could be established based on the size of the loop and distance from the end of the molecule. These measurements indicated that both Sp1 and E2 had specifically recog-

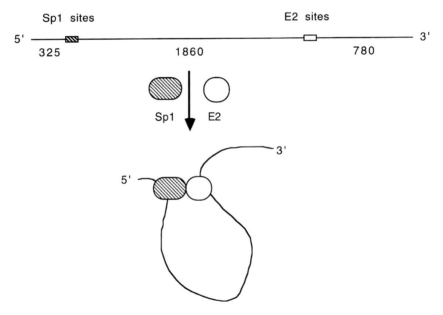

FIGURE 2-4. Formation of DNA loops by protein-protein interactions in vitro. Line drawing at top shows location of four Sp1 (hatched box) and five E2 (open box) binding sites, and the distances (in bp) between sites and ends of DNA. Electron microscopy at bottom shows formation of looped structures by Sp1 (hatched circle) and E2 (open circle) bound to DNA. (Based on data from Li et al., 1991.)

nized their cognate binding sites on the DNA fragment and had interacted with one another to create the loop. As described in Chapter 3, the formation of DNA loops may be facilitated by the ability of some bound transcription factors to bend DNA.

Negative Regulatory Elements

DNA sequences that function primarily to inhibit expression of a gene within certain cell types or under specific developmental or physiological conditions are defined as negative regulatory elements. These elements bind factors (repressors) that decrease the rate of transcription by adversely affecting either initiation or elongation.

Silencer Elements

Silencers restrict expression in a position- and orientation-independent manner, much like enhancers but to opposite effect (reviewed by Renkawitz, 1990). Factors binding to silencers are believed to interfere with formation of the transcription initiation complex. Silencers provide a mechanism for restricting expression of a gene to a limited number of cell types. For example, expression of the thyroid stimulating hormone β (TSHβ) gene is restricted to cells in the anterior pituitary and is activated at least in part by the binding of the pituitary-specific transcriptional activator PIT-1 to sites in the promoter between 128 and 80 bp 5' to the transcription initiation site (Steinfelder et al., 1992). However, PIT-1 is expressed in all cells of the anterior pituitary, whereas TSHβ is expressed only in thyrotrophs, and the PIT-1 binding sites do not provide sufficient information to direct thyrotroph-specific expression. DNA sequences located between 128 and 480 bp 5' to the transcription initiation site were shown to function as a silencer that prevented reporter gene expression in both TSHβ-expressing and nonexpressing cells (Kim et al., 1996). The presence of an enhancer element located in the distal flanking region (between 1.2 and approximately 10 kb 5' to the initiation site) was sufficient to overcome the effects of the silencer in TSHβ-expressing but not in TSHβ-nonexpressing cells. These results suggest that only TSHβ-expressing cells contain an enhancer-binding activator whose positive effects are greater than the negative effects of the putative repressor that binds to the silencer. The silencer DNA sequence was shown to be associated with the nuclear matrix in TSHβ-nonexpressing cells, but unfortunately TSHβ-expressing cells were not analyzed for this property, and thus the relationship between nuclear matrix attachment and silencing is unknown. Silencing may involve the gene assuming an inactive chromatin configuration, but this was also not determined. The silencer contained features characteristic of matrix attachment regions, including high AT content, multiple sequences matching the topoisomerase II consensus binding site, and multiple AT-rich palindromic sequences capable of forming cruciform DNA structures (Kim et al., 1996). Other *cis*-acting regulatory elements such as boundary elements (described later in this chapter) also share characteristics of matrix attachment regions.

Position-Dependent Negative Regulatory Elements

Position-dependent negative regulatory elements are often located between promoter and enhancer elements and appear to bind repressors that prevent factors bound at the enhancer from interacting with the transcription initiation complex. The functional properties of positive and negative regulatory elements described thus far are illustrated by a description of the gene complex that encodes α-fetoprotein (AFP) and albumin, the major serum proteins in fetal and adult mammals, respectively. As shown in Figure 2.5, the mouse albumin and AFP genes are contiguous in genomic DNA, with the albumin gene located 13.5 kb 5' to the AFP gene in the same transcriptional orientation (Hammer et al., 1987). AFP gene expression is restricted to yolk sac, fetal liver, and fetal gastrointestinal tract. In addition, the level of expression is very high in yolk sac and fetal liver (accounting for 20% and 5% of total RNA, respectively) and more modest in the gut (less than 0.1% of total RNA). This highly regulated pattern of AFP gene expression is determined by three enhancers located in the 5'-flanking region of the AFP gene: EI (located 2.5 kb 5' to the gene) directs expression to yolk sac, fetal liver, and gastrointestinal tract; EII (−5.0 kb) directs expression to yolk sac and liver; and EIII (−6.5 kb) directs expression to yolk sac only (Hammer et

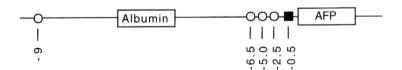

FIGURE 2-5. *Cis*-acting transcriptional regulatory elements controlling expression of the albumin and α-fetoprotein genes. The albumin and α-fetoprotein (AFP) genes are indicated as boxes. Enhancer (EI, EII, and EIII) and negative regulatory elements are depicted by ovals and square, respectively, with coordinates given relative to the downstream transcription initiation site.

al., 1987). Thus, the number of enhancers contributing to expression in the various tissues corresponds to the relative levels of expression.

Expression of AFP and albumin is developmentally regulated such that after birth AFP gene expression is repressed and albumin gene expression increases in the liver. Repression of AFP gene expression in the liver was shown to require sequences located within the first 1 kb of 5'-flanking sequences, between the proximal promoter and the three enhancers (Vacher and Tilghman, 1990). The negative regulatory element was not functional when it was placed 5' to the enhancers. The use of a position-dependent negative regulatory element in this context appears to be related to the fact that although an enhancer is located 9 kb 5' to the albumin gene that directs expression to the liver (Pinkert et al., 1987), the AFP enhancer elements also contribute to the high level of albumin gene expression in the liver (Vacher and Tilghman, 1990). Thus, the position-dependent negative regulatory element allows selective repression of AFP gene expression whereas a silencer would repress both AFP and albumin gene transcription. Because this element has no effect on expression prior to birth, it is likely to bind a repressor that is expressed specifically in postnatal liver. The complex regulatory phenomena involving multiple *cis*-acting elements described above may also explain why these two genes have remained in close proximity to one another since they arose by a gene duplication event several hundred million years ago (Hammer et al., 1987).

Transcription Arrest Sites

Negative regulatory elements that affect elongation rather than initiation of transcription have been identified within the first several hundred base pairs 3' to the transcription initiation site. These elements presumably bind repressors that block elongation of the nascent primary RNA transcript, a mechanism that has been termed promoter-proximal attenuation. This mechanism may allow certain genes to remain poised for rapid transcription in response to physiologic stimuli. Genes that are regulated by this mechanism include the immediate-early response genes *C-FOS* and *C-MYC* (reviewed by Krumm and Groudine, 1995). In the case of *C-MYC* , when proliferating HL60 cells are exposed to retinoic acid, which induces cellular differentiation, transcription is prematurely terminated at two sites, located 371 and 421 nucleotides downstream of the major *C-MYC* transcription initiation site, which are preceded by a thymidine-rich sequence and a GC-rich sequence capable of forming a stem-loop structure (Krumm et al., 1993). *Trans*-acting factors involved in transcription arrest have not been identified to date.

Chromosomal Domain Elements

Most recently, *cis*-acting elements have been described that exert their effects over very large distances that may encompass entire clusters of genes. Additional distinguishing characteristics of these elements are that (1) their effects on transcription may not be easily classified as positive or negative; (2) they may affect DNA replication as well as transcription; and (3) they may affect the chromatin structure over hundreds of kilobases of DNA in a cell-type-specific and developmentally regulated manner.

Locus Control Regions

The presence of a powerful, positive *cis*-acting locus control region (LCR) appears to be a necessary prerequisite for the expression of certain genes that are expressed at high levels in a cell-type-specific manner. These elements appear to direct the establishment of a milieu within chromatin, termed a domain, in which transcription factors are able to access their binding sites and activate gene transcription. The first LCR described spans a region located 6 to 18 kb 5' to the human ε-globin gene (Fig. 2.6) and exerts its effect over the downstream 50 kb of the β-globin gene cluster (Forrester et al., 1986; Tuan et al., 1985; reviewed by Townes and Behringer, 1990). The proximal promoter regions of the ε, ^{G}γ, ^{A}γ, δ and β-globin genes are hypersensitive to DNase I digestion specifically in nuclei isolated from erythroid progenitor cells, indicating an altered chromatin structure associated with transcription factor binding (see Chapter 1). In contrast, the LCR contains four regions that are super-hypersensitive to DNase I (i. e., digestion occurs at much lower concentrations of DNase I) in erythroid cells, indicating an even more marked degree of cell-type-specific chromatin remodeling within this element.

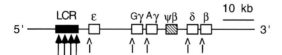

FIGURE 2-6. The structure of the β-globin gene cluster. Shown are the functional ε,^{G}γ, ^{A}γ, δ, and β-globin genes, the nonfunctional ψβ pseudogene, and the locus control region (LCR), which is required for erythroid-specific expression of each gene in the cluster. The location of erythroid-specific DNase hypersensitive sites (open arrows) and super-hypersensitive sites (closed arrows) in the gene promoters and LCR, respectively, are also indicated.

Several properties of the LCR have been defined by studies utilizing transgenic mice. In the presence of the LCR, a β-globin transgene was expressed specifically in erythroid cells and the level of expression was dependent on the number of copies of the transgene that had integrated into the mouse germline and was not dependent on the site of integration (Grosveld et al., 1987). In contrast, the level of expression of most transgenes is not correlated with copy number and is highly influenced by integration site, which can result in a lack of expression in the appropriate tissue and/or inappropriate expression in tissues where the endogenous gene is not expressed. In addition, transfection of constructs containing the LCR cloned 5' to a heterologous Thy-1 gene, which was not normally expressed in erythroid cells, resulted in erythroid cell–specific expression (Blom van Assendelft et al., 1989). The LCR contains multiple copies of three core motifs: 5'-CACCC-3', 5'-GATA-3', and 5'-TGA(C/G)TCA-3', which represent binding sites for three essential erythroid-specific transcription factors: EKLF, GATA-1, and NF-E2, respectively (reviewed by Orkin, 1995). These same transcription factor binding sites are also present in the promoters of erythroid-specific genes and thus the unique function of the LCR has yet to be understood at the molecular level.

The human α-globin gene cluster contains the embryonic ζ2– and adult α2– and α1–globin genes. An LCR was identified approximately 40 kb 5' to the ζ2–globin gene (Jarman et al., 1991). Deletion of the LCR from the α- or β-globin gene cluster results in loss of expression of all globin genes located in *cis* to the mutation as described in Chapter 4.

Several other genes have been shown to possess LCRs, including the human CD2 gene (Greaves et al., 1989), human red and green visual pigment genes (Wang et al., 1992), and the immunoglobulin heavy chain locus (Madisen and Groudine, 1994). In the case of the human CD2 gene, studies in transgenic mice have demonstrated that the LCR functions to establish and/or maintain an open chromatin configuration regardless of the integration site (Festenstein et al., 1996). As in the case of the β-globin gene cluster, the LCR controlling the visual pigment genes is located 5' to the 5'-most gene of the cluster that encodes the red pigment, and the downstream green pigment gene is inactivated by deletions that remove the LCR and red pigment gene but leave intact the green pigment gene, which is normally located 42 kb 3' to the LCR (Wang et al., 1992). Transcriptional regulation of both pigment genes by a single LCR may assure that a single cone cell expresses only a single pigment gene. It is not yet clear whether all genes or clusters of genes have LCRs that are essential in *cis* for their regulated transcription. Given the fact that clustered genes would otherwise be dispersed throughout the genome during evolution, it is likely that such clusters are maintained by selection because of the presence of shared *cis*-acting transcriptional regulatory elements.

Boundary Elements

A second type of chromosomal domain element that has been described is the boundary element. These elements in and of themselves have neither a positive nor a negative effect on the rate of transcription. Instead, they function to insulate the gene they flank from the potential effects of any positive or negative regulatory elements of neighboring genes (reviewed by Eissenberg and Elgin, 1991). The first boundary elements described were the scs and scs' sites flanking the *Drosophila 87A7* heat shock locus (Kellum and Schedl, 1991a,b). In the polytene chromosomes of the *Drosophila* salivary gland, the conversion of chromatin from a closed to an open configuration can be visualized under the microscope as the formation of chromosome puffs. The boundary elements localized to the boundaries of the puff associated with expression of the *hsp70* gene at locus *87A7*, suggesting that these elements might function to limit the region of chromatin conversion.

The A elements identified in the chicken lysozyme gene also function as boundary elements (Stief et al., 1989). The DNA bounded by the A elements is in a DNase I–sensitive, open chromatin configuration within cells that express the lysozyme gene, whereas DNA outside the elements is in a DNase I–resistant, closed chromatin configuration suggesting that, as in the case of the LCR, the A elements may participate in the establishment of a chromosomal domain. Like the LCR, and unlike the scs elements, the A elements have enhancer activity when reporter constructs are assayed for expression in stably transformed cell lines.

A boundary element was subsequently identified 5' to the LCR of the chicken β-globin gene cluster such that the LCR has no effect on sequences 5' to the boundary element (Chung et al., 1993). Remarkably, the element functions as an insulator when transgenes are introduced into chicken, human, or *Drosophila* cells. The presence of the insulator is consistent with the observation that in erythroid cells, chromatin over more than 200 kb 3' to the LCR is in an open chromatin configuration, whereas chromatin 5' to the LCR is in a condensed state (Chung et al., 1993). Analysis of the human CD2 gene LCR revealed that it could be dissected into two regions, one of which functioned as a classical enhancer and the other as a boundary element (Festenstein et al., 1996). Based on these results, it seems safe to predict that many chromosomal domain elements will turn out to be composite structures containing sequences that mediate both enhancer and insulator functions.

The biochemical basis for insulator function has not been determined. Some chromosomal domain elements, such as the A elements, contain a matrix attachment region (MAR), which is believed to be a site at which chromatin is attached to the nuclear matrix. According to one model that attempts to relate chromsomal organization to gene regulation, chromatin loops extend out from the MAR–nuclear matrix attachment sites and constitute domains of expression that are insulated from the effects of *cis*-acting elements and *trans*-acting factors present within other nearby chromatin loops (reviewed by Chung et al., 1993; Garrard, 1990; Gasser and Laemmli, 1987; Laemmli et al., 1992). Recently, a *trans*-acting factor, BEAF-32 (boundary element–associated factor of 32 kDa), was identified that bound to a palindromic sequence 5'-CGATAGTATCG-3' within the *cis*-acting scs' boundary element of the *Drosophila hsp70* gene at locus *87A7* (Zhao et al., 1995). BEAF-32 was shown to localize to one edge of many different chromosome puffs, indicating that BEAF-32 plays a general role in the establishment of chromosomal domains and that at least one other *trans*-acting boundary element–binding factor must exist. The binding of BEAF-32 to only one edge of a puff suggests that chromosomal domains may have a polar organization (Zhao et al., 1995). These studies provide the first glimpse of the molecular mechanisms by which chromosomal domains are established and suggest that the same general principles of *cis*-acting sequences and *trans*-acting factors may provide a useful framework for constructing models of higher order chromatin structure and function.

References

Blom van Assendelft, G., O. Hanscombe, F. Grosveld, and D. R. Greaves. The β-globin dominant control region activates homologous and heterologous promoters in a tissue-specific manner. *Cell* 56:969–977, 1989.

Breathnach, R., and P. Chambon. Organization and expression of eucaryotic split genes coding for proteins. *Annu. Rev. Biochem.* 50:349–383, 1981.

Chung, J. H., M. Whitely, and G. Felsenfeld. A 5' element of the chicken β-globin domain serves as an insulator in human erythroid cells and protects against position effects in Drosophila. *Cell* 74:505–514, 1993.

Emami, K. H., W. W. Navarre, and S. T. Smale. Core promoter specificities of the Sp1 and VP16 transcriptional activation domains. *Mol. Cell. Biol.* 15:5906–5916, 1995.

Eissenberg, J. C., and S. C. R. Elgin. Boundary functions in the control of gene expression. *Trends Genet.* 7:335–340, 1991.

Festenstein, R., M. Tolaini, P. Corbella, C. Mamalaki, J. Parrington, M. Fox, A. Miliou, M. Jones, and D. Kioussis. Locus control region function and heterochromatin-induced position effect variegation. *Science* 271:1123–1125, 1996.

Forrester, W. C., C. Thompson, J. T. Elder, and M. Groudine. A developmentally stable chromatin structure in the human β-globin gene cluster. *Proc. Natl. Acad. Sci. U.S.A.* 83:1359–1363, 1986.

Garrard, W. T. Chromosomal loop organization in eukaryotic genomes. In *Nucleic Acids and Molecular Biology*, F. Eckstein and D. M. J. Lilley, eds. Berlin: Springer-Verlag, pp. 163–175, 1990.

Gasser, S. M., and U. K. Laemmli. A glimpse at chromosomal order. *Trends Genet.* 3:16–22, 1990.

Greaves, D. R., F. D. Wilson, G. Lang, and D. Kioussis. Human CD2 3'-flanking sequences confer high-level, T cell-specific, position-independent gene expression in transgenic mice. *Cell* 56:979–986, 1989.

Grosveld, F. G., G. Blom van Assendelft, D. R. Greaves, and G. Kollias. Position-independent, high-level expression of the human β-globin gene in transgenic mice. *Cell* 51:975–985, 1987.

Hammer, R. E., R. Krumlauf, S. A. Camper, R. L. Brinster, and S. M. Tilghman. Diversity of alpha-fetoprotein gene expression in mice is generated by a combination of separate enhancer elements. *Science* 235:53–58, 1987.

Jarman, A. P., W. G. Wood, J. A. Sharpe, G. Gourdon, H. Ayyub, and D. R. Higgs. Characterization of the major regulatory element upstream of the human α-globin gene cluster. *Mol. Cell. Biol.* 11:4679–4689, 1991.

Kaufmann, J., and S. T. Smale. Direct recognition of initiator elements by a component of the transcription factor TFIID complex. *Genes Dev.* 8:821–829, 1994.

Kellum, R., and P. Schedl. A position-effect assay for boundaries of higher order chromosomal domains. *Cell* 64:941–950, 1991a.

Kellum, R., and P. Schedl. A group of scs elements function as domain boundaries in an enhancer-blocking assay. *Mol. Cell. Biol.* 12:2424–2431, 1991b.

Kim, M. K., L. A. Lesoon-Wood, B. D. Weintraub, and J. H. Chung. A soluble transcription factor, Oct-1, is also found in the insoluble nuclear matrix and possesses silencing activity in its alanine-rich domain. *Mol. Cell. Biol.* 16:4366–4377, 1996.

Krumm, A., and M. Groudine. Tumor suppression and transcription elongation: the dire consequences of changing partners. *Science* 269:1400–1401, 1995.

Krumm, A., T. Meulia, and M. Groudine. Common mechanisms for the control of eukaryotic transcriptional elongation. *Bioessays* 15:659–665, 1993.

Laemmli, U. K., E. Kas, L. Poljak, and Y. Adachi. Scaffold-associated regions: cis-acting determinants of chromatin structural loops and functional domains. *Curr. Opin. Genet. Dev.* 2:275–285, 1992.

Li, R., J. D. Knight, S. P. Jackson, R. Tjian, and M. R. Botchan. Direct interaction between Sp1 and the BPV enhancer E2 protein mediates synergistic activation of transcription. *Cell* 65:493–505, 1991.

Madisen, L., and M. Groudine. Identification of a locus control region in the immunoglobulin heavy-chain locus that deregulates c-myc expression in plasmacytoma and Burkitt's lymphoma cells. *Genes Dev.* 8:2212–2226, 1994.

Orkin, S. H. Transcription factors and hematopoietic development. *J. Biol. Chem.* 270:4955–4958, 1995.

Pinkert, C. A., D. M. Ornitz, R. L. Brinster, and R. D. Palmiter. An albumin enhancer located 10 kb upstream functions along with its promoter to direct efficient, liver-specific expression in transgenic mice. *Genes Dev.* 1:268–276, 1987.

Ptashne, M. How eukaryotic transcriptional activators work. *Nature* 335:683–689, 1988.

Renkawitz, R. Transcriptional repression in eukaryotes. *Trends Genet.* 6:192–197, 1990.

Roy, A. L., M. Meisterernst, P. Pognonec, and R. G. Roeder. Cooperative interaction of an initiator-binding transcription factor and the helix-loop-helix activator USF. *Nature* 354:245–248, 1991.

Seto, E., Y. Shi, and T. Shenk. YY1 is an initiator sequence-binding protein that directs and activates transcription in vitro. *Nature* 354:241–245, 1991.

Smale, S. T. Core promoter architecture for eukaryotic protein-coding genes. In *Transcription: Mechanisms and Regulation*, R. C. Conaway and J. W. Conaway, eds. New York: Raven Press, pp. 63–81, 1994.

Smale, S. T., and D. Baltimore. The "initiator" as transcription control element. *Cell* 57:103–113, 1989.

Steinfelder, H. J., S. Radovick, M. A. Mroczynski, P. Hauser, J.H. McClaskey, B. D. Weintraub, and F. E. Wondisford. Role of a pituitary-specific transcription factor (Pit1/GHF-1) or a closely related protein in cAMP regulation of human thyrotropin-ß subunit gene expression. *J. Clin. Invest.* 89:409–419, 1992.

Stief, A., D. M. Winter, W. H. Stratling, A. E. Sippel. A nuclear DNA attachment element mediates elevated and position-independent gene activity. *Nature* 341:343–345, 1989.

Thompson, C. C., and S. L. McKnight. Anatomy of an enhancer. *Trends Genet.* 8: 232–236, 1992.

Townes, T., and R. R. Behringer. Human globin locus activation region (LAR): role in temporal control. *Trends Genet.* 6:219–223, 1990.

Tuan, D., W. Solomon, L. Qiliang, and I. M. London. The "β-like-globin" gene domain in human erythroid cells. *Proc. Natl. Acad. Sci. U.S.A.* 82:6384–6388, 1985.

Vacher, J., and S. M. Tilghman. Dominant negative regulation of the mouse α-fetoprotein gene in adult liver. *Science* 250: 1732–1735, 1990.

van Ooij, C., R. S. Snyder, B. W. Paeper, and G. Duester. Temporal expression of the human alcohol dehydrogenase gene family during liver development correlates with differential promoter activation by hepatocyte nuclear factor 1, CCAAT/enhancer-binding protein α, liver activator protein, and D-element-binding protein. *Mol. Cell. Biol.* 12:3023–3031, 1992.

Wang, Y., J. P. Macke, S. L. Merbs, D. J. Zack, B. Klaunberg, J. Bennett, J. Gearhart, and J. Nathans. A locus control region adjacent to the human red and green visual pigment genes. *Neuron* 9:429–440, 1992.

Zawel, L., and D. Reinberg. Initiation of transcription by RNA polymerase II: a multistep process. *Prog. Nucl. Acids Res. Mol. Biol.* 44:67–108, 1993.

Zhao, K., C. M. Hart, and U. K. Laemmli. Visualization of chromosomal domains with boundary element-associated factor BEAF-32. *Cell* 81:879–889, 1995.

3 *Trans*-Acting Factors

Transcription factors are *trans*-acting proteins that affect the rate of transcription by specific interactions with DNA and/or other proteins (see Chapter 1). Transcriptional activators and repressors have positive and negative effects, respectively, on the rate of transcription. Transcriptional regulators may affect the rate of transcription initiation and/or mRNA elongation. In addition to DNA-binding activators and repressors, a variety of coactivators, corepressors, and other cofactors have been identified that do not bind to DNA directly but instead interact with the DNA-binding proteins and mediate their effects on transcription. Some of these co-factors have enzymatic activities that allow them to modify other cofactors, Pol II, or histones. Each of the transcription factor classes listed in Table 3.1 will be described in this chapter, followed by a discussion of pathways that transduce signals (e.g., cytokines, growth factors, and small molecules) at the cell surface to transcription factors that alter gene expression in the nucleus.

Transcriptional Activators

Modular Model of Transcription Factor Function

Trans-acting factors that have a positive effect on the rate of transcription (transactivators) have been studied most intensively. The structural analysis of these proteins suggested that they were modular in design, containing domains that were structurally and functionally discrete so that domains could be experimentally swapped between factors and retain their functional characteristics (Keegan et al., 1986). At the most basic level of design, transcriptional activators can be viewed as bipartite molecules containing DNA-binding and transactivation domains. A DNA-

Table 3.1. Transcription Factors

1. Activators
2. Coactivators
3. Architectural factors
4. Repressors and corepressors
5. Chromatin remodeling factors
6. Transcription elongation factors

binding domain targets the factor to specific DNA sequences, thus positioning the factor to interact with specific target proteins in a manner that stimulates transcription initiation or elongation. Most transcriptional activators are dimeric proteins, and for these factors protein dimerization is a necessary prerequisite for DNA binding. The dimerization domain is thus a third functional structure within many transcriptional activators and is usually contiguous with the DNA-binding domain in the primary structure of the protein. Finally, additional signal sequences are involved in the regulation of transcription factor function, such as nuclear localization sequences and sites of posttranslational modification that may affect dimerization, DNA binding, transactivation, subcellular localization, or protein stability. Each of these aspects of transcription factor structure and function will be described in subsequent sections of this chapter.

Although transcription factors show remarkable modularity of structure in that the DNA-binding domain from one factor can be fused to the transactivation domain of another factor and each domain may retain its respective function, there is also overlap of function between these domains in vivo. For example, whereas the specific structural motifs (DNA-binding domains) that are described below are necessary and in some cases sufficient to impart sequence-specific DNA-binding activity to the proteins in which they reside, it has become apparent that these domains support additional functions that involve protein-protein interactions. Indeed, for several transcription factors, including the zinc finger factor GATA-1 (Visvader et al., 1995) and the bHLH protein MYOD (Tapscott et al., 1988), forced expression of the DNA-binding domain alone can induce programs of cellular differentiation. In the case of GATA-1, the carboxyl-terminal zinc finger is required for sequence-specific DNA binding, whereas the amino-terminal finger interacts with other transcription factors (Tsang et al., 1997). In addition to zinc finger and bHLH domains, homeodomains have also been implicated in protein-protein interactions (Zhang et al., 1996; see below). Conversely, recent experiments indicate that protein-protein interactions between transactivation domains of factors bound to adjacent DNA sequences can result in cooperative DNA binding (Tanaka, 1996; see below). Thus, the compartmentalization of function implied by the modular model is an oversimplification of the elegant and complex molecular mechanisms of transcriptional regulation that have evolved over a billion years of eukaryotic existence.

DNA-Binding and Dimerization Domains

The DNA-binding domain is that part of the protein that interacts with DNA. Most DNA binding domains contain an amphipathic alpha helix with basic residues that establish noncovalent interactions with the bases and negatively charged phosphate backbone of the DNA double helix. In contrast to bacterial restriction endonucleases, which usually bind to a unique DNA sequence, most eukaryotic transcription factors can bind with varying affinity to multiple sequences. Transcription factors exist as families of related proteins that, by virtue of similar DNA-binding domains, can bind to related or identical DNA sequences. Thus, a single factor can bind to multiple sequences, and a single DNA sequence can be bound by multiple (related or even unrelated) transcription factors. For this reason, scanning nucleotide sequences for transcription factor binding sites can be uninformative or misleading. Factor binding and transcription assays must be performed to establish sites of factor binding that are relevant to the regulation of gene expression in vivo. Different factors may bind to the same DNA sequence under different developmental or physiological conditions so that the identification of a transcription factor binding site depends on the cellular context.

Many transcription factors are members of families of proteins that share in common a specific DNA-binding motif. In most transcription factors, the DNA-binding domain constitutes the most highly conserved sequences within the protein when comparing family members within a species or homologous proteins in different species. In contrast, transcriptional activation domains do not represent homology units that are usually highly conserved within transcription factor families or between species. These observations suggest that the DNA-binding domain represents the key structural and functional component of transcriptional activators. For this reason, the presentation of specific transcription factors in Chapters 5 through 11 is organized according to DNA binding motifs.

Analysis of the nucleotide sequence of cDNAs encoding transcription factors allowed prediction of the amino acid sequence of these proteins. Comparison of the DNA-binding domains has revealed that greater than 80% of transcription factors fall into one of four groups, defined by related sequences that establish a tertiary protein structure capable of binding to DNA (Papavassiliou, 1995). These four sequence motifs are the basic helix-loop-helix, basic leucine zipper, zinc finger, and the helix-turn-helix motif present in the homeodomain (Fig. 3.1). The structural properties of each of these DNA binding motifs and representative examples of transcription factors containing them are described below.

The homeodomain motif. The homeodomain is a 60-amino-acid-residue motif that shows remarkable sequence similarity among transcription factors spanning 600 million years of evolutionary divergence from *Drosophila melanogaster* to *Homo sapiens*. The homeodomain is encoded by a 180-bp DNA sequence, the homeobox (this nomenclature is often misused in the literature). The homeodomain creates a tertiary structure that most closely resembles the helix-turn-helix DNA-binding motif (Fig. 3.1) of prokaryotic transcription factors (Gehring et al., 1990). Structural studies of homeodomain proteins from yeast, flies, and humans revealed that the homeodomain consists of three α helices preceded by an amino-terminal arm and that it interacts with DNA such that the third α helix inserts into the major groove and the amino-terminal arm contacts bases in the minor groove of the DNA (reviewed by Li et al., 1995).

The first homeodomain proteins identified were shown to play a key role in the establishment of the basic body plan during *Drosophila* embryogenesis. They were isolated as targets of homeotic mutations that transform one body segment of the fly into another (e.g., formation of an additional thoracic segment in place of an abdominal segment). Remarkably, these *Drosophila* genes cross-hybridized with mouse and human DNA sequences, thus allowing the isolation of homologous mammalian genes (reviewed by McGinnis and Krumlauf, 1992). The *Drosophila* genetic system that specifies anterior-posterior positional identity is both structurally and functionally conserved in other organisms, including mice and humans. There are 39 mammalian *HOX* genes that are related to the *Drosophila HOM-C* genes, including the prototypic member, *Antennapedia*. These mammalian genes are arranged in four clusters (*HOX-A, HOX-B, HOX-C,* and *HOX-D*) that are located on four different chromosomes (Scott, 1992). In both *Drosophila* and mammals, there is a relationship between gene order within a cluster and the temporospatial pattern of expression during development, with genes at the 5' end of each cluster being expressed at the posterior end of the embryo (reviewed by McGinnis and Krumlauf, 1992; Shashikant et al., 1991). This multigene organization is reminiscent of the temporospatial organization of the β-globin gene cluster, which was described in Chapter 2.

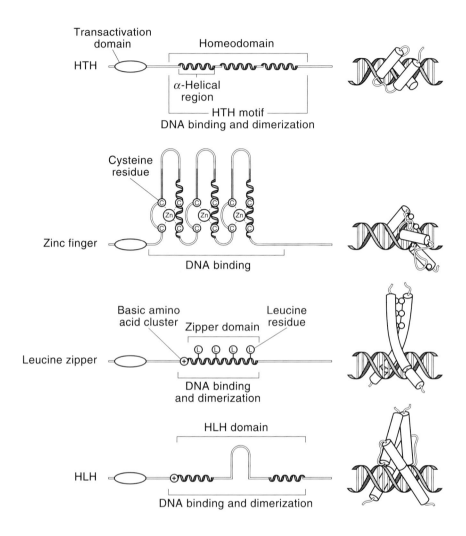

FIGURE 3-1. DNA-binding domains. At left are shown the structures of four DNA-binding motifs, the helix-turn-helix (HTH) homeodomain, zinc finger, basic leucine zipper, and basic helix-loop-helix (HLH) domain. At right are shown the interactions of these domains with DNA as determined by crystallographic analyses. C, cysteine; L, leucine; Zn, zinc. (Reproduced with permission from Papavassiliou, 1995. Copyright ©1995 by Massachusetts Medical Society. All rights reserved.)

In addition to the *HOM-C* and *HOX* gene products, additional homeodomain-containing transcription factors have been identified. Among these, the *PAX* genes represent a family of nine different transcription factors in mammals that are related to the protein product of the *Drosophila paired* gene (Gruss and Walther, 1992). DNA binding by the PAIRED protein requires both the homeodomain and a second conserved motif, the paired domain (Table 3.2). Another group of homeodomain proteins that contain a bipartite DNA-binding domain are the POU proteins, so named because the first three recognized members were the transcription factors PIT-1, OCT-1, and UNC-86 (Herr et al., 1988). Despite the fact that some homeodomain proteins require an additional domain for DNA binding, homeodomain proteins in general appear to have specialized over evolutionary time as transcriptional regulators that are involved in developmental processes by determining cell fate, either with respect to positional identity (HOX) or cell type (PAX, POU). Specific functions of these transcription factors will be described in greater detail in Chapters 7, 9, and 11.

The zinc finger motif. The zinc finger is a motif in which four amino acids, most commonly either four cysteine or two cysteine and two histidine residues, are involved in the formation of a tetrahedral coordination complex with Zn(II) that creates a tertiary structure with DNA-binding properties (Fig. 3.1). Most zinc finger proteins must contain at least two such fingers in order to bind to DNA effectively. Zinc finger proteins probably constitute the largest group of transcription factors and may number several thousand in the human genome (reviewed by Berg and Shi, 1996). For the Cys_2His_2 type, each zinc finger consists of two antiparallel β sheets followed by an α helix (Berg, 1988). The mouse factor ZIF268 (also known as EGR-1) contains three zinc fingers and determination of the crystal structure of ZIF268 bound to DNA revealed that the zinc fingers interact with DNA in the major groove of the double helix via amino acids within the α helix (Pavletich and Pabo, 1991). Each zinc

TABLE 3.2. Homeodomain transcription factors

Transcription Factor Family	Additional DNA-Binding Domain	Described in Chapter
HOX	None	7
PAX	Paired domain	9
POU	POU-specific domain	11

finger was shown to contact a 3-bp sequence (Fig. 3.2), such that each finger domain interacted with DNA essentially independently of the other fingers (Berg and Shi, 1996; Pavletich and Pabo, 1991). The binding sites for zinc finger factors are often rich in guanine residues that interact with arginine residues in the fingers (Fig. 3.2). Important examples of proteins that contain two Cys$_4$ zinc fingers are the members of the nuclear receptor superfamily (reviewed by Evans, 1988; Mangelsdorf et al., 1995) and the GATA family of transcription factors (reviewed by Orkin, 1992). Zinc finger transcription factors are described in detail in Chapters 5 and 6.

The basic leucine zipper motif. Basic leucine zipper (bZIP) transcription factors contain a heptad repeat motif in which every seventh amino acid is leucine or, less frequently, another hydrophobic amino acid (isoleucine, valine, or methionine) (Landschulz et al., 1988). These hydrophobic residues mediate dimerization of bZIP monomers (Fig. 3.1). The leucine zipper represents an amphipathic α helix in which the hydrophobic residues are arrayed along one face, thus facilitating dimeric association via a parallel coiled-coil interaction. The process of dimerization juxtaposes basic amino acid residues that are located just amino-terminal to the leucine zipper in each bZIP monomer to create a functional DNA-binding domain (reviewed by Busch and Sassone-Corsi, 1990). Thus, dimerization is absolutely required for DNA binding of bZIP proteins (Kouzarides and Ziff, 1988; Vinson et al., 1989).

Important bZIP factors include the members of the AP-1 superfamily, which include the related proteins of the FOS and JUN families (Ta-

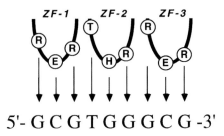

FIGURE 3-2. DNA binding by the zinc fingers of ZIF268. Specific contacts between amino acid residues of the three zinc fingers (ZF-1, ZF-2, and ZF-3) of ZIF268 and one strand of its DNA binding-site nucleotide sequence are shown, using the single-letter code for amino acids: E, glutamic acid; H, histidine; R, arginine; T, threonine.

TABLE 3.3. Dimerization specificity of bZIP and
bHLH proteins

	Homodimers or Heterodimers	Heterodimers Only
bZIP	*JUN Family*	*FOS Family*
	C-JUN	C-FOS
	JUNB	FOSB
	JUND	FRA-1
		FRA-2
bHLH	*Class I*	*Class II*
	E12	MYOD, MYOGENIN, MYF5,
	E47	and MRF4 (myogenic)
	E2-2	TAL-1 (hematopoietic)
	HEB	MASH-1 (neurogenic)

ble 3.3). Members of the FOS and JUN families have been implicated as playing key roles in the transcriptional regulation of cellular proliferation (Angel and Karin, 1991). Genes expressed in response to the phorbol ester mitogen TPA contain a *cis*-acting TPA response element 5'-TGA(C/G)TCA-3' to which AP-1 binds (Fig. 3.3), indicating that this transcription factor family plays an important role in cellular responses to mitogens. Members of the JUN subfamily can homodimerize, dimerize with other members of the JUN family, or heterodimerize with members of the FOS family. In contrast, members of the FOS family can only effectively heterodimerize with members of the JUN family (Table 3.3). The presence of multiple dimerization partners provides an opportunity for generating diversity by combinatorial association, with each dimer having the potential for different DNA sequence recognition and binding affinity, different transactivation activity, and different regulatory properties.

ATF/CREB, a second bZIP family, includes the proteins CREB, CREM, ATF-1, ATF-2, ATF-3, and ATF-4. The prototypical binding site for members of this family contains the sequence 5'-TGACGTCA-3', which is identical to the AP-1 binding site except for an additional nucleotide in the middle of the palindrome. ATF and CREB proteins participate in homodimeric and heterodimeric interactions and can also heterodimerize with C-JUN family members, providing even greater combinatorial diversity. Several members of the ATF/CREB family are regulated by cyclic AMP-dependent protein kinase (protein kinase A) and play essential roles in the transcriptional activation of cAMP-inducible genes that are involved in a variety of biological processes including establishment of circadian rhythms, gluconeogenesis, opiate

5'-TGACTCA-3'

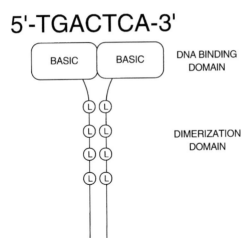

FIGURE 3-3. DNA binding by bZIP proteins. Dimerization of the bZIP proteins C-FOS and C-JUN is mediated by the leucine (L) zipper motifs and results in the juxtaposition of basic amino acid residues to form a functional DNA-binding domain capable of recognizing the AP-1 binding site sequence 5'-TGACTCA-3'. The binding site sequence is palindromic and the basic domains are arrayed in an anti-parallel orientation so that each domain binds to the half-site sequence 5'-TGA-3' present on one strand of the DNA double helix.

tolerance, pituitary development, and responses to neuronal stimulation (reviewed by Papavassiliou, 1995).

The basic helix-loop-helix motif. The properties of the basic helix-loop-helix (bHLH) motif are very similar to those of the bZIP motif. The bHLH domain consists of two stretches of amino acids capable of forming an α helix separated by a nonhelical loop (Fig. 3.1). The α-helices were predicted to mediate protein dimerization that juxtaposes 14-amino-acid basic regions from the two monomers to form a functional DNA-binding domain (reviewed by Blackwell and Weintraub, 1990), a hypothesis that has been confirmed by structural analyses (Ellenberger et al., 1994).

In addition to the presence of adjacent DNA binding and dimerization domains, a second similarity between the bHLH and bZIP proteins is the existence of families of related factors. The bHLH proteins can be subdivided into two classes based on their dimerization potential (Murre et al., 1989a, b). Class I bHLH proteins include E12, E47, E2-2, and HEB (Henthorn et al., 1990, Hu et al., 1992; Murre et al., 1989a). Class I proteins are ubiquitously expressed and can homodimerize or heterodimerize with class II proteins (Table 3.3). In contrast, the class II proteins are expressed in a tissue-specific pattern and can only hetero-dimerize with class I proteins. Thus, the dimerization potentials of the bHLH class I and II proteins are similar to those of the bZIP, JUN, and FOS families, respectively. The class II bHLH proteins MYOD, MY-OGENIN, MYF5, and MRF4 are key regulators of myogenesis. They function as transcription factors only after heterodimerization with E12 or E47 (Weintraub et al., 1991). In addition to interacting with the my-ogenic bHLH proteins, the E12 and E47 proteins also heterodimerize with TAL-1 and MASH-1, which are hematopoietic- and neural-specific bHLH proteins, respectively (reviewed by Zhuang et al., 1992). Almost all bHLH proteins recognize the consensus sequence 5'-CANNTG-3', which is designated as the E-box (reviewed by Kadesch, 1992). As in the case of the binding sites for AP-1 proteins described above, the E-box sequence is a palindrome consisting of two half sites each of which is recognized by one of the basic domains of the bHLH dimer (Blackwell and Weintraub, 1990). Several bHLH proteins are described in greater detail in Chapter 8.

There are two additional families of bHLH proteins, the bHLH-ZIP and bHLH-PAS families, which are distinguished by the fact that in these proteins the HLH domain is insufficient to mediate dimerization. The bHLH-ZIP transcription factors contain an α-helical leucine zipper do-main immediately carboxy-terminal to the helix-loop-helix domain. The bHLH-ZIP family includes the C-MYC protein, which, like C-FOS and C-JUN, plays a key role in cellular proliferation. Binding of C-MYC (and the other members of its family, N-MYC and L-MYC) to DNA requires dimerization with MAX, another bHLH-ZIP protein (Blackwood and Ei-senman, 1991). Two other bHLH-ZIP proteins, USF (Gregor et al., 1990) and TFE3 (Beckmann et al., 1990), bind to the same DNA sequence as the C-MYC/MAX heterodimer, 5'-CACGTG-3'. However, despite related bHLH-ZIP sequences, these proteins are unable to heterodimerize. The ZIP domain amino acid sequence determines the specificity of dimeri-zation (Beckmann and Kadesch, 1991). TFE3 and three proteins with vir-tually identical bHLH domains, TFEB, TFEC, and MITF, represent a sub-set of bHLH-ZIP proteins that are able to homodimerize or heterodimerize with each other (but not with MAX, MYC, or USF) and bind to the sequence 5'-CA(C/T)GTG-3' (reviewed by Moore, 1995).

The bHLH-PAS proteins constitute another family of bHLH proteins that contain a second dimerization domain. In these proteins, both the HLH and PAS domains are required for dimerization (Dolwick et al., 1993; Jiang et al., 1996; Lindebro et al., 1995; Reisz-Porszasz et al., 1994). The PAS domain is approximately 300 amino acids in length and was first identified in the proteins PER, ARNT, and SIM (Hoffman et al., 1991;

Nambu et al., 1991). PER and SIM regulate *Drosophila* circadian rhythms and neurogenesis, respectively (Citri et al., 1987; Nambu et al., 1991). ARNT (aryl hydrocarbon nuclear translocator) and AHR (aryl hydrocarbon receptor), another PAS protein, are heterodimeric partners that form the mammalian AHR complex or dioxin receptor, a ligand-activated transcription factor (Burbach et al., 1992; Reyes et al., 1992). Additional members of this family include HIF-1α (hypoxia-inducible factor 1α), a mammalian transcription factor that controls homeostatic responses to hypoxia (Wang et al., 1995), and TRH (trachealess), which regulates development of the *Drosophila* respiratory tract (Isaac and Andrew, 1996; Wilk et al., 1996). ARNT can heterodimerize with AHR, HIF-1α, or SIM, and can also homodimerize (Reyes et al., 1992; Sogawa et al., 1995; Swanson et al., 1995; Wang et al., 1995). ARNT, or a related protein ARNT-2 (Hirose et al., 1996), appears to be a common subunit of all bHLH-PAS proteins, similar to the role of class I bHLH proteins.

Transactivation Domains

Compared to the extensive structural and functional studies that have been performed to analyze dimerization and DNA-binding domains, much less is understood about the structure and function of transactivation domains. In contrast to the elegant molecular structures that have been determined for several DNA-binding domains, biophysical data obtained on transactivation domains indicate that most of these domains appear unstructured when analyzed as isolated proteins in solution (reviewed by Triezenberg, 1995). This apparent lack of structure may imply a plasticity that allows transactivation domains to participate in multiple protein-protein interactions that vary from one promoter to another. Four types of activation domains have been proposed, consisting of polypeptide sequences rich in glutamine, proline, serine/threonine, or acidic amino acid residues (reviewed by Mitchell and Tjian, 1989; Triezenberg, 1995) as exemplified by the transcription factors SP1 (Courey and Tjian, 1989), CTF/NF-1 (Mermod et al., 1989), PIT-1 (Theill et al., 1989), and GATA-1 (Martin and Orkin, 1990), respectively. Many transcription factors contain more than one activation domain, as in the case of the bHLH-ZIP protein TFE3, which contains both acidic and proline-rich activation domains (Artandi et al., 1995).

Several comments are in order regarding the classification scheme for transactivation domains described above. First, many transactivation domains do not fall into any of these categories. Second, this simplistic categorization based on the predominant amino acid present within the domain provides no information about the mechanism of action. This latter point is illustrated by studies of acidic activation domains. These domains were proposed to exist as unstructured "acid blobs" (Sigler, 1988) or as amphipathic α helices (Ptashne, 1988). Studies of the yeast activators GAL4 and GCN4 and the mammalian activator VP16 indicated that the degree of transactivation correlated with the number of negatively charged residues (Cress and Treizenberg, 1991; Gill and Ptashne, 1987; Gill et al., 1990; Hope et al., 1988; Sadowski et al., 1988; Triezenberg et al., 1988). When random fragments of *E. coli* genomic DNA were tested for their ability to encode transactivation domains, about 1% were functional in the assay and most of these contained an excess of acidic residues (Ma and Ptashne, 1987). However, mutational analysis of the VP16 activation domain revealed that specific hydrophobic residues were as important for function as the acidic residues (Regier et al., 1993). A functional requirement for hydrophobic residues in the glutamine-rich transactivation domain of SP1 was also demonstrated (Gill et al., 1994). Genetic studies of the GAL4 acidic activation domain indicated that most of the acidic residues could be substituted by nonacidic residues without loss of function and that the key structural requirement appeared to be the ability to form a β sheet (Leuther et al., 1993; Van Hoy et al., 1993), demonstrating a level of complexity that was not apparent from the primary structure.

Given the lack of information regarding the structure of transactivation domains, it is nonetheless reasonable to assume that these undetermined and possibly fluid structures provide a basis for protein-protein interactions. What then are the protein targets of the transactivation domains? The finding that mammalian transactivation domains rich in acidic and serine/threonine residues activated transcription in yeast cells, whereas domains rich in glutamine residues did not (Berger et al., 1992), pointed to a multiplicity of targets (and to a certain degree provided some legitimacy for the categories of transactivation domains that were maligned in the preceding discussion). Transcriptional activators may function by one or more of several different mechanisms (reviewed by Triezenberg, 1995). First, they may disrupt the nucleosomal structure of chromatin by displacing histone and nonhistone proteins that have a repressive effect on transcription. Second, they may recruit general transcription factors into the transcription initiation complex, either by direct interaction or by interacting with TAFs. Third, they may stimulate transcript elongation and/or inhibit premature termination. In many cases, these transactivator functions are mediated by interactions with coactivators, as will be described in a subsequent section of this chapter.

Regulation of Transcription Factor Activity by Posttranslational Modification

The activity of transcriptional regulatory proteins can be regulated at the level of synthesis, which most commonly occurs with respect to developmental regulators. In contrast, physiological regulators are often regulated by posttranslational modifications that allows for a more rapid response, and several examples of such modifications are presented in this section. Additional regulatory mechanisms, including interactions with small molecule ligands and with repressor proteins, are described in later sections of this chapter.

Redox regulation of DNA binding. As described above, the bZIP proteins C-FOS and C-JUN heterodimerize to form the transcription factor AP-1, which binds to the DNA sequence 5'-TGA(C/G)TCA-3' and activates transcription of genes whose products are required for cellular proliferation. Treatment of C-FOS or C-JUN protein prior to heterodimerization with N-ethylmaleimide (NEM), which alkylates sulfhydryl groups, inhibited DNA-binding activity, indicating that modification of cysteine residues in both proteins affected DNA binding (Abate et al., 1990). All FOS and JUN family proteins contain an invariant Lys-Cys-Arg sequence in the basic domain, whereas the transforming protein v-JUN, which is a constitutively active form of C-JUN, contains a Cys-to-Ser substitution at this location. A Cys-to-Ser substitution in C-JUN resulted in increased DNA-binding activity in the absence or presence of NEM, suggesting that the Cys residue may allow regulation of DNA binding. This hypothesis was further supported by the discovery of REF-1, a nuclear protein that in the presence of thioredoxin, an enzyme that reduces cysteine residues, increased AP-1 DNA-binding activity (Abate et al., 1990; Xanthoudakis and Curran, 1992). These results suggest that regulation of REF-1 activity in response to various extracellular signals may determine the proportion of C-JUN and C-FOS molecules that are in a reduced state that is competent for DNA binding.

NF-κB designates a family of transcription factors whose activity is induced in response to a variety of extracellular stimuli including interleukin-1, tumor necrosis factor, mitogens, oxidative stress, ultraviolet and ionizing radiation, bacterial lipopolysaccharide, and viral double-stranded RNA, resulting in the transcriptional activation of genes involved in immune and inflammatory responses (reviewed by Bauerle and Henkel, 1994; Thanos and Maniatis, 1995). NF-κB has also been implicated in atherogenesis and AIDS pathogenesis (Brand et al., 1996; Griffin et al., 1989; reviewed by Sen and Packer, 1996). In contrast to the bHLH, bZIP, homeodomain, and zinc finger proteins described above, members of this transcription factor family contain a Rel homology domain of approximately 300 amino acids that is required for dimerization, nuclear localization, and DNA binding. The DNA binding domains of Rel family members conform to the consensus sequence RXXRXRXXC (C, cysteine; R, arginine; X, any amino acid) (Kumar et al., 1992). As in the case of C-FOS and C-JUN, oxidation of the conserved cysteine residue inhibited DNA binding. Cellular redox status appears to play an important role in modulating the signal transduction pathways that result in the expression of genes encoding components of NF-κB and AP-1 as well as in the direct modification of these proteins (reviewed by Sen and Packer, 1996).

Regulation of DNA binding by phosphorylation. In addition to redox regulation, the DNA-binding activity of AP-1 is also affected by the phosphorylation status of C-JUN. In nonstimulated cells, C-JUN is phosphorylated at three serine and threonine residues immediately amino-terminal to the DNA binding domain and dephosphorylation at these sites increases DNA-binding activity (Boyle et al., 1991). The DNA-binding activity of a variety of other transcription factors has been shown to be either inhibited or, less frequently, stimulated by phosphorylation (reviewed by Hunter and Karin, 1992). In most of these cases, however, there is less evidence that phosphorylation status is modulated by developmental or physiological signals. In addition to the regulation of DNA binding, phosphorylation is also employed as a means to regulate other aspects of transcription factor function, including dimerization, transactivation, and protein stability. Examples of these regulatory mechanisms are provided elsewhere in this chapter. In particular, a detailed description of several kinase pathways that transduce signals from the cell surface to the nucleus is presented at the end of the chapter.

Regulation of nuclear localization by dephosphorylation. Most transcription factors contain specific sequences that target the protein for nuclear localization. These nuclear localization signals usually consist of several clusters of arginine and lysine residues that allow interaction with specific transporter molecules associated with the nuclear pore complex (reviewed by Boulikas, 1993). In the case of the transcription factor NF-AT (nuclear factor of activated T cells), nuclear import is regulated by the opposing action of kinases and phosphatases. In nonstimulated cells, NF-AT is phosphorylated on serine residues by glycogen synthase kinase-3 (GSK-3), which targets the protein for nuclear export and cytoplasmic sequestration (Beals et al., 1997). When T cells are immunologically stimulated, intracellular concentrations of calcium increase, resulting in the

activation of the calcium-dependent protein serine/threonine phosphatase calcineurin (Jain et al., 1993). Calcineurin dephosphorylates NF-AT
and remains associated with the factor as it is transported into the nucleus (Shibasaki et al., 1996), indicating that the continued presence of
the phosphatase is required to counteract ongoing phosphorylation. In
addition, phosphorylation of NF-AT by C-JUN N-terminal kinase (JNK)
at serine residues distinct from those phosphorylated by GSK-3, can also
oppose the effects of calcineurin (Chow et al., 1997). Thus, the net effect
of kinase and phosphatase activity within the cell will determine the
amount of NF-AT that is transported to the nucleus, where it can exert
its biological effects via transcriptional activation.

Cofactors for Dimerization and DNA Binding

Cofactor for dimerization. The homeodomain transcriptional activator hepatocyte nuclear factor 1α (HNF- 1α) binds to DNA as a homodimer.
Dimerization of HNF-1α is facilitated by the cofactor DCoH (Mendel et
al., 1991). Whereas the mechanism by which DCoH functions as a dimerization cofactor remains unknown despite the determination of its
crystal structure (Endrizzi et al., 1995), several other remarkable discoveries have been made regarding this protein. DCoH was also shown to
catalyze the dehydration of the biopterin cofactor for phenylalanine hydroxylase (Citron et al., 1992; Zhao et al., 1994). Thus DCoH functions
both as a transcriptional cofactor and as an enzyme. Phenylalanine hydroxylase is a liver-specific enzyme that may be transcriptionally regulated by HNF-1α. This hypothesis was supported by the equally remarkable discovery of a bacterial protein, phhB, which is approximately
30% identical to DCoH and which is required for expression of other
genes in the *phh* operon including the *phhA* gene encoding phenylalanine
hydroxylase (Zhao et al., 1994). Expression of DCoH in bacterial cells
containing a mutant *phhB* gene restored expression of the *phhA* gene
(Endrizzi et al., 1995). DCoH is thus a remarkable evolutionarily conserved bifunctional protein.

Cooperative DNA binding. DNA binding proteins do not function in isolation and, in many cases, cooperative interactions between transcription
factors bound at adjacent sites are essential for establishing high-affinity,
sequence-specific binding. Whereas the example provided below involves homeodomain proteins that play key roles in development, cooperative binding is also essential for the function of transcription factors
that respond to physiological signals, as the *cis*-acting elements to which
they bind ("response elements") are usually composite sites to which at

least two different factors bind in a cooperative manner. Cooperative binding allows transcription factors to bind to short nucleotide sequences in a specific manner. For example, if factor A recognizes a specific 5-bp sequence, ATCGA, this sequence is expected to occur by chance once every 3125 bp. Likewise, the binding site for factor B, GCTAG, will also occur by chance approximately once every 3125 bp, or approximately one million times per haploid genome. However, if factor A binds with high affinity only at sites adjacent to binding sites for factor B, then such tandem sites will occur by chance only once every 9,765,625 bp. Cooperativity also provides a basis for combinatorial regulation, with a given factor interacting cooperatively with a subset of other transcription factors, each of which is subject to a unique pattern of regulation. As a result, it is possible for 5,000 to 10,000 DNA binding proteins to direct the transcription of 50,000 to 100,000 genes under all possible developmental and physiological conditions.

The homeodomain proteins encoded by the invertebrate *HOM-C* and vertebrate *HOX* genes play key roles in establishing the basic body plan of the organism, and the local expression pattern of these homeodomain proteins is hypothesized to determine segmental identity within the developing embryo (see Chapter 9). This program of segmental specialization is presumably the result of transcriptional regulation of genes containing binding sites for specific *HOM-C/HOX* genes. Despite the fact that genetic analyses indicated that the HOM-C proteins are each functionally unique, studies of DNA binding suggested that they all recognized similar sequences with similar affinities. A clue to the resolution of this apparent paradox came from the discovery that mutations in the *extradenticle (exd)* gene result in homeotic transformations, similar to those observed due to mutations in *HOM-C* genes, without changing *HOM-C* gene expression, suggesting that EXD modulates the function of HOM-C proteins (Peifer and Wieschaus, 1990). EXD was shown to increase the DNA binding specificity of the HOM-C proteins UBX, ABD-A, and EN, but not ABD-B or ANTP, for specific target sites by binding to adjacent DNA sequences (Chan et al., 1994; van Dijk and Murre, 1994). EXD is also a homeodomain protein and removal of residues amino-terminal to the homeodomain eliminated interactions with UBX and ABD-A, whereas removal of residues carboxyl-terminal to the homeodomain eliminated interactions with EN (van Dijk and Murre, 1994). Three human homologues of EXD have been identified, PBX1, PBX2, and PBX3, which have greater than 70% amino acid identity with EXD (Monica et al., 1991; Rauskolb et al., 1993). Thus, during evolution, the one *exd* and eight *HOM-C* genes of *Drosophila* increased in number to three *PBX* and thirty-nine *HOX* genes found in mammals, with this increased genetic complexity presumably representing one underlying basis for the increased complexity of the mammalian developmental program.

Coactivators

Transcription factors may interact directly with the basal components of the transcription initiation complex including TBP, TFIIA, TFIIB, TFIIF, and TFIIH (Chi et al., 1995; reviewed by Triezenberg, 1995). However, it appears that many important functional effects of activators are mediated by adapter proteins or coactivators. Whereas transactivators participate in DNA-protein and protein-protein interactions, the coactivators participate only in protein-protein interactions and provide a physical connection between the transcriptional activators and the basal factors of the transcription initiation complex (see Fig. 1.2).

Three classes of coactivators have been identified as multiprotein complexes. The TAFs were biochemically isolated as components of the TFIID complex, whereas the SRB and SWI/SNF proteins were identified as components of the Pol II holoenzyme complex (see Chapter 1). In addition, individual proteins (e.g., CBP and P300) have been identified through directed searches for coactivators of specific transcription factors, and the possibility that these coactivators are also components of larger complexes has not been excluded. Coactivators appear to function by at least two different mechanisms (reviewed by Guarente, 1995). The first mechanism is as an adapter that physically connects the sequence-specific transcription factors bound at distal sites to the basal factors of the transcription initiation complex. The second mechanism by which coactivators stimulate transcription is by counteracting the repressive effects of histones and possibly nonhistone chromatin proteins on transcription. Histone displacement may be necessary to allow the binding of transcriptional activators or basal factors and/or to allow transcript elongation.

TAFs

A large number of studies have demonstrated specific interactions between transactivation domains and proteins of the transcription initiation complex, especially the TAF components of TFIID. Several examples of interactions between activation domains of sequence-specific transcription factors and TAFs are provided below. Because TAFs were originally purified and cloned from *Drosophila*, many of the initial studies analyzed interactions between dTAFs and mammalian transcription factors. Thus far, nine TAF_{II} subunits have been identified in *Drosophila.* They have been designated (based on their estimated molecular masses as determined by polyacrylamide gel electrophoresis): $dTAF_{II}250$ (also known as $dTAF_{II}230$), $dTAF_{II}150$, $dTAF_{II}110$, $dTAF_{II}80$ (also known as $dTAF_{II}85$), $dTAF_{II}60$ (also known as $dTAF_{II}62$), $dTAF_{II}42$ (also known as $dTAF_{II}40$), $dTAF_{II}$ 30α and $dTAF_{II}$ 30β (also known as $dTAF_{II}$ 28α and $dTAF_{II}28β$, respectively) and $dTAF_{II}$ 22 (reviewed by Burley and Roeder, 1996; Goodrich and Tjian, 1994; Verrijzer and Tjian, 1996).

$dTAF_{II}110$. The mammalian zinc finger factor SP1, which contains two glutamine-rich transactivation domains, was shown to interact with $dTAF_{II}110$, and point mutations in the SP1 transactivation domains interfered with binding to $dTAF_{II}110$ and activation of transcription (Goodrich et al., 1993; Gill et al., 1994; Hoey et al., 1993). The finding that the glutamine-rich domains of SP1 interacted with $dTAF_{II}110$ (but none of the other dTAFs), whereas selected proline-rich and acidic transactivation domains did not interact with $dTAF_{II}110$, provided further evidence for the association of particular transactivation domains with specific coactivators (Chen et al., 1994; Goodrich et al., 1993; Hoey et al., 1993). Some, but not all, other glutamine-rich domains interact with $dTAF_{II}110$, demonstrating the limitations of the present classification system for understanding transactivation domain function (Chen et al., 1994; Ferreri et al., 1994; Hoey et al., 1993).

$dTAF_{II}40$. $dTAF_{II}40$ interacts with the acidic activation domain of the viral transactivator VP16 but not with the glutamine-rich domain of SP1 or the proline-rich domain of CTF-1 (Goodrich et al., 1993). In addition, both VP16 and $dTAF_{II}40$ (and its human homologue, $hTAF_{II}31$) were shown to interact with TFIIB (Goodrich et al., 1993; Klemm et al, 1995; Lin and Green, 1991), providing evidence for multivalent interactions between transcriptional activators and general transcription factors.

$hTAF_{II}30$. The AF-2 transactivation domain in the estrogen receptor, which is not particularly rich in glutamine, proline, serine/threonine, or acidic amino acid residues, was shown to interact with human $TAF_{II}30$ (which is not homologous to either of the 30-kDa TAFs isolated from *Drosophila* cells) (Jacq et al., 1994). $hTAF_{II}30$ was also shown to interact with human TBP and $hTAF_{II}250$, which also interact with one another (Jacq et al., 1994), providing further evidence that complex, multivalent protein-protein interactions occur during the formation of the transcription initiation complex. In contrast to AF-2, the AF-1 domain of the estrogen receptor did not interact with $hTAF_{II}30$, suggesting that interaction of these two transactivation domains with different target proteins

may account for their observed synergistic effects on transcriptional activation (Jacq et al., 1994).

dTAF$_{II}$150. The transcriptional activator NTF-1 (neurogenic element-binding transcription factor 1) can bind to dTAF$_{II}$150, and NTF-1 can activate in vitro transcription in the presence of general transcription factors and recombinant TBP, dTAF$_{II}$150, and dTAF$_{II}$250 as the only TFIID components (Chen et al., 1994). NTF-1 can also activate transcription in the presence of TBP, dTAF$_{II}$250, and dTAF$_{II}$60 as the only TFIID components. NTF-1 forms complexes with both dTAF$_{II}$150 and dTAF$_{II}$60 in vitro (Chen et al., 1994). These results suggest that either dTAF$_{II}$150 or dTAF$_{II}$60 may serve as a coactivator for NTF-1. The NTF-1 transactivation domain also does not fit into one of the four categories described above (acidic, glutamine-, proline-, or serine/threonine-rich), but instead is rich in hydrophobic residues, particularly isoleucine (Attardi and Tjian, 1993).

dTAF$_{II}$60. The *Drosophila* zinc finger protein HUNCHBACK (HB) can also bind to dTAF$_{II}$60 (Sauer et al., 1995b). An HB binding site is present in the *hb* gene promoter and in vitro transcription from the *hb* promoter was stimulated in the presence of TBP, dTAF$_{II}$250, and dTAF$_{II}$60 as the only TFIID components. The *hb* promoter also contains binding sites for the homeodomain protein bicoid (BCD), which binds to dTAF$_{II}$110 via a glutamine-rich transactivation domain. In vitro transcription from the *hb* promoter was activated by BCD but not by HB in the presence of TBP, dTAF$_{II}$250, and dTAF$_{II}$110, whereas synergistic activation of transcription by HB and BCD occurred in the presence of TBP, dTAF$_{II}$250, and d-TAF$_{II}$110, and dTAF$_{II}$60 (Sauer et al., 1995b). The *hb* promoter contains three BCD binding sites, and in vitro transcription increased synergistically as the number of BCD binding sites present in the promoter construct were increased (Sauer et al., 1995a). The synergistic effect of BCD on transcription was the result of the fact that, in addition to the glutamine-rich transactivation domain that interacts with dTAF$_{II}$110, BCD also has a second transactivation domain that interacts with dTAF$_{II}$60 (Sauer et al., 1995a). The multiple protein-DNA and protein-protein interactions that occur at the *hb* promoter are illustrated in Figure 3.4.

In addition to cataloguing protein-protein interactions from the point of view of the TAFs, it is also possible to determine the interactions between a single transcriptional activator and different general transcription factors and TAFs. In the case of P53, direct interactions have been demonstrated with TBP and TFIIH (Liu et al., 1993; Martin et al., 1993; Seto et al., 1992; Xiao et al., 1994) as well as with dTAF$_{II}$40 and dTAF$_{II}$60

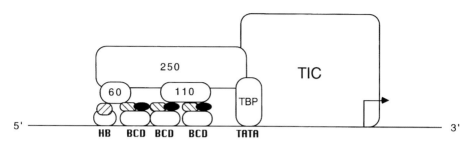

FIGURE 3-4. Multiple interactions between activators, DNA, and TBP-associated factors (TAFs). Sequence-specific binding of BCD, HB, and TBP to the *hb* promoter is illustrated. Transactivation domains of HB and BCD (hatched) interact specifically with dTAF$_{II}$60, whereas a second transactivation domain of BCD (solid) interacts specifically with dTAF$_{II}$110. Both dTAF$_{II}$60 and dTAF$_{II}$110 interact with dTAF$_{II}$250, which in turn interacts with TBP, the subunit of the transcription initiation complex (TIC) that binds to the TATA box sequence located immediately 5' to the transcription initiation site (bent arrow). Relative protein sizes and distances along the DNA are not drawn to scale in this schematic illustration.

and their human homologues hTAF$_{II}$31 and hTAF$_{II}$70 (Lu and Levine, 1995; Thut et al., 1995). P53 can activate transcription in the presence of general transcription factors plus dTBP, dTAF$_{II}$40, dTAF$_{II}$60, and d-TAF$_{II}$250 and missense mutations that affect the transactivation function of P53 also affect its interaction with TAFs (Thut et al., 1995).

Several important conclusions can be drawn from these studies. First, the transactivation domains of transcription factors make specific contacts with TAFs that are functionally relevant. Second, a single transcription factor (through one or more transactivation domains) can interact with multiple TAFs and such interactions may have synergistic effects. Third, the binding of multiple transcription factors to promoter or enhancer sequences provides further opportunity for the establishment of multiple transactivation domain–TAF contacts that can have synergistic effects on transcription. Fourth, the multiplicity of interactions that have already been documented between transcription factors and TAFs suggest that the latter play an important role in determining the rate of transcription initiation. Interactions of TAFs with sequence-specific transcriptional activators may be required for the recruitment of TFIID to the TATA box, which may represent the rate-limiting step in the formation of the transcription initiation complex. Fifth, TAFs have enzymatic activities that indicate a role in transcription-associated chromatin remodeling, as will be described in a later section of this chapter.

Most of the studies described above investigated the involvement of TAFs using in vitro transcription assays. Recent in vivo studies have provided a different view of TAF function (Moqtaderi et al., 1996; Walker et al., 1996). *Saccharomyces cerevisiae* also contain TAFs, many of which are homologous to human and *Drosophila* TAFs (reviewed by Struhl, 1995). Yeast strains were generated that were either constitutively or conditionally deficient in one or more TAFs, including y-TAF$_{II}$145 (also known as yTAF$_{II}$130), the homologue of human and *Drosophila* TAF$_{II}$250, which in all three species is the core subunit of the TAF complex and the only TAF that binds directly to TBP (Sauer et al., 1995b; reviewed by Struhl, 1995). In TAF-deficient yeast, basal and induced expression of a number of genes was unaffected (Moqtaderi et al., 1996; Walker et al., 1996). The transcription of two genes with nonconsensus TATA box elements was decreased (Moqtaderi et al., 1996), but the number of genes assayed was insufficient to assume a causal relationship. The fact that several of the yeast TAFs were required for viability suggests either that the TAFs have subtle effects on a large number of genes that cumulatively affect viability or that TAFs are required only for the activation of a subset of genes (Moqtaderi et al., 1996), such as those involved in cell cycle regulation because this process is perturbed in TAF-deficient yeast cells (Walker et al., 1996). The discrepancy between the results obtained by in vivo and in vitro transcription assays may be due to the absence in the latter of other components of the transcription initiation complex (such as the SRB and SWI/SNF proteins) or other coactivators (such as CBP, P300, and P/CAF) whose functions may overlap with those of the TAFs, as described in subsequent sections of this chapter. This functional redundancy may apply either to specific interactions with transcriptional activators and basal transcription factors, to specific enzymatic activities involved in transcription-associated chromatin remodeling, or both.

Recent experiments suggest rather convincingly, however, that for some genes TAF function does appear to be essential for transcriptional activation mediated by specific DNA-binding proteins in vivo. In particular, dTAF$_{II}$60 and dTAF$_{II}$110 function have been shown to be required for transcription mediated by the activator BCD during *Drosophila* eye development (Sauer et al., 1996). Thus, the absence of redundancy in at least some transcriptional systems may explain the lethality associated with loss of TAF function. Further complicating the analysis has been the recent demonstration of a tissue-specific TAF. Human TAF$_{II}$105, which is similar to hTAF$_{II}$130 and dTAF$_{II}$110 in its carboxyl-terminal domain, is present in 5% to 10% of TFIID complexes isolated from B lymphocytes and may specifically interact with DNA-binding proteins that activate transcription of B-cell–specific genes (Dikstein et al., 1996b). It goes without saying that having found a B-cell–specific TAF, it is likely that other TAFs with restricted patterns of expression will be identified in the future.

SRB Proteins

A second class of coactivators was identified originally in yeast, both by co-purification with Pol II and by genetic studies, and some members of this class have also been identified in mammalian cells (reviewed by Guarente, 1995). A holoenzyme complex (see Chapter 1) purified from yeast extracts and shown to contain Pol II and a collection of approximately 20 proteins (including SRB2, SRB4, SRB5, and SRB6) termed the mediator was capable of responding to transcriptional activators in vitro, whereas transactivators had no effect in the presence of Pol II alone (Kim et al., 1994). *SRB* genes were identified in a screen for suppressors of cold sensitivity associated with mutations of the Pol II large subunit truncated in the C-terminal heptapeptide repeat domain (Nonet and Young, 1989). SRB proteins were shown to associate directly with the C-terminal domain (Kim et al., 1994). In these experiments, SRBs mediated the effects of transactivators in the absence of TAFs, and TAFs were able to activate transcription in the absence of SRBs, suggesting that SRBs and TAFs may have overlapping functions.

Other Non-TAF Coactivators

In contrast to the multiprotein complexes described above, a steadily growing list of individual proteins have been identified that function as coactivators for important mammalian transcription factors. However, further analysis of these mammalian coactivators, which were isolated by virtue of their ability to physically interact with specific transcriptional activators, has revealed that they also appear to function through multiple interactions with activators, other coactivators, and basal transcription factors. Several illustrative examples are provided below.

CBP. As described in a later section of this chapter, CBP was originally identified as a coactivator of the bZIP protein CREB (Kwok et al., 1994). Subsequently, CBP was shown to be involved in transcriptional activation mediated by a wide variety of sequence-specific DNA-binding proteins, including C-FOS, C-JUN, C-MYB, and nuclear receptors (reviewed by Janknecht and Hunter, 1996). Thus, whereas the original studies suggested a specific role for CBP in phosphorylation-dependent transactivation by CREB, the large number of transcription factors with which it interacts suggests a more general role similar to that of the TAFs. As in the case of the TAFs, CBP appears to possess two important types of functional activity. First, CBP contains a glutamine-rich domain at its carboxyl terminus that can interact with TFIIB (Kwok et al., 1994), thus providing a physical connection with the transcription initiation complex. Second, CBP contains a protein motif known as the bromodomain, which is also present in SWI2 and $TAF_{II}250$ (reviewed by Guarente, 1995). A proposed function of the SWI/SNF complex (described below) is to counteract the repressive effects of histone and nonhistone chromatin proteins on transcription, suggesting that CBP might also participate in this process. Indeed, there are currently no data that address the possibility that CBP might exist in vivo as a component of the mammalian SWI/SNF complex. Most recently, CBP and the related protein P300 (see below) were shown to have histone acetyltransferase activity, providing evidence that these coactivators are directly involved in chromatin remodeling (Bannister and Kouzarides, 1996; Ogryzko et al., 1996).

P300. Another coactivator whose primary amino acid sequence is highly related to that of CBP was isolated independently as a protein that interacts with the E1A transforming protein of adenovirus (Eckner et al., 1994). All of the domains in CBP that contact activators are also present in P300 and when the biological or biochemical activity of CBP and P300 have been compared, they have functioned equivalently (Arany et al., 1994, 1995; Kamei et al., 1996; Lundblad et al., 1995). However, the demonstration that mutations in the *CBP* gene result in disease, as described in Chapter 13, indicates that either CBP performs unique functions that cannot be provided by P300 or that a reduction in the combined concentrations of CBP and P300 adversely affects cellular processes. P300 was co-immunoprecipitated from human cells with antibodies against TBP (Abraham et al., 1993), suggesting that P300 and CBP may be part of the TAF complex described above.

XH2. An X-linked gene encoding a member of the helicase II superfamily with sequence similarity to yeast and human SNF2 has been identified (Gibbons et al., 1995). As in the case of *CBP*, mutations in the *XH2* gene are associated with a human malformation/mental retardation syndrome (Gibbons et al., 1995) (see Chapter 13).

OBF-1. All of the coactivators described above are ubiquitously expressed in human cells. In contrast, expression of OBF-1 (also known as

BOB-1 and OCA-B) is restricted to B lymphocytes (Gstaiger et al., 1995; Luo and Roeder, 1995; Strubin et al., 1995). Immunoglobulin genes are expressed specifically within B cells and this cell-type-specific transcription is directed by *cis*-acting promoter and enhancer elements that contain variants of an 8-bp consensus sequence, 5'-ATTTGCAT-3', known as the octamer motif (reviewed by Staudt and Lennardo, 1991). However, the octamer motif alone cannot determine B cell–specific transcription because it is also found in ubiquitously expressed genes such as those encoding histone H2B and various small nuclear RNAs (reviewed by Strubin et al., 1995). Two octamer binding proteins, OCT-1 and OCT-2, were identified in B cells, and whereas OCT-2 is expressed only in B cells, OCT-1 is ubiquitously expressed (Muller et al., 1988; Staudt et al., 1986; Sturm et al., 1988). Both OCT-1 and OCT-2 are members of the POU family of transcription factors (see Chapter 11), which contain a bipartite DNA-binding domain consisting of a homeodomain and a POU domain (Sturm et al., 1988).

These results indicated that neither the known *cis*-acting elements nor *trans*-acting factors could account for B cell type–specific immunoglobulin gene transcription. However, in vitro transcription from immunoglobulin gene promoters was more efficient when B cell, as opposed to non–B cell, extracts were utilized (Luo et al., 1992), suggesting the existence of other B cell–specific *trans*-acting factors. OBF-1, which was cloned on the basis of its ability to interact with OCT-1 and OCT-2, is expressed specifically within B cells (Gstaiger et al., 1995; Luo and Roeder, 1995; Strubin et al., 1995). OBF-1 interacts specifically with the POU domain of OCT-1 and OCT-2 and not with other POU proteins. Furthermore, whereas OCT-1 and OCT-2 bind to a variety of octamer sequences, ternary complexes containing OBF-1 form only on specific DNA sequences (Gstaiger et al., 1996), thus providing a mechanism for the selective activation of B cell–specific genes. The same amino acid residues of OCT-1 and OCT-2 are involved in DNA sequence recognition and OBF-1 interaction, suggesting either that OBF-1 influences site selection by OCT-1 and OCT-2 or that the DNA sequence determines activator-coactivator interactions. OBF-1 form more stable complexes with OCT-1 and OCT-2 in the presence than in the absence of DNA, supporting the latter hypothesis (Gstaiger et al., 1996). The investigations of immunoglobin gene expression that have been conducted over the past ten years provide a paradigm for the evolution of transcriptional regulation studies, starting with the identification of *cis*-acting DNA sequences, followed by cognate *trans*-acting DNA-binding proteins and then activator-binding proteins, and, finally, the identification of cell-type-specific DNA-activator-coactivator complexes.

Architectural Transcription Factors

In addition to transcriptional activators and repressors, a third class of DNA-binding proteins has been identified. These transcription factors affect transcription by binding to *cis*-acting DNA regulatory sequences and bending DNA. This alteration of tertiary structure has a profound effect on the ability of other transcription factors to bind to DNA and to interact with one another and with the transcription initiation complex. The most important family of architectural transcription factors are proteins that contain a DNA-binding domain not previously described, the HMG (high mobility group) domain, an evolutionarily conserved 80-amino-acid motif that has been identified in DNA-binding proteins from yeast to humans (Harley et al., 1992; Laudet et al., 1993). Most or all HMG domain proteins bend DNA by binding in the minor groove of the double helix (in contrast to the majority of DNA binding proteins, which occupy the major groove). For example, binding of the lymphoid enhancer factor LEF-1 to the enhancer of the T-cell receptor α gene induces a sharp bend in the DNA that allows factors binding on either side of LEF-1 to functionally interact with one another (Travis et al., 1991; Waterman et al., 1991). LEF-1 cannot activate transcription of a basal promoter directly but instead facilitates functional interactions between other enhancer-bound factors (Giese et al., 1992). Thus, LEF-1 assembles a higher-order nucleoprotein complex by bringing nonadjacent transcription factor binding sites into close proximity (Giese et al., 1995). Similarly, the protein HMG I(Y) plays an essential role in the synergistic activation of human interferon ß gene transcription by promoter-bound factors. In this case, binding of HMG I(Y) at three different sites in the promoter facilitates the binding of ATF-2 and NF-κB at adjacent sites such that they interact with one another and with general transcription factors to form a stable higher-order transcription complex (Du et al., 1993). Specific mammalian HMG domain proteins are described in greater detail in Chapter 10.

The function of several HMG-domain proteins must be reassessed in the light of recent discoveries. The protein β-catenin has been shown to associate with lymphoid enhancer factor (LEF) and T cell factor (TCF) family members and activate transcription of genes containing binding sites for these factors (Molenaar et al., 1996). Thus, it appears that LEF or TCF supply the DNA-binding domain, β-catenin provides the transactivation domain, and neither protein can activate transcription without the other. The association between β-catenin and LEF or TCF is regulated by cellular signaling mechanisms. Under basal conditions, β-catenin is detected at the cell membrane in a complex with the adenomatous polyposis coli (APC) tumor suppressor protein and the serine-threonine kinase glycogen synthase kinase-3β (GSK-3β) and has a short half-life, whereas in response to extracellular signals, β-catenin dissociates from APC and GSK-3β and accumulates in the nucleus (Korinek et al., 1997; Morin et al., 1997; Rubinfeld et al., 1996, 1997). Proper regulation of β-catenin by APC appears to be essential for normal development (Molenaar et al., 1996) and, in colon carcinoma cells, transcription mediated by the TCF4/β-catenin complex is constitutively activated due to loss-of-function mutations in APC or activating mutations in β-catenin (Korinek et al., 1997; Morin et al., 1997).

Repressors and Corepressors

Repressors can interfere with the function of transcriptional activators by a large variety of mechanisms. In some cases, the repressor complexes with the activator and prevents it from reaching its site of action in the nucleus. Other repressors substitute for one subunit of a heterodimeric factor and prevent it from binding to DNA or activating transcription. Other repressors bind to the transactivation domain and in doing so may prevent interactions with coactivators or may actually mediate destabilizing interactions with components of the transcription initiation complex, thus functioning as corepressors. Transcriptional activators can also function as repressors under certain circumstances. Illustrative examples of mechanisms of transcriptional repression are described below and are summarized in Table 3.4.

TABLE 3.4. Repressors of transcriptional activators

Repressor	Activator	Mechanism of Repression	Mechanism of Derepression
I-κB	NF-κB	Blocks nuclear transport	Phosphorylation and degradation
HSP90	GR	Blocks nuclear transport	Ligand binding
IP-1	FOS/JUN	Blocks DNA binding	Phosphorylation
ID	E2A/MYOD	Blocks DNA binding	?Decreased synthesis
ΔFOSB	FOSB/JUN	Blocks transactivation	Alternative splicing
LIP	LAP	Blocks transactivation	Alternative translation initiation
MAD	MYC/MAX	Active transrepression	?Decreased synthesis
HES	E2A/MYOD	Active transrepression	?Decreased synthesis

Regulation of Nuclear Transport

IκB and NF-κB. Under basal conditions, NF-κB is sequestered in the cytosol by the repressor IκB and cannot bind to DNA, although treatment of cytosolic extracts with deoxycholate and other detergents can release NF-κB DNA-binding activity (Bauerle and Baltimore, 1988a, b). When cells are exposed to one of the inducing agents (described above), NF-κB is released from IκB and translocates to the nucleus where it can activate transcription of genes containing its cognate binding site. The signal transduction pathway that is activated by inducing agents is not fully characterized (Anderson et al., 1994; Cao et al., 1996) but results in the phosphorylation of IκB on serine residues 32 and 36 (Beg et al., 1993; Brown et al., 1995; Chen et al., 1995; Traenckner et al., 1995) by a specific IκB kinase (DiDonato et al., 1997). Phosphorylation of IκB targets the protein for ubiquitination and degradation by the proteasome pathway (Henkel et al., 1993; Lin et al., 1995; Palombella et al., 1994; Traenckner et al., 1994). Thus, a phosphorylation-dependent modulation of the repressor half-life (Sun et al., 1994) determines NF-κB activity.

HSP90. The 90-kDa heat shock protein/chaperone HSP90 was originally considered a repressor like IκB because of its ability to sequester several ligand-inducible transcription factors in the cytoplasm, but recent experiments suggest that it actually plays a dual role. In the absence of ligand, glucocorticoid receptors are sequestered in the cytoplasm in a multiprotein complex that includes HSP90 (reviewed by Beato et al., 1995; Pratt, 1993). After ligand binding, the receptor is released from the complex, translocates to the nucleus, and activates transcription of genes containing the *cis*-acting hormone-response element. Similarly, the unliganded aryl hydrocarbon receptor (AHR), a bHLH-PAS monomer, is also part of a cytosolic multiprotein complex that includes HSP90. After binding of aryl hydrocarbons such as dioxin, the AHR is translocated to the nucleus where it heterodimerizes with the aryl hydrocarbon nuclear translocator (ARNT), another bHLH-PAS monomer (which despite its name does not translocate AHR to the nucleus) to form the transcriptionally active AHR complex (Pollenz et al., 1994). HSP90 functions as more than just a repressor, however, as it appears necessary to maintain both the glucocorticoid receptor and AHR in a conformation that allows ligand binding (Pratt, 1993; Whitelaw et al., 1995). If HSP90 were functioning simply as a repressor, then loss of function should result in constitutive (ligand independent) activity of the receptors. However, the glucocorticoid receptor and AHR can each activate transcription via their cognate binding sites in a ligand-inducible manner when expressed in wild-type yeast but not when the yeast *hsp90* gene has been disrupted (Bohen and Yamamoto, 1993; Carver et al., 1994). Thus HSP90 can now be more properly considered a cofactor for ligand binding.

Regulation of DNA Binding by Heterodimers

Id and bHLH proteins. ID is a repressor that contains an HLH dimerization domain but lacks the basic domain required for DNA binding. ID can therefore heterodimerize with other HLH proteins but the resulting heterodimer lacks DNA-binding activity. The expression of ID competitively inhibits the formation of active heterodimers between myogenic class II bHLH proteins, such as MYOD and MYOGENIN, and class I proteins, such as E47 and E12 (Benezra et al., 1990). The onset of myogenesis is associated with downregulation of ID expression and upregulation of myogenic bHLH proteins, and overexpression of ID can inhibit myocyte differentiation (Jen et al., 1992), suggesting that the relative levels of ID and the myogenic bHLH proteins may play an important role in the transition from determined myoblast to differentiated myocyte.

IP-1 and bZIP proteins. An analogous situation exists with respect to the bZIP proteins: IP-1 contains the leucine zipper dimerization domain but lacks the basic domain and can heterodimerize with members of the C-FOS and C-JUN families of bZIP factors, thus inhibiting the formation of AP-1 heterodimers with DNA-binding activity (Auwerx and Sassone-Corsi, 1991). IP-1 can heterodimerize with bZIP proteins only when it is nonphosphorylated, thus providing a mechanism for regulation of repression via signal transduction pathways leading to protein kinase activation. IP-1 was shown to be phosphorylated and inactivated by protein kinase A. Because AP-1 activity is thought to be activated via the protein kinase C cascade, whereas CREB activity is activated via the protein kinase A cascade, this finding suggested the existence of cross talk between these two major pathways transducing signals to the nucleus (Auwerx and Sassone-Corsi, 1991).

Regulation of Transactivation by Heterodimers

In the examples provided thus far the repressors are products of genes distinct from the activators that they regulate. In other cases, however, activators and repressors are differentially expressed from a single gene by posttranscriptional regulation. Thus, although gene expression is regulated primarily at the level of transcription, the transcription factors are themselves the products of genes that are often regulated at posttranscriptional levels, as illustrated below.

Alternative splicing: FOSB and ΔFOSB. FOSB is a member of the FOS family of basic leucine zipper (bZIP) transcription factors that heterodimerize with JUN family members to form AP-1 proteins that can activate transcription of genes containing a TPA response element (TRE). ΔFOSB (also known as FOSB2) is an alternatively spliced isoform that lacks the last 101 amino acids at the carboxyl terminus of FOSB (Mumberg et al., 1991; Nakabeppu and Nathans, 1991; Yen et al., 1991). Whereas ΔFOSB contains the bZIP domain that mediates dimerization and DNA binding, it lacks the transactivation domain identified in FOSB. ΔFOSB forms dimers with JUN family members that are unable to activate transcription. Thus, in any cell the relative levels of the repressor ΔFOSB and the activators FOSB and C-FOS will determine the degree of transcriptional activation of genes containing a TRE. Functional antagonism was also demonstrated at the level of cellular transformation, as ΔFOSB suppressed the ability of FOSB to transform cotransfected cultured mouse or rat fibroblasts (Mumberg et al., 1991; Yen et al., 1991). Alternative splicing events that affect transactivation have also been reported for the transcription factors CREM (Foulkes et al., 1991) and TFE3 (Roman et al., 1991).

Alternative translation initiation: LAP and LIP. LAP (liver activator protein; also known as NF-IL6) is another bZIP transcriptional activator. As in the case of FOSB, the mRNA sequences encoding the transactivation domain are located 5' to the sequences encoding the bZIP domain. Utilization of an internal AUG translation initiation codon results in the synthesis of LIP, a repressor that can dimerize, bind to DNA, and inhibit transcriptional activation mediated by LAP (Descombes and Schibler, 1991). LAP activates transcription of hepatocyte-specific genes including albumin, and the LAP/LIP ratio increases fivefold during liver differentiation, suggesting that the relative levels of activator and repressor determine the rate of transcription of target genes.

Active repression mediated by corepressors. For the preceding examples, repressor function appears to involve formation of a transcriptionally inactive heterodimer, and these proteins thus block activation rather than actively repressing transcription. The bHLH-ZIP protein C-MYC heterodimerizes with MAX to form a transcriptional activator in actively proliferating cells (Amati et al., 1992, 1993; Blackwood and Eisenman, 1991; Blackwood et al., 1992; Kretzner et al., 1992). The MAD proteins (MAD1,

MXI1, MAD3, and MAD4) are bHLH-ZIP proteins that can also hetero-dimerize with MAX and bind to the same sequence (5'-CACGTG-3') as the C-MYC/MAX heterodimer, but MAD/MAX heterodimers repress transcription (Ayer et al., 1993; Hurlin et al., 1995; Zervos et al., 1993). The ratio of C-MYC/MAX to MAD/MAX heterodimers may be an important determinant of cellular proliferation, as differentiation of cells in the monocyte/macrophage line is associated with a transition from predominance of C-MYC/MAX to MAD/MAX heterodimers (Ayer and Eisenman, 1993). Screens to identify proteins that interact with MAD and MXI1 lead to the cloning of mouse cDNA sequences encoding two proteins with homology to SIN3, a yeast protein involved in the transcriptional repression of a wide variety of genes (Ayer et al., 1995; Schreiber-Agus et al., 1995). Both yeast and mouse SIN3 proteins do not bind to DNA directly but function as corepressors by forming ternary complexes with DNA-bound repressors. The region of SIN3 that interacts with MAD1 is highly conserved between yeast and mouse such that yeast SIN3 can also specifically interact with MAD1 and repress transcription (Kasten et al., 1996). SIN3 is recruited to MAD1, MXI1, and also to unliganded nuclear receptor proteins (see Chapter 5) in concert with the corepressor NCoR, and these proteins in turn recruit a histone deacetylase HD1 (Alland et al., 1997; Hassig et al., 1997; Heinzel et al., 1997; Laherty et al., 1997; Nagy et al., 1997; Zhang et al., 1997). As described in detail below, histone deacetylase mediates chromatin remodeling and transcriptional silencing.

Additional examples of bHLH repressors are the *Drosophila* HAIRY and ENHANCER OF SPLIT proteins (Delidakis and Artavanis-Tsakonas, 1992; Giebel et al., 1997; Klambt et al., 1989; Knust et al. 1992; Ohsako et al., 1994) and the homologous mammalian HES proteins (Akazawa et al., 1992; Feder et al., 1993; Ishibashi et al., 1994; Sasai et al., 1992; Takebayashi et al., 1995). In mammalian cells, forced expression of the bHLH activator MYOD can result in myogenic differentiation (Davis et al., 1987; reviewed by Rudnicki and Jaenisch, 1995; Weintraub, 1993). However, coexpression of HES-1 blocks MYOD-mediated myogenesis (Akazawa et al., 1992). Similarly, neurogenesis directed by the bHLH activator MASH-1 (Guillemot et al., 1993) is blocked by coexpression of HES-1 in vivo (Ishibashi et al., 1994). A four-amino-acid sequence, WRPW (Trp-Arg-Pro-Trp), is found at the carboxyl terminus of all of the bHLH repressors but none of the bHLH activators described above (Ohsako et al., 1994). This tetrapeptide sequence is necessary for interaction of HAIRY with the corepressor GROUCHO (Paroush et al., 1994). When this tetrapeptide is transferred to a heterologous GAL4 DNA-binding protein with no inherent activator or repressor activity, the resulting fu-

sion protein is a strong transcriptional repressor and can bind GROU-
CHO or the human homologue TLE-1, demonstrating that this motif is
sufficient for repressor activity (Fisher et al., 1996). Furthermore, expression of a GAL4-GROUCHO fusion protein results in repression of reporter genes bearing GAL4 binding sites. These results indicate that the
corepressors GROUCHO and TLE-1 are recruited to DNA by protein-
protein interactions with the WRPW motif of HAIRY and HES-1, respectively. GROUCHO family members are active repressors in that they
are able to repress basal as well as activator-induced transcription and
can thus be distinguished from the passive inhibition of activation
achieved by the transcriptionally inactive HLH and bZIP proteins described above. Genetic studies indicate that GROUCHO is required for
neurogenesis, segmentation (establishment of the basic body plan), and
sex determination, emphasizing the key role played by transcriptional
repressors in development.

Direct Repression of Transcription Initiation Complex Formation

Many transcriptional repressors do not target a specific transcriptional
activator for repression by sequestration or heterodimerization but instead appear to target the transcription initiation complex, either directly
or indirectly through corepressors, and are required for proper execution
of the genetic programs that provide the molecular basis for development. Additional examples of developmentally regulated repressors include the zinc finger protein WT-1 (Madden et al., 1991), which is required for normal genitourinary development (Bruening et al., 1992) (see
Chapter 6) and the homeodomain proteins MSX1 (Catron et al., 1995)
and MSX2 (Semenza et al., 1995), which are required for normal craniofacial development (Jabs et al., 1993; Satokata and Maas, 1994) (see
Chapter 15). MSX1 has been shown to interact directly, via its homeodomain, with the TATA binding protein (TBP) of the transcription initiation complex and the same homeodomain sequences are required for
TBP interaction and transcriptional repression (Zhang et al., 1996). Both
MSX1 and MSX2 can repress transcription of reporter genes that lack a
cognate binding site (Catron et al., 1995; Semenza et al., 1995), providing
further evidence that they directly target one or more components of the
transcription initiation complex. The available experimental data do not
provide a clear indication as to whether MSX proteins repress transcription by binding to DNA directly, or by binding to general or sequence-
specific transcription factors as a corepressor, or whether they require
both DNA and protein interactions similar to the PBX proteins described
above. The transcriptional repressor WT-1 and the transcriptional acti-

vator EGR-1 are both zinc finger proteins that bind to the same DNA sequence and the relative amounts of EGR-1 and WT-1 may be a determinant of the balance between cellular proliferation and differentiation (Madden et al., 1991), similar in principle (but not in mechanism of action, because WT-1 and EGR-1 do not compete for a dimerization partner) to the relationship between the C-MYC and MAD proteins described above.

Signal-Dependent Corepressor Interactions

In addition to GROUCHO, HLE-1, and SIN3, another corepressor is the retinoblastoma protein, RB. The interaction of RB with the DNA-binding protein E2F converts E2F from an activator to a repressor (Hiebert et al., 1992; Weintraub et al., 1992, 1995). The interaction of RB with E2F is regulated by cyclin dependent kinases during the cell cycle, such that phosphorylation of RB during S phase prevents its interaction with E2F (Chellappan et al., 1991). E2F is thus free to activate transcription of genes whose protein products are required for DNA synthesis, which is presumably mediated by the interaction of E2F with one or more coactivators. The adenovirus transforming protein E1A binds to RB and by doing so prevents RB from interacting with E2F (reviewed by Dyson and Harlow, 1992; Moran, 1993). As a result, E2F is unopposed as a transcriptional activator of genes encoding proteins required for DNA synthesis, thus resulting in cellular proliferation. The nomenclature becomes a little tortured in this case: if RB is a corepressor, then E1A must be an anti-corepressor.

The thyroid and retinoid acid receptors, like E2F, are constitutively bound to DNA. In the absence of the proper physiological signal (ligand binding), the receptors interact with corepressor TRAC proteins (Chen and Evans, 1995; Horlein et al., 1995), which dissociate on ligand binding and allow interactions with coactivators including CBP and steroid receptor coactivator-1 (Kamei et al., 1996; Onate et al., 1995).

Chromatin Remodeling Factors

As described in Chapter 1, decompaction of chromatin is required for transcription of DNA to occur. In particular, the hyperacetylation of lysine residues within the amino-terminal domains of the core histones is associated with actively transcribed chromatin (reviewed by Brownell and Allis, 1996; Wolffe and Pruss, 1996). Acetylation of lysine residues neutralizes the positive charge of the side chain, which is predicted to destabilize the interaction of the histone with negatively charged DNA.

Destabilization of the nucleosome would then facilitate access of transcription factors to the DNA. In addition to histone acetylation, other events such as DNA uncoiling may occur before and during transcription. An increasing number of proteins have been implicated in this process of chromatin remodeling, including the SWI/SNF and GCN5 proteins that are conserved from yeast to humans, the nucleosome remodeling factor (NURF) identified in *Drosophila*, and the mammalian proteins CBP, P300, and P300/CBP-associated factor (P/CAF). Consistent with the multiple lines of experimental evidence that indicate that chromatin remodeling involves histone acetylation, recent data indicate that several proteins implicated in chromatin remodeling have histone acetyltransferase (HAT) activity.

GCN5

A genetic selection in *Saccharomyces cerevisiae* allowed the identification and isolation of the genes *ADA2, ADA3, ADA5,* and *GCN5,* encoding proteins that functionally interact with the acidic activation domain of VP16, a transcriptional activator encoded by the herpes simplex virus (Berger et al., 1992; Marcus et al., 1994, 1996; Pina et al., 1993). These proteins were shown to physically interact with one another, with transactivators, and with general transcription factors, suggesting that they functioned as a coactivator complex (Horiuchi et al., 1995). GCN5 was subsequently shown to have HAT activity (Brownell et al., 1996). Human GCN5 was also shown to possess HAT activity and an amino acid substitution within the HAT domain was shown to reduce both HAT activity and transcription, thus providing a convincing link between histone acetylation and transcriptional activation (Wang et al., 1997). The fact that GCN5 is required only for transcription mediated by a subset of activators in yeast suggested the possibility of multiple histone acetyltransferases, each interacting with different activators (Brownell et al., 1996). As described below, this prediction has now been confirmed.

SWI/SNF Proteins

Studies of the yeast and human Pol II holoenzymes have identified, in addition to the SRB complex described above, another multiprotein coactivator complex that contains at least 11 polypeptides, including the proteins SWI1, SWI2/SNF2, SWI3, SNF5, SNF6, and SNF11 (reviewed by Guarente, 1995; Kingston et al., 1996; Krude and Elgin, 1996; Winston and Carlson, 1992). As in the case of the SRB proteins, the yeast SWI/SNF complex was found to associate with Pol II by interacting with the carboxyl-terminal domain of the large subunit (Wilson et al., 1996). Genetic studies were consistent with the hypothesis that SWI/SNF proteins form a complex that alters chromatin structure during transcriptional activation. The genes encoding these proteins were identified in two independent screens for mutations that either (1) prevent activation of the *HO* gene so that the yeast do not switch mating type or (2) prevent activation of the *SUC2* gene in glucose-deprived cells. Suppressor mutations were then identified in genes encoding histone and nonhistone chromatin proteins, suggesting that the SWI/SNF proteins may disrupt the nucleosomal structure of chromatin so that sequence-specific and/or general transcription factors can bind to DNA and initiate transcription (Cote et al., 1994; Hirschhorn et al., 1992; Kruger et al., 1995). For example, when transcription of the *SUC2* gene is activated, the chromatin structure of the *SUC2* promoter is altered, as determined by sensitivity to digestion by micrococcal nuclease. However, in yeast containing *snf5* or *swi2/snf2* mutations, neither full transcriptional activation nor chromatin alteration occurs (Hirschhorn et al., 1992). Mutations in yeast that decrease expression of histones H2A and H2B partially restore *SUC2* transcriptional activation and chromatin alteration, suggesting that the SWI/SNF proteins are required for chromatin remodeling and transcriptional activation. In the presence of a bound transactivator, the purified yeast SWI/SNF complex was shown to remove histones from nucleosomes in vitro in an ATP-dependent manner (Cote et al., 1994; Owen-Hughes et al., 1996).

Analysis of the SWI2/SNF2 amino acid sequence revealed homology to a superfamily of proteins with conserved DNA-dependent ATPase and DNA helicase domains (Bork and Koonin, 1993; Gorbalenya and Koonin, 1993). Members of this family perform a variety of biological functions including DNA recombination and repair, mitotic chromosome segregation, and transcriptional regulation (reviewed by Carlson and Laurent, 1994).

Two human homologues of SWI2/SNF2, BRG1 and HBRM, have been identified (Chiba et al., 1994; Khavari et al., 1993; Muchardt and Yaniv, 1993). BRG1 was present in a multiprotein complex of approximately 2 MDa, similar to the size of the yeast SWI/SNF complex (Khavari et al., 1993). By assaying fractionated extracts for BRG1 immunoreactivity, a mammalian SWI/SNF complex was partially purified and shown to mediate ATP-dependent nucleosome disruption and transactivator binding (Kwon et al., 1994), demonstrating evolutionary conservation of both structure and function. Using immunoaffinity chromatography, complexes containing BRG1 or HBRM were purified and shown to contain (depending on the cellular source of the extracts) 9 to 12 polypeptides ranging from 47 to 250 kDa, which were designated as BRG1 associated factors or BAFs (Wang et al., 1996a). Remarkable similarities were noted when the amino acid sequences of the mammalian proteins BAF190, BAF170, BAF155, BAF60, and BAF47 were compared with the yeast proteins SNF2/SWI2, SWI3, SWI3, SWP73, and SNF5, respectively (Wang et al., 1996a, 1996b). However, a variety of different complexes were identified in different mammalian cell types. For example, BAF60 proteins were encoded by a multigene family and whereas BAF60A was ubiquitously expressed, BAF60B and BAF60C were expressed preferentially in muscle and pancreas, respectively (Wang et al., 1996b). Furthermore, whereas BAF60A was present in the 2-MDa BRG1 complex, BAF60B was present in a 1-MDa complex containing some but not all BAFs present in the 2-MDa complex (Wang et al., 1996b).

There is as yet no convincing experimental data to indicate whether the SWI/SNF proteins function as essential coactivators by interacting specifically with DNA-binding transcriptional activators in mammalian cells. However, the fact that mutations in genes encoding these proteins have selective effects on the transcription of a limited number of genes suggests that this is likely to be the case. The diversity of mammalian SWI/SNF homologues suggest that they may participate in chromatin remodeling processes that are cell-type, developmental-stage, and/or gene-specific.

NURF

In *Drosophila,* an ATP-dependent nucleosome remodeling factor (NURF), consisting of four polypeptides of 215, 140, 55, and 38 kDa, has been shown to interact with the GAGA DNA-binding protein to alter chromatin structure in the region of the *hsp70* gene promoter (Tsukiyama and Wu, 1995). NURF ATPase activity is stimulated by nucleosomes but not by free DNA or histones, suggesting that NURF directly alters nucleosome structure. Cloning of the 140-kDa ATPase subunit of NURF (designated ISWI for imitation switch protein) revealed amino acid sequence similarity to members of the SWI2/SNF2 family of ATPases (Tsukiyama et al., 1995). However, NURF is not part of the SWI/SNF complex, the ATPase activity of which is stimulated by free DNA but not by nucleosomes (Cote et al., 1994). These results suggest that whereas both the SWI/SNF and NURF complexes may disrupt nucleosomes, they may do so by different mechanisms. One possible explanation is that NURF is involved in the initial disruption of nucleosome structure required for transcription factor binding, whereas SWI/SNF proteins are involved in the extension of nucleosome-free regions required for transcription initiation and/or elongation. For example, the 30-nm chromatin fiber is at least partially disrupted during transcription, probably through the depletion of histone H1 and possibly the unfolding or sliding of the octamer core on the DNA template (reviewed by Felsenfeld, 1992).

The human *hSNF2L* gene (Okabe et al., 1992) encodes a protein that is 75% identical to ISWI over its entire length, suggesting that it is the homologue of ISWI rather than SNF2. A yeast homologue of ISWI has also been identified (Tsukiyama et al., 1995), indicating that ISWI has been conserved throughout eukaryotic evolution. The observation that the ATPases of the NURF (ISWI) and SWI/SNF (SWI2/SNF2) complexes have been conserved from yeast to humans suggest that these chromatin remodeling factors play important biological roles. However, unlike the yeast *HO* and *SUC1* genes, thus far there are no mammalian genes that have been shown to require SWI/SNF or NURF complexes for transcription in vivo (Kingston et al., 1996). The further analysis of SWI/SNF and NURF proteins will provide an essential link between the models of transcription based on plasmid DNA templates, which are utilized in the transient transfection experimental paradigm, and transcription of chromatin templates as it actually occurs in vivo.

It should also be noted that just as there are proteins that are necessary to maintain chromatin in an open, transcriptionally active state, there appear to be proteins that maintain chromatin in a closed, transcriptionally repressed state. Thus far, the systems that have been studied most extensively involve the SSN6/TUP1 and PC-G proteins of yeast and *Drosophila*, respectively (reviewed by Kingston et al., 1996). Similar chromatin-compacting factors are also likely to participate in the transcriptional repression of mammalian genes.

P/CAF

The first direct connection between mammalian transcriptional activators/coactivators and chromatin remodeling factors was the identification of a P300/CBP-associated factor (P/CAF) that was shown to interact directly with the carboxyl-terminal transactivation domain of CBP and P300 (Yang et al., 1996). P/CAF was shown to have three remarkable qualities. First, the carboxyl-terminal half of P/CAF was homologous to the yeast protein GCN5, and both proteins demonstrated histone acetyltransferase activity, although P/CAF was active on both free histone and nucleosome templates whereas GCN5 only acetylated free histones. Second, P/CAF interacted with the same region of CBP and P300 as the adenovirus-transforming protein E1A in a competitive manner. Third, forced expression of E1A and P/CAF had opposite effects on the cell cycle. Compared to control cells, a greater proportion of cells over-expressing E1A and a lesser proportion of cells overexpressing P/CAF were in S phase. These results suggest that in addition to RB (see above), P/CAF is another cellular protein that is inactivated by interaction with E1A, thus accounting for the ability of E1A to cause cellular transformation. P/CAF could thus be recruited to specific promoters by interaction with CBP or P300 and contribute to promoter activation by decompacting chromatin via histone acetylation (Yang et al., 1996).

These results are significant for several reasons. First, they provide a connection between transcription factors, coactivators, transforming proteins, and cellular growth control. Second, they provide a connection between the models of *trans*-acting factors binding to *cis*-acting sequences, elucidated through the study of plasmid DNA templates in transient transfection experiments, with the reality of chromatin templates in vivo. Having said that, the model is, at least at first glance, somewhat problematic. Many of the transcriptional activators that are recognized by CBP, such as C-JUN, C-FOS, and perhaps SRF or ELK-1/TCF, appear to promote cellular proliferation, and P/CAF is proposed to facilitate transcriptional activation of promoters recognized by these factors by histone acetylation, yet overexpression of P/CAF inhibits cell cycle progression. One possible explanation is that P/CAF binds to CBP/P300 only when these coactivators have bound to certain activators, so that P/CAF is not involved in transcriptional activation mediated by growth-promoting factors such as C-JUN but is instead involved in transcriptional activation mediated by (unknown) growth suppressing factors. Another intriguing possibility is that the histone acetylase activity of P/CAF may be cell-cycle or growth-factor regulated. Determining how P/CAF expression and activity are regulated and whether P/CAF associates with other proteins in addition to CBP and P300 (e.g., other coactivators, SWI/SNF family members, general transcription factors) are likely to be areas of active experimental investigation in the near future.

CBP and P300

As described in an earlier section of this chapter, CBP and P300 are proteins, consisting of more than 2400 amino acids each, that function as coactivators that interact both with DNA-binding transcriptional activators and with components of the transcription initiation complex such as TBP. In addition, CBP and P300 interact with P/CAF, a histone acetyltransferase, as described above. Remarkably, both CBP and P300 also have histone acetyltransferase activity (Bannister and Kouzarides, 1996; Ogryzko et al., 1996). Whereas P/CAF acetylates histone H3 and, to a lesser degree, H4, P300 and CBP acetylate all four core histones in nucleosomes. In contrast to yeast and human GCN5 and P/CAF, which contain a putative acetyl-CoA binding site that is conserved in all other known histone acetyltransferases, this motif cannot be detected in CBP and P300 by standard algorithms (Ogryzko et al., 1996). Thus, the mechanism of histone acetylation by CBP and P300 may differ from that employed by GCN5 and P/CAF, which may imply differences with respect to substrates and/or regulation of activity.

These striking results indicate that CBP and P300 do not function merely as adaptor molecules linking DNA-binding transcription factors to the transcription initiation complex. In addition, their role in transcriptional regulation also involves chromatin remodeling. This latter process may require the combined substrate specificities of CBP or P300 and P/CAF. It is possible that histone acetylation is promoter-specific and that the specificity is mediated by the interaction of specific histone acetyltransferases with specific DNA-binding proteins.

$TAF_{II}250$

As described in Chapter 1, the amino-terminal regions of $dTAF_{II}42$ and $dTAF_{II}62$ bear remarkable structural similarity to the carboxyl-terminal core domains of histones H3 and H4, respectively, and $dTAF_{II}42$ and $dTAF_{II}62$ form heterotetramers with structural similarity to the H3/H4 heterotetramer that forms the histone core (Hoffmann et al., 1996; Nakatani et al., 1996; Xie et al., 1996). Furthermore, $dTAF_{II}28\alpha$ resembles H2B, such that TFIID may form a structure similar to the histone octamer consisting of two dimers of H2B-like TAFs and a tetramer of H3/H4–like TAFs and therefore may constitute a nucleosome-like structure on DNA binding (Hoffmann et al., 1996). As if these findings were not remarkable enough, the *Drosophila*, human, and yeast $TAF_{II}250$ homologues were shown to possess histone acetyltransferase activity that is specific for H3 and H4 (Mizzen et al., 1996). These results suggest the possibility that histone acetylation by $TAF_{II}250$ may facilitate nucleosome displacement and possibly the replacement of histones with TAFs to form a nucleoprotein complex (the TAFosome?) in which DNA is accessible for transcription by Pol II. In addition, the finding that $TAF_{II}250$, GCN5, CBP, P300, and P/CAF all have histone acetyltransferase activity suggests that these proteins may each act only on a subset of transcribed genes.

HD1 and Rpd3

Given the existence of histone acetylases, it should come as little surprise that histone deacetylases are also present in eukaryotic cells. The cloning of cDNA sequences encoding the human histone deacetylase HD1 revealed that the protein is 60% identical to the yeast protein Rpd3, a putative transcriptional repressor (Taunton et al., 1996). Rpd3 may bind to the corepressor Sin3 (reviewed by Wolffe, 1996), creating two remarkably parallel and complementary systems for mediating transcriptional activation and repression via changes in chromatin structure: (1) activator—co-activator (CBP/P300)—histone acetylase (P/CAF)→ chromatin decondensation→ transcriptional activation and (2) repressor—core-

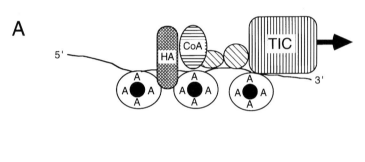

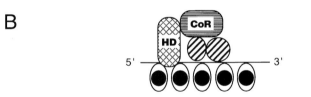

FIGURE 3-5. Chromatin remodeling and transcriptional regulation. (A) Transcriptional activation. Sequence-specific transcriptional activators (hatched) bind to DNA and, via protein-protein interactions, recruit a coactivator (CoA; horizontally striped) that interacts with the transcription initiation complex (TIC; vertically striped) and with a histone acetyltransferase (HA; cross-hatched). Addition of acetyl groups (A) to the amino terminal tails of core histones (filled) results in an open chromatin configuration that allows transcription factor binding to DNA and Pol II transcription of the DNA template into RNA. (B) Transcriptional repression. Sequence-specific transcriptional repressors (hatched) bind to DNA and, via protein-protein interactions, recruit a co-repressor (CoR; horizontally striped) that interacts with a histone deacetylase (HD; cross-hatched). Removal of acetyl groups from the amino terminal tails of core histones (filled) results in a closed chromatin configuration (indicated by tighter loops of DNA around histones) that prevents transcription factor binding to DNA and Pol II transcription of the DNA template into RNA.

pressor (Sin3)—histone deacetylase (Rpd3)→ transcriptional inactivation (Fig. 3.5).

Direct Remodeling by Sequence-Specific Transcriptional Activators

Although many DNA binding proteins may affect chromatin structure indirectly by recruiting coactivators, other sequence-specific transcription factors may alter chromatin directly. As described in Chapter 1, the DNA binding domain of the liver-specific transcription factor HNF-3 bears a close structural resemblance to the linker histone H5 (Clark et al., 1993). In addition to structural similarity, functional similarities have also been noted. Analysis of the albumin gene enhancer revealed that nucleosomes were precisely positioned with respect to the enhancer DNA sequence in liver nuclei where the gene is transcribed and the enhancer is bound by transcriptional activators, whereas the nucleosomes were positioned randomly in nuclei where the gene is not expressed and transcriptional activators are not bound (McPherson et al., 1993). Two HNF-3 binding sites in the enhancer were shown to be essential for the formation of the phased nucleosomal array, suggesting that HNF-3, as in the case of histone H1, may be able to interact with the histone core octamer and thus stabilize the position of specific nucleosomes with respect to the enhancer DNA sequence. Such nucleosome phasing may be necessary for the subsequent binding of other sequence-specific DNA-binding proteins to the enhancer (Archer et al., 1991; Pina et al., 1990).

Transcription Elongation Factors

Although transcription factors primarily influence the rate of transcription initiation, some factors also exert effects on transcription elongation (Yankulov et al., 1994). RNA Pol II pauses periodically during the process of transcription elongation and the frequency and duration of such pauses is an important determinant of the time required for transcription of a full-length primary RNA transcript (Krumm and Groudine, 1995). Several transcriptional activators have been shown to increase the processivity of transcription by Pol II and allow efficient elongation through pausing and arrest sites (Yankulov et al., 1994). The general transcription factor TFIIF also has a dual role in transcription initiation and elongation, as described in Chapter 1. Association of TFIIF with Pol II during elongation increases processivity by preventing transient pausing (Aso et al., 1995). No direct interaction between a transactivation domain and TFIIF has been demonstrated, leaving open the possibility that "co-elongators"

perform this function. The ability of $TAF_{II}250$ to specifically phosphorylate the RAP74 subunit of TFIIF (Dikstein et al., 1996a; see Chapter 1)
is notable in this regard. Decreased processivity in the absence of transcriptional activators may provide a mechanism that allows genes whose
transcription is induced by physiological stimuli to remain poised for
transcriptional activation (Yankulov et al., 1994), as described in Chapter
2 with respect to the *C-MYC* gene. The effect of activators on transcription is thus amplified by increases in both the rate of initiation and elongation.

Another *trans*-acting factor that has been implicated in the regulation
of elongation, but which is not a DNA-binding protein that affects transcription initiation, is the product of the von Hippel-Lindau (*VHL*) tumor
suppressor gene, which disrupts the formation of Elongin (also known
as SIII), a heterodimeric transcription-elongation factor (Aso et al., 1995;
Duan et al., 1995; Kibel et al., 1995). Elongin, as in the case of TFIIF,
stimulates elongation by suppressing pausing of Pol II (Aso et al., 1995).
Although VHL was shown to disrupt the formation of the Elongin het-
erotrimer in vitro (Kibel et al., 1995), it remains to be determined whether
changes in VHL levels result in changes in the rate of transcription and
steady-state levels of specific mRNA species. A recent study demonstrated that in cells cultured at high density, VHL was present predominantly in the cytoplasm, whereas in cells cultured at low density, VHL
localized to the nucleus (Lee et al., 1996), raising the possibility that VHL
may regulate transcription in response to physiological signals. However, much more work is required to establish the functional interactions
between VHL and Elongin in vivo. SII is another transcription elongation
factor, which contains a protein domain with sequence similarity to the
A subunit of Elongin, that allows Pol II to transcribe through protein-
bound regions of DNA including transcription arrest sites (Aso et al.,
1995). Future studies may provide functional connections between *trans*-
acting elongation factors such as Elongin, SII, and VHL and *cis*-acting
transcription arrest sites such as those identified within the *C-MYC* gene
(see Chapter 2) and thus provide a molecular basis for this transcriptional regulatory mechanism.

Signal Transduction from the Cell Surface to the Nucleus

The Role of CBP in Signal Transduction Via Kinase Cascades

Many transcription factors are not constitutively active but instead respond to specific cellular signals that are transmitted by protein kinases
and small molecule ligands. Recent studies indicate that the coactivator

CBP plays an important role in the process by which these signals affect gene transcription. The following discussion of CBP provides an opportunity to emphasize two important concepts. First, the activity of transcription factors is regulated by protein phosphorylation. Second, several important protein kinase cascades have been identified in mammalian cells, including the protein kinase A, protein kinase C, and MAP kinase cascades that allow extracellular and cytosolic signals to be transmitted to the nucleus, where long-lasting cellular responses are initiated via changes in gene expression (reviewed by Karin and Hunter, 1995).

The binding of many polypeptide hormones to their cognate cell surface receptors results in the activation of adenylate cyclase, which synthesizes the second messenger cyclic AMP (cAMP). The binding of cAMP to the regulatory subunit of the cAMP-dependent protein kinase (protein kinase A) results in the release of an active catalytic subunit that then translocates to the nucleus (Nigg et al., 1985). Protein kinase A phosphorylates serine (S) and threonine (T) residues that occur within a consensus sequence (K/R)(K/R)X(S/T) in which two lysine (K) or arginine (R) residues are separated from the phosphorylation site by a single residue, which may be any amino acid (X). One of the targets for phosphorylation by protein kinase A is a bZIP transcription factor, cAMP response element binding protein (CREB), which binds to the cAMP response element (CRE) present in the 5'-flanking region of many genes whose expression is regulated by cellular cAMP levels. CREB is not transcriptionally active unless it is phosphorylated by protein kinase A on a serine residue (S133) in its activation domain (Gonzalez and Montminy, 1989). When CREB is phosphorylated at S133, it is able to directly interact with a coactivator, the CREB binding protein (CBP) (Chrivia et al., 1993; Parker et al., 1996). CBP is essential for the activation of transcription mediated by the CRE because microinjection of anti-CBP antibodies blocked transcription from a cAMP-responsive promoter (Arias et al., 1994).

A second major signal transduction pathway in all eukaryotic cells is the mitogen-activated protein (MAP) kinase cascade (Fig. 3.6). Growth factors such as epidermal growth factor (EGF) and platelet-derived growth factor (PDGF) stimulate cellular proliferation by binding to their cognate receptors, which are protein tyrosine kinases. Ligand binding induces receptor dimerization and transphosphorylation that allows the formation of a multiprotein complex that includes the adaptor protein GRB2, the guanine nucleotide-exchange factor SOS, guanine nucleotide-binding protein RAS, and the serine/threonine protein kinase RAF (reviewed by Davis, 1994). RAF phosphorylates MEK-1, a MAP kinase kinase, which in turn phosphorylates the extracellular signal regulated

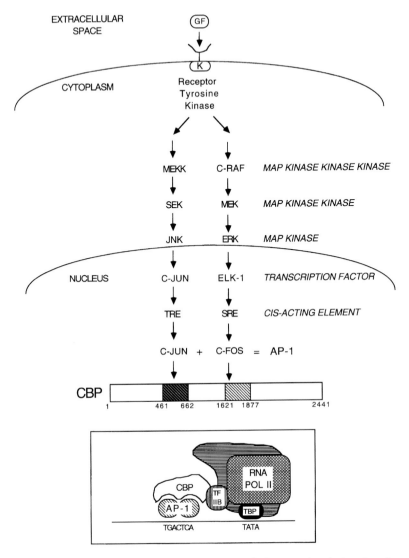

FIGURE 3-6. Proliferative responses to growth factor stimulation involve signal transduction pathways that lead to transcriptional activation mediated by AP-1 and CBP. Binding of growth factors (GF) to their cognate receptors, many of which have an intracellular kinase domain (K), initiates a cascade of phosphorylation events that transduces growth signals to the nucleus via binding of phosphorylated C-JUN to the TPA response element (TRE) and ELK-1 to the serum response element (SRE) located in the 5'-flanking region of the *C-JUN* and *C-FOS* genes, respectively. C-JUN and C-FOS dimerize to form the transcription factor AP-1, which activates transcription by binding to the sequence 5'-TGA(C/ G)TCA-3' and interacting with the coactivator CBP (interaction sites with C-JUN and C-FOS are indicated by hatched boxes), which in turn interacts directly with TFIIB and perhaps other components of the transcription initiation complex.

kinase-1 (ERK-1) and ERK-2, which are MAP kinases that phosphorylate serine and threonine residues that occur within the proline (P)-directed consensus sequence $PX_{1-2}(S/T)P$ (Davis, 1994). Several mitogen-activated genes, including *C-FOS*, contain a *cis*-acting DNA sequence, the serum response element (SRE). The serum response factor (SRF) binds to the SRE, but has little transactivating ability (reviewed by Treisman, 1990). Instead, it recruits the ternary complex factor ELK-1 to cooperatively bind to the SRE (Shaw et al., 1989). However, binding of SRF and ELK-1 to the SRE occurs in the absence of mitogenic stimulation and does not result in transcription. Instead, growth factor binding results in the phosphorylation of ELK-1 by ERK-1 or ERK-2 within its transactivation domain (Marais et al., 1993), thus allowing ELK-1 to mediate the effects of this MAP-kinase signal-transduction pathway on gene expression. CBP is also essential for the activation of transcription mediated by the SRE: microinjection of anti-CBP antibodies blocked transcription from a serum-responsive promoter (Arias et al., 1994). Studies demonstrating a selective interaction between CBP and the ERK-phosphorylated form of the ELK-1 transactivation domain have not been reported.

Another protein kinase cascade results in the activation of the MAP kinase JNK1 (JUN N-terminal kinase), which is also known as SAPK (stress-activated protein kinase). Whereas ERK is activated via the MAP kinase kinase kinase RAF and the MAP kinase kinase MEK, MEKK-1 and SEK-1 are the kinases that lead to activation of JNK1 (Fig. 3.6). JNK1 phosphorylates serine residues (S63 and S73) in the transactivation domain of C-JUN, an event that is required for transcriptional activation (Derijard et al., 1994; Smeal et al., 1991). C-JUN is a component of the bZIP transcription factor AP-1, which activates transcription in response to growth factors or exogenous mitogens such as TPA through a *cis*-acting DNA sequence, the TPA response element (TRE), which is present in the 5'-flanking region of many mitogen-responsive genes. The *C-JUN* gene contains a TRE that can be bound by C-JUN homodimers whose transcriptional activity is stimulated by JNK1 in response to mitogens. Mitogens thus result in the synthesis of C-FOS (via the SRE-SRF+ELK−1-ERK pathway) and C-JUN (via the TRE—C-JUN—JNK pathway) and the formation of the highly active form of AP-1, the C-FOS/C-JUN heterodimer. CBP is also essential for the activation of transcription mediated by the TRE because microinjection of anti-CBP antibodies blocked transcription from a TRE-containing promoter (Arias et al., 1994). CBP may therefore also recognize the phosphorylated form of C-JUN. CBP also appears to interact directly with C-FOS but this interaction does not require phosphorylation (Bannister and Kouzarides, 1995). However, phosphorylation of C-FOS at threonine-232 (by a kinase distinct from the ERK and JNK proteins) in response to growth factor stimulation also increases the transcriptional activity of AP-1 by an undetermined mechanism (Deng and Karin, 1994). Thus, CBP may stimulate AP-1 transcriptional activity by at least three different mechanisms involving interactions with C-FOS, C-JUN, and possibly ELK-1.

Signal Transduction Via Ligand Binding by Nuclear Receptors

In the signal transduction pathways described above, transcription factor activation is many steps removed from the original stimulus. In contrast, other transcription factors are directly activated by ligand binding. The largest and most biologically important group of ligand-activated transcription factors is the nuclear receptor superfamily (see Chapter 5). Included within this superfamily are the steroid hormone receptor, retinoid receptor, and orphan receptor families, each of which contains five or more members (reviewed by Beato et al., 1995; Mangelsdorf et al., 1995). Transactivation by nuclear receptors requires a conserved AF2 domain located on the carboxyl-terminal side of the ligand-binding domain. Several candidate coactivators have been identified that exhibit ligand-dependent binding to the carboxyl terminus of nuclear receptors. Steroid receptor coactivator-1 (SRC-1) was shown to stimulate the transcriptional activity of all steroid and retinoid receptors tested (Onate et al., 1995) and to possess histone acetyltransferase activity (Spencer et al., 1997). A second coactivator, P160, was shown to be encoded by an alternative transcript from the same gene as SRC-1 (Kamei et al., 1996). CBP was shown to interact with multiple steroid and retinoid receptors in a ligand-dependent manner that required an intact AF2 domain. Separate domains within CBP interacted with the ligand-binding domain of nuclear receptors and with the P160 coactivator, which in turn interacted with the nuclear receptor AF2 domain, resulting in a transcriptionally active DNA–nuclear receptor–CBP–P160 quaternary complex (Kamei et al., 1996). As might be predicted from the preceding analyses, microinjection of anti-CBP antibodies blocked ligand-dependent transcriptional activation by nuclear receptors.

A fascinating discovery regarding the many functions of CBP was its potential role as an integrator of signals converging on the AP-1 and nuclear receptor transcriptional regulatory pathways. Previous studies had demonstrated that several different nuclear receptors could repress AP-1–dependent gene transcription in a ligand-dependent manner (reviewed by Beato et al., 1995). The inhibition of AP-1 transcriptional activity was shown to result from competition by nuclear receptors for limiting amounts of CBP (Kamei et al., 1996). Several important conclusions can be drawn from these data. First, these results indicate that within each cell, CREB, AP-1, nuclear receptors, and other transcription factors, including E2F1 (Trouche and Kouzarides, 1996), may compete for binding to limiting amounts of CBP. Second, provided that the concentration of CBP is limiting, both the relative and the absolute concentration of each factor will determine its degree of transcriptional activity. Third, the expression of one transcription factor may affect the transcription of a large number of genes that do not even contain binding sites for that factor but instead contain binding sites for other CBP-interacting factors. These observations provide a fascinating glimpse into the complex, interrelated functioning of transcriptional regulators in mammalian cells. They also provide a caveat for investigators to consider regarding the limits of reductionist experimentation in providing an understanding of biological processes.

The JAK-STAT Pathway: Signal Transduction Via Direct Transcription Factor Phosphorylation at the Cell Membrane

Several examples have already been provided in this chapter of transcriptional activators and repressors whose activity is regulated by phosphorylation events. There are now numerous examples of phosphorylation or dephosphorylation events that affect each aspect of transcription factor function, including nuclear localization, dimerization, DNA binding, transactivation, and protein stability. Important roles for the protein kinase C, protein kinase A (PKA), and MAP kinase cascades in transcription factor regulation were described earlier in this chapter. Whereas the modification of transcriptional activators such as CREB and C-JUN by the serine/threonine protein kinases PKA and JNK, respectively, occurs within the nucleus, another major signal transduction pathway, the JAK-STAT pathway, results in the direct tyrosine phosphorylation of transcription factors at the cell membrane, as first discovered by studies of interferon-inducible genes described below.

The binding of interferon α (IFN-α) to its receptor at the cell membrane results in the rapid transcriptional activation of genes containing a *cis*-acting regulatory element, the interferon-stimulated response element (ISRE), which is bound by the *trans*-acting interferon-stimulated gene factor 3 (ISGF-3) (Levy et al., 1988). Most IFN-α–inducible genes contain an ISRE, which has the consensus sequence 5'-AGTTTCNNTTTCNY-3' (N, any nucleotide; Y, C or T), within 200 bp of the transcription initiation site (Darnell et al., 1994). Assays of DNA-binding activity indicated that ISGF-3 activity was induced within minutes after cells were exposed to IFN-α and the induction did not

A

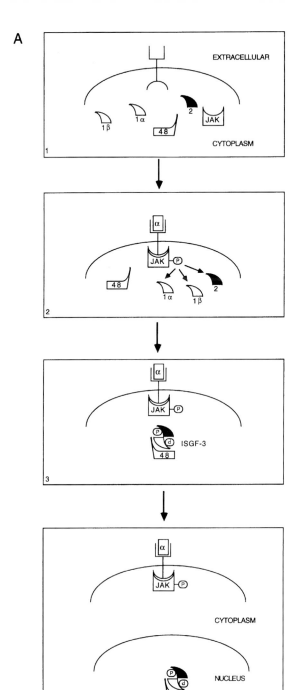

B

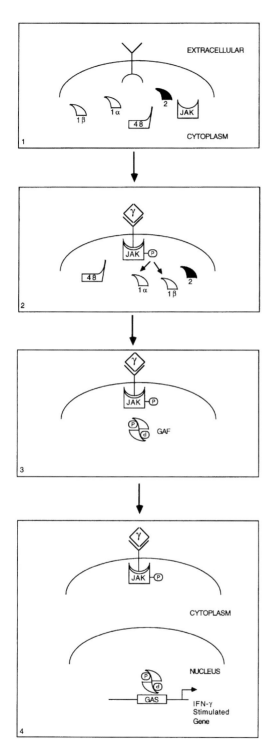

FIGURE 3-7. Interferon stimulated gene expression: the JAK-STAT pathway. (A) Interferon α and interferon-stimulated gene factor 3 (ISGF-3). In the absence of binding of interferon α to its receptor, the JAK and STAT proteins are free in the cytoplasm (panel 1). Binding of interferon α leads to a change in the conformation of the intracellular receptor domain that allows binding of JAK1 and TYK2 kinases that become activated by transphosphorylation and then phosphorylate STAT1 and STAT2 proteins (panel 2). Phosphorylation results in dimerization of STAT1 and STAT2 (to form STAT1α/STAT2 and STAT1β/STAT2 heterodimers) and association with the 48-kDa DNA-binding subunit to form ISGF-3 (panel 3). ISGF-3 translocates to the nucleus, binds to genes containing an interferon-stimulated response element (ISRE) in the promoter region, and activates transcription (panel 4). (B) Interferon gamma (IFN-γ) and IFN-γ activating factor (GAF). In the absence of binding of interferon gamma to its receptor, the JAK and STAT proteins are free in the cytoplasm (panel 1). Binding of interferon gamma results in phosphorylation of STAT1 by JAK1 and JAK2 (panel 2). Phosphorylated STAT1α homodimerizes to form GAF (panel 3). GAF translocates to the nucleus, binds to genes containing a interferon-γ activation site (GAS) in the promoter region, and activates transcription (panel 4). (Adapted from Darnell et al., 1994.)

89

require *de novo* protein synthesis (Levy et al., 1988). All components of ISGF-3 were present in the cytoplasm of uninduced cells, and IFN-α stimulation resulted in a posttranslational modification that allowed subunit association and nuclear translocation (Levy et al., 1989). Purified ISGF-3 was shown to consist of polypeptide subunits of 113, 91, 84, and 48 kDa, only the last of which actually contacts DNA (Fu et al., 1990). cDNA cloning revealed that the 91- and 84-kDa subunits were isoforms encoded by the same gene, the 113-kDa subunit was encoded by a closely related gene, and the DNA-binding 48-kDa subunit was encoded by a third gene (Fu et al., 1992; Schindler et al., 1992a). The 84-, 91-, and 113-kDa subunits all contained an SH2 domain, a motif by which proteins interact with protein tyrosine kinases. At the same time, a mutant cell line that was unresponsive to IFN-α stimulation was shown to lack expression of the TYK2 nonreceptor protein tyrosine kinase (Velazquez et al., 1992). Furthermore, the 84-, 91–, and 113-kDa proteins were shown to be phosphorylated on tyrosine residues in response to IFN-α stimulation leading to the formation of an active ISGF-3 complex capable of binding to the ISRE of IFN-α–inducible genes (Fu, 1992; Schindler et al., 1992a, b). These observations provided a connection between the binding of IFN-α to its receptor at the cell surface and the activation of ISGF-3 (Fig. 3.7A).

Interferon γ (IFN-γ) binds to a cell surface receptor that is unique from that bound by IFN-α and stimulates the transcription of genes containing a different *cis*-acting element, the IFN-γ activation site (GAS) which has the consensus sequence 5'-TTNCNNNAA-3 and is bound by the *trans*-acting IFN-γ activated factor (GAF) (Darnell et al., 1994). Remarkably, GAF was shown to consist of the 91-kDa subunit of ISGF-3, which on IFN-γ stimulation is phosphorylated by either JAK1 or JAK2, nonreceptor protein tyrosine kinases that are closely related to TYK2. The phosphorylated 91-kDa protein dimerizes, translocates to the nucleus, and binds directly to the GAS (Darnell et al., 1994; Shuai et al., 1992) (Fig. 3.7B).

Subsequent studies revealed that a large number of cytokines that bind to nonkinase cell surface receptors, including granulocyte-macrophage colony-stimulating factor, interleukin (IL)-3, IL-5 and IL-10, transduce signals via TYK/JAK kinases to the same polypeptides identified as components of ISGF-3 and GAF (Larner et al., 1993). The 91-, 84-, and 113-kDa transcription factors were renamed as STAT (signal transduction and activator of transcription) 1α, STAT1β, and STAT2, respectively, and additional members of this family—STAT3, STAT4, and STAT5—were subsequently identified (reviewed by Darnell, 1997; Darnell et al., 1994). Specific interactions between receptors, JAK kinases, and STATs were demonstrated (Stahl et al., 1995), providing a molecular basis for transcriptional responses to cytokine stimulation. Growth factors such as epidermal growth factor and platelet-derived growth factor, which bind to receptors with intrinsic tyrosine kinase activity that results in activation of MAP kinase pathways, also activate JAK/STAT pathways (Ruff-Jamison et al., 1993; Sadowski et al., 1993; Silvennoinen et al., 1993; Zhong et al., 1994). Transcriptional activation by STAT3 in response to IL-6 stimulation was shown to require, in addition to JAK kinase-mediated tyrosine phosphorylation, serine phosphorylation at a site that matched the consensus sequence (Pro-X-Ser/Thr-Pro) for phosphorylation by MAP kinases (Zhang et al., 1995). These results established a direct genetic connection between responses to cytokines and growth factors and between the receptor tyrosine kinase/MAP kinase and JAK/STAT pathways, thus elucidating another mechanism by which extracellular signals are integrated at the transcriptional level.

Transcription Factor Phosphorylation by Pol II–Associated Factors

A recent discovery that further demonstrates the complexity of transcriptional regulation is the finding that the AF-1 transcriptional activation domain of the zinc finger transcription factor RARα (see Chapter 5) is phosphorylated by the serine/threonine protein kinase CDK7, a component of TFIIH (Rochette-Egly et al., 1997). Thus, not only do the transcriptional activators interact with the general transcription factors and affect their function, but reciprocal regulation of the activators by the general factors also appears to occur, because the CDK7-dependent phosphorylation is required for transcriptional activity of AF-1. These observations provide further evidence of the multiple enzymatic activities that precede the actual polymerization of ribonucleosides into the primary RNA transcript.

References

Abate, C., L. Patel, F. J. Rauscher III, and T. Curran. Redox regulation of Fos and Jun DNA-binding activity in vitro. *Science* 249:1157–1161, 1990.

Abraham, S. E., S. Lobo, P. Yaciuk, H. G. Wang, and E. Moran. p300, and p300-associated proteins, are components of TATA-binding protein (TBP) complexes. *Oncogene* 8:1639–1647, 1993.

Akazawa, C., Y. Sasai, S. Nakanishi, and R. Kageyama. Molecular characterization of a rat negative regulator with a basic helix-loop-helix structure predominantly expressed in the developing nervous system. *J. Biol. Chem.* 267: 21879–21885, 1992.

Alland, L., R. Muhle, H. Hou, Jr., J. Potes, L. Chin, N. Schreiber-Agus, and R. A. DePinho. Role for N-CoR and histone deacetylase in Sin3-mediated transcriptional repression. *Nature* 387:49–55, 1997.

Amati, B., M. W. Brooks, N. Levy, T. D. Littlewood, G. I. Evans, and H. Land. Oncogenic activity of the c-Myc protein requires dimerization with Max. *Cell* 72:233–245, 1993.

Amati, B., S. Dalton, M. W. Brooks, T. D. Littlewood, G. I. Evans, and H. Land. Transcriptional activation by the human c-Myc oncoprotein in yeast requires interaction with Max. *Nature* 359:423–426, 1992.

Anderson, M. T., F. J. T. Staal, C. Gitler, L. A. Herzenberg, and L. A. Herzenberg. Separation of oxidant-initiated and redox-regulated steps in the NF-κB signal transduction pathway. *Proc. Natl. Acad. Sci. U.S.A.* 91:11527–11531, 1994.

Angel, P. and M. Karin. The role of Jun, Fos, and the AP-1 complex in cell proliferation and transformation. *Biochim. Biophys. Acta* 1072:129–157, 1991.

Arany, Z., W. R. Sellers, D. M. Livingston, and R. Eckner. E1A-associated p300 and CREB-associated CBP belong to a conserved family of coactivators. *Cell* 77:799–800, 1994.

Arany, Z., D. Newsome, E. Oldread, D. M. Livingston, and R. Eckner. A family of transcriptional adaptor proteins targeted by the E1A oncoprotein. *Nature* 374:81–84, 1995.

Archer, T. K., M. G. Cordingley, R. G. Wolford, and G. L. Hager. Transcription factor access is mediated by accurately positioned nucleosomes on the mouse mammary tumor virus promoter. *Mol. Cell. Biol.* 11:688–698, 1991.

Arias, J., A. Alberts, P. Brindle, F. Claret, T. Smeal, M. Karin, J. Feramisco, and M. Montminy. Activation of cAMP and mitogen responsive genes relies on a common nuclear factor. *Nature* 370:226–228, 1994.

Artandi, S. E., K. Merrell, N. Avitahl, K.-K. Wong, and K. Calame. TFE3 contains two activation domains, one acidic and the other proline-rich, that synergistically activate transcription. *Nucleic Acids Res.* 23:3865–3871, 1995.

Aso, T., W. S. Lane, J. W. Conaway, and R. C. Conaway. Elongin (SIII): a multisubunit regulator of elongation by RNA polymerase II. *Science* 269:1439–1443, 1995.

Attardi, L. D., and R. Tjian. Drosophila tissue-specific transcription factor NTF-1 contains a novel isoleucine-rich activation motif. *Genes Dev.* 7:1341–1353, 1993.

Auwerx, J., and P. Sassone-Corsi. IP-1: A dominant inhibitor of Fos/Jun whose activity is modulated by phosphorylation. *Cell* 64: 983–993, 1991.

Ayer, D. E., and R. N. Eisenman. A switch from Myc:Max to Mad:Max heterocomplexes accompanies monocyte/macrophage differentiation. *Genes Dev.* 7: 2110–2119, 1993.

Ayer, D. E., L. Kretzner, and R. N. Eisenman. Mad: a heterodimeric partner for Max that antagonizes Myc transcriptional activity. *Cell* 72:211–222, 1993.

Ayer, D. E., Q. A. Lawrence, and R. N. Eisenman. Mad-Max transcriptional repression is mediated by ternary complex formation with mammalian homologs of yeast repressor Sin3. *Cell* 80:767–776, 1995.

Bannister, A. J., and T. Kouzarides. CBP-induced stimulation of c-Fos activity is abrogated by E1A. *EMBO J.* 14:4758–4762, 1995.

Bannister, A. J., and T. Kouzarides. The CBP co-activator is a histone acetyltransferase. *Nature* 641–643, 1996.

Bauerle, P. A., and D. Baltimore. Activation of DNA-binding activity in an apparently cytoplasmic precursor of the NF-κB transcription factor. *Cell* 53:211–217, 1988a.

Bauerle, P. A., and D. Baltimore. IκB: a specific inhibitor of the NF-κB transcription factor. *Science* 242:540–546, 1988b.

Bauerle, P. A., and T. Henkel. Function and activation of NF-κB in the immune system. *Annu. Rev. Immunol.* 12:141–179, 1994.

Beals, C. R., C. M. Sheridan, C. W. Turck, P. Gardner, and G. R. Crabtree. Nuclear export of NF-ATc enhanced by glycogen synthase kinase-3. *Science* 275:1930–1933, 1997.

Beato, M., P. Herrlich, and G. Schutz. Steroid hormone receptors: many actors in search of a plot. *Cell* 83:851–857, 1995.

Beckmann, H., and T. Kadesch. The leucine zipper of TFE3 dictates helix-loop-helix dimerization specificity. *Genes Dev.* 5:1057–1066, 1991.

Beckmann, H., L.-K. Su, and T. Kadesch. TFE3: a helix-loop-helix protein that activates transcription through the immunoglobulin enhancer μE3 motif. *Genes Dev.* 4:167–179, 1990.

Beg, A. A., T. S. Finco., P. V. Nantermet, and A. S. Baldwin. Tumor necrosis factor and interleukin-1 lead to phosphorylation and loss of IκB: a mechanism of NF-κB activation. *Mol. Cell. Biol.* 13:3301–3310, 1993.

Benezra, R., R. L. Davis, D. Lockshon, D. L. Turner, and H. Weintraub. The protein Id: a negative regulator of helix-loop-helix DNA binding proteins. *Cell* 61:49–59, 1990.

Berg, J. M. Proposed structure for the zinc-binding domains from transcription factor IIIA and related proteins. *Proc. Natl. Acad. Sci. U.S.A.* 85:99–102 , 1988.

Berg, J. M., and Y. Shi. The galvanization of biology: a growing appreciation for the roles of zinc. *Science* 271:1081–1085, 1996.

Berger, S. L., B. Pina, N. Silverman, G. A. Marcus, J. Agapite, J. L. Regier, S. J. Triezenberg, and L. Guarente. Genetic isolation of ADA2: a potential transcriptional adaptor required for function of certain acidic activation domains. *Cell* 70:251–265, 1992.

Blackwell, T. K., L. Kretzner, E. M. Blackwood, R. N. Eisenman, and H. Weintraub. Sequence-specific DNA binding by the c-Myc protein. *Science* 250:1149–1151, 1990.

Blackwell, T. K., and H. Weintraub. Differences and similarities in DNA-binding preferences of MyoD and E2A protein complexes revealed by binding site selection. *Science* 250:1104–1110, 1990.

Blackwood, E. M., and R. N. Eisenman. Max: a helix-loop-helix zipper protein that forms a sequence-specific DNA-binding complex with myc. *Science* 251:1211–1217, 1991.

Blackwood, E. M., B. Luscher, and R. N. Eisenman. Myc and Max associate in vivo. *Genes Dev.* 6:71–80, 1992.

Blobel, G. A., M. C. Simon, and S. H. Orkin. Rescue of GATA-1-deficient embryonic stem cells by heterologous GATA-binding proteins. *Mol. Cell. Biol.* 15:626–633, 1995.

Bohen, S. P., and K. R. Yamamoto. Isolation of Hsp90 mutants by screening for decreased steroid receptor function. *Proc. Natl. Acad. Sci. U.S.A.* 90:11424–11428, 1993.

Bork, P., and E. V. Koonin. An expanding family of helicases within the 'DEAD/H' superfamily. *Nucleic Acids Res.* 21:751–752, 1993.

Boulikas, T. Nuclear localization signals (NLS). *Crit. Rev. Eukaryotic Gene Expression* 3:193–227, 1993.

Boyle, W. J., T. Smeal, L. H. K. Defize, P. Angel, J. R. Woodgett, M. Karin, and T. Hunter. Activation of protein kinase C decreases phosphorylation of c-Jun at sites that negatively regulate its DNA-binding activity. *Cell* 64:573–584, 1991.

Brand, K., S. Page, G. Rogler, A. Bartsch, R. Brandl, R. Knuechel, M. Page, C. Kaltschmidt, P. A. Bauerle, and D. Neumeier. Activated transcription factor nuclear factor-kappa B is present in the atherosclerotic lesion. *J. Clin. Invest.* 97:1715–1722, 1996.

Brown, K., S. Gerstberger, L. Carlson, G. Franzoso, and U. Siebenlist. Control of IκB-α proteolysis by site-specific, signal-induced phosphorylation. *Science* 267:1485–1488, 1995.

Brownell, J. E., and C. D. Allis. Special HATs for special occasions: linking histone acetylation to chromatin assembly and gene activation. *Curr. Opin. Genet. Dev.* 6:176–184, 1996.

Brownell, J.E., J. Zhou, T. Ranalli, R. Kobayashi, D. Edmondson, S. Roth, and C. D. Allis. Tetrahymena histone acetyltransferase A: a homolog to yeast Gcn5p linking acetylation to gene activation. *Cell* 84:843–851, 1996.

Bruening, W., N. Bardeesy, B. L. Silverman, R. A. Cohn, G. A. Machin, A. J. Aronson, D. Housman, and J. Pelletier. Germline intronic and exonic mutations in the Wilms' tumor gene (WT1) affecting urogenital development. *Nat. Genet.* 1:144–148, 1992.

Burbach, K. M., A. Poland, and C. A. Bradfield. Cloning of the Ah-receptor cDNA reveals a distinctive ligand-activated transcription factor. *Proc. Natl. Acad. Sci. U.S.A.* 89:8185–9189, 1992.

Burley, S. K., and R. G. Roeder. Biochemistry and structural biology of transcription factor IID (TFIID). *Annu. Rev. Biochem.* 65:769–799, 1996.

Busch, S. J., and P. Sassone-Corsi. Dimers, leucine zippers and DNA binding domains. *Trends Genet.* 6:36–40, 1990.

Cao, Z., W. J. Henzel, and X. Gao. IRAK: a kinase associated with the interleukin-1 receptor. *Science* 271:1128–1131, 1996.

Carlson, M., and B. C. Laurent. The SNF/SWI family of global transcriptional activators. *Curr. Opin. Cell Biol.* 6:396–402, 1994.

Carver, L. A., V. Jackiw, and C. A. Bradfield. The 90-kDa heat shock protein is essential for Ah receptor signalling in a yeast expression system. *J. Biol. Chem.* 269:30109–30112, 1994.

Catron, K. M., H. Zhang, S. C. Marshall, J. A. Inostroza, J. M. Wilson, and C. Abate. Transcriptional repression by Msx-1 does not require homeodomain DNA-binding sites. *Mol. Cell. Biol.* 15:861–871, 1995.

Chan, S.-K., L. Jaffe, M. Capovilla, J. Botas, and R. S. Mann. The DNA binding specificity of ultrabithorax is modulated by cooperative interactions with extradenticle, another homeoprotein. *Cell* 78:603–615, 1994.

Chellappan, S. P., S. Hiebert, M. Mudryj, J. M. Horowitz, and J. R. Nevins. The E2F transcription factor is a cellular target for the RB protein. *Cell* 65:1053–1061, 1991.

Chen, J. D., and R. M. Evans. A transcriptonal co-repressor that interacts with nuclear hormone receptors. *Nature* 377:454–457, 1995.

Chen, J.-L., L. D. Attardi, C. P. Verrijzer, K. Yokomori, and R. Tjian. Assembly of recombinant TFIID reveals differential coactivator requirements for distinct transcriptional activators. *Cell* 79:93–105, 1994.

Chen, Z., J. Hagler, V. J. Palombella, F. Melandri, D. Scherer, D. Ballard, and T. Maniatis. Signal-induced site-specific phosphorylation targets IκBa to the ubiquitin-proteasome pathway. *Genes Dev.* 9:1586–15597, 1995.

Chi, T., P. Lieberman, K. Ellwood, and M. Carey. A general mechanism for transcriptional synergy by eukaryotic activators. *Nature* 377:254–257, 1995.

Chiba, H., M. Muramatsu, A. Nomoto, and H. Kato. Two human homologues of Saccharomyces cerevisiae SWI2/SNF2 and Drosophila brahma are transcriptional coactivators cooperating with the estrogen receptor and the retinoic acid receptor. *Nucleic Acids Res.* 22:1815–1820, 1994.

Chow, C.-W., M. Rincon, J. Cavanagh, M. Dickens, and R. J. Davis. Nuclear accumulation of NFAT4 opposed by the JNK signal transduction pathway. *Science* 278:1638–1641, 1997.

Chrivia, J. C., R. P. Kwok, N. Lamb, M. Hagiwara, M. R. Montminy, and R. H. Goodman. Phosphorylated CREB binds specifically to the nuclear protein CBP. *Nature* 365:855–859, 1993.

Citri, Y., H. V. Colot, A. C. Jacquier, Q. Yu, J. C. Hall, D. Baltimore, and M. Rosbash. A family of unusually spliced biologically active transcripts encoded by a Drosophila clock gene. *Nature* 326:42–47, 1987.

Citron, B. A., M. D. Davis, S. Milstien, J. Gutierrez, D. B. Mendel, G. R. Crabtree, and S. Kaufman. Identity of 4a-carbinolamine dehydratase, a component of the phenylalanine hydroxylation system, and DCoH, a transregulator of homeodomain proteins. *Proc. Natl. Acad. Sci. U. S. A.* 89:11891–11894, 1992.

Clark, K. L., E. D.Halay, E. Lai, and S. K. Burley. Co-crystal structure of the HNF-3/fork head DNA-recognition motif resembles histone H5. *Nature* 364:412–420, 1993.

Cote, J., J. Quinn, J. Workman, and C. L. Peterson. Stimulation of Gal4 derivative binding to nucleosomal DNA by the yeast SWI/SNF complex. *Science* 265:53–60, 1994.

Courey, A. J., and R. Tjian. Analysis of Sp1 in vivo reveals multiple transcriptional domains, including a novel glutamine-rich activation motif. *Cell* 55:887–898, 1989.

Cress, W. D., and S. J. Triezenberg. Critical structural elements of the VP16 transcriptional activation domain. *Science* 251:87–90, 1991.

Darnell, J. E., Jr. STATs and gene regulation. *Science* 277:1630–1635, 1997.

Darnell, J. E., Jr., I. M. Kerr, and G. R. Stark. Jak-STAT pathways and transcriptional activation in response to IFNs and other extracellular signaling proteins. *Science* 264:1415–1421, 1994.

Davis, R. MAPKs: new JNK expands the group. *Trends Biochem. Sci.* 19:470–473, 1994.

Davis, R. L., H. Weintraub, and A. B. Lassar. Expression of a single transfected cDNA converts fibroblasts to myoblasts. *Cell* 51:987–1000, 1987.

Delidakis, C., and S. Artavanis-Tsakonas. The Enhancer of split [E(spl)] locus of

Drosophila encodes seven independent helix-loop-helix proteins. *Proc. Natl. Acad. Sci. U.S.A.* 89:8731–8735, 1992.

Deng, T., and M. Karin. c-Fos transcriptional activity stimulated by H-Ras-activated protein kinase distinct from JNK and ERK. *Nature* 371:171–175, 1994.

Derijard, B., M. Hibi, I.-H. Wu, T. Barrett, B. Su, T. Deng, M. Karin, and R. Davis. JNK1: a protein kinase stimulated by UV light and Ha-Ras that binds and phosphorylates the c-Jun activation domain. *Cell* 76:1025–1037, 1994.

Descombes, P., and U. Schibler. A liver-enriched transcriptional activator protein, LAP, and a transcriptional inhibitory protein, LIP, are translated from the same mRNA. *Cell* 67:569–579, 1991.

DiDonato, J. A., M. Hayakawa, D. M. Rothwarf, E. Zandi, and M. Karin. A cytokine-responsive IκB kinase that activates the transcription factor NF-κB. *Nature* 388:548–554, 1997.

Dikstein, R., S. Ruppert, and R. Tjian. TAF$_{II}$250 is a bipartite protein kinase that phosphorylates the basal transcription factor RAP74. *Cell* 84:781–790, 1996a.

Dikstein, R., S. Zhou, and R. Tjian. Human TAF$_{II}$105 is a cell type-specific TFIID subunit related to h TAF$_{II}$130. *Cell* 87:137–146, 1996b.

Dolwick, K. M., H. I. Swanson, and C. A. Bradfield. In vitro analysis of Ah receptor domains involved in ligand-activated DNA recognition. *Proc. Natl. Acad. Sci. U.S.A.* 90:8566–8570, 1993.

Du, W., D. Thanos, and T. Maniatis. Mechanisms of transcriptional synergism between distinct virus-inducible enhancer elements. *Cell* 74:887–898, 1993.

Duan, D. R., A. Pause, W. H. Burgess, T. Aso, D. Y. T. Chen, K. P. Garrett, R. C. Conaway, J. W. Conaway, W. M. Linehan, and R. D. Klausner. Inhibition of transcription elongation by the VHL tumor suppressor protein. *Science* 269:1402–1406, 1995.

Dyson, N., and E. Harlow. Adenovirus E1A targets key regulators of cell proliferation. In *Cancer Surveys, Vol 12. Tumor Suppressor Genes: The Cell Cycle and Cancer*, A. Levine, ed. Cold Spring Harbor, New York: Cold Spring Harbor Laboratory Press, 1992, pp. 161–195

Eckner, R., M. E. Ewen, D. Newsome, M. Gerdes, J. A. DeCaprio, J. B. Lawrence, and D. M. Livingston. Molecular cloning and functional analysis of the adenovirus E1A-associated 300-kD protein (p300) reveals a protein with properties of a transcriptional adaptor. *Genes Dev.* 8:869–884, 1994.

Ellenberger, T. D. Fass, M. Arnaud, and S. C. Harrison. Crystal structure of transcription factor E47: E-box recognition by a basic region helix-loop-helix dimer. *Genes Dev.* 8:970–980, 1994.

Endrizzi, J. A., J. D. Cronk, W. Wang, G. R. Crabtree, and T. Alber. Crystal structure of DCoH, a biofunctional, protein-binding transcriptional coactivator. *Science* 268:556–559, 1995.

Evans, R. M. The steroid and thyroid hormone receptor superfamily. *Science* 240:889–895, 1988.

Feder, J. N., L. Y. Jan, and Y. N. Jan. A rat gene with sequence homology to the Drosophila gene hairy is rapidly induced by growth factors known to influence neuronal differentiation. *Mol. Cell. Biol.* 13:105–113, 1993.

Felsenfeld, G. Chromatin as an essential part of the transcription mechanism. *Nature* 355:219–224, 1992.

Ferreri, K., G. Gill, and M. Montminy. The cAMP-regulated transcription factor

CREB interacts with a component of the TFIID complex. *Proc. Natl. Acad. Sci. U.S.A.* 91:1210–1213, 1994.

Fisher, A. L., S. Ohsako, and M. Caudy. The WRPW motif of the hairy-related basic helix-loop-helix repressor proteins acts as a 4-amino-acid transcription repression and protein-protein interaction domain. *Mol. Cell. Biol.* 16:2670–2677, 1996.

Foulkes, N. S., E. Borrelli, and P. Sassone-Corsi. CREM gene: use of alternative DNA-binding domains generates multiple antagonists of cAMP-induced transcription. *Cell* 64:739–749, 1991.

Fu, X.-Y. A transcription factor with SH2 and SH3 domains is directly activated by an interferon α-induced cytoplasmic protein tyrosine kinase(s). *Cell* 70: 323–335, 1992.

Fu, X.-Y., D. S. Kessler, S. A. Veals, D. E. Levy, and J. E. Darnell, Jr. ISGF3, the transcription activator induced by interferon α, consists of multiple interacting polypeptide chains. *Proc. Natl. Acad. Sci. U.S.A.* 87:8555–8559, 1990.

Fu, X.-Y., C. Schindler, T. Improta, R. Aebersold, and J. E. Darnell, Jr. The proteins of ISGF-3, the interferon α-induced transcriptional activator, define a gene family involved in signal transduction. *Proc. Natl. Acad. Sci. U.S.A.* 89: 7840–78743, 1992.

Gehring, W. J., M. Muller, M. Affolter, A. Percival-Smith, M. Billeter, Y. Q. Qian, G. Otting, and K. Wuthrich. The structure of the homeodomain and its functional implications. *Trends. Genet.* 6:323–329, 1990.

Gibbons, R. J., D. J. Picketts, L.Villard, and D. R. Higgs. Mutations in a putative global transcriptional regulator cause X-linked mental retardation with α-thalassemia. *Cell* 80:837–845, 1995.

Giebel, B., and J. A. Campos-Ortega. Functional dissection of the Drosophila enhancer of split protein, a suppressor of neurogenesis. *Proc. Natl. Acad. Sci. U. S. A.* 94:6250–6254, 1997.

Giese, K., J. Cox, and R. Grosschedl. The HMG domain of lymphoid enhancer factor 1 bends DNA and facilitates assembly of functional nucleoprotein structures. *Cell* 69:185–189, 1992.

Giese, K., C. Kingsley, J. R. Kirshner, and R. Grosschedl. Assembly and function of a TCR α enhancer complex is dependent on LEF-1 induced DNA bending and multiple protein-protein interactions. *Genes Dev.* 9:995–1008, 1995.

Gill, G., E. Pascal, Z. H. Tseng, and R. Tjian. A glutamine-rich hydrophobic patch in transcription factor Sp1 contacts the dTAF$_{II}$110 component of the Drosophila TFIID complex and mediates transcriptional activation. *Proc. Natl. Acad. Sci. U.S.A.* 91:192–196, 1994.

Gill, G., and M. Ptashne. Mutants of GAL4 protein altered in an activation function. *Cell* 51:121–126, 1987.

Gill, G., I. Sadowski and M. Ptashne. Mutations that increase the activity of a transcriptional activator in yeast and mammalian cells. *Proc. Natl. Acad. Sci. U.S.A.* 87:2127–2131, 1990.

Goodrich, J. A., T. Hoey, C. J. Thut, A. Admon, and R. Tjian. Drosophila TAF$_{II}$40 interacts with both a VP16 activation domain and the basal transcription factor TFIIB. *Cell* 75:519–530, 1993.

Goodrich, J. A., and R. Tjian. TBP-TAF complexes: selectivity factors for eukaryotic transcription. *Curr. Opin. Cell Biol.* 6:403–409, 1994.

Gonzalez, G. A., and M. R. Montminy. Cyclic AMP stimulates somatostatin gene transcription by phosphorylation of CREB at serine 133. *Cell* 59:675–680, 1989.

Gorbalenya, A. E., and E. V. Koonin. Helicases: amino acid sequence comparisons and structure-function relationships. *Curr. Opin. Struct. Biol.* 3:419–429, 1993.

Gregor, P., M. Sawadogo, and R. G. Roeder. The adenovirus major late transcription factor USF is a member of the helix-loop-helix group of regulatory proteins and binds to DNA as a dimer. *Genes Dev.* 4:1730–1740, 1990.

Griffin, G. E., K. Leung, T. M. Folks, S. Kunkel, and G. J. Nabel. Activation of HIV gene expression during monocyte differentiation by induction of NF-κB. *Nature* 339:70–73, 1989.

Gruss, P., and C. Walther. Pax in development. *Cell* 69:719–722, 1992.

Gstaiger, M., O. Georgiev, H. van Leeuwen, P. van der Vliet, and W. Schaffner. The B cell coactivator Bob1 shows DNA sequence-dependent complex formation with Oct-1/Oct-2 factors, leading to differential promoter activation. *EMBO J.* 15:2781–2790, 1996.

Gstaiger, M., L. Knoepfel, O. Georgiev, W. Schaffner, and C. M. Hovens. A B-cell coactivator of octamer-binding transcription factors. *Nature* 373:360–362, 1995.

Guarente, L. Transcriptional coactivators in yeast and beyond. *Trends Biochem. Sci.* 20:517–521, 1995.

Guillemot, F., L.-C. Lo, J. E. Johnson, A Auerbach, D. J. Anderson, and A. L. Joyner. Mammalian achaete-scute homolog 1 is required for the early development of olfactory and autonomic neurons. *Cell* 75:463–476, 1993.

Harley, V. R., D. I. Jackson, P. J. Hextall, J. R. Hawkins, G. D. Berkovitz, S. Sockanathan, R. Lovell-Badge, and P. N. Goodfellow. DNA-binding activity of recombinant SRY from normal males and XY females. *Science* 255:453–456, 1992.

Hassig, C. A., T. C. Fleischer, A. N. Billin, S. L. Schreiber, and D. E. Ayer. Histone deacetylase activity is required for full transcriptional repression by mSin3A. *Cell* 89:341–347, 1997.

Heinzel, T., R. M. Lavinsky, T.-M. Mullen, M. Soderstrom, C. D. Laherty, J. Torchia, W.-M. Yang, G. Brard, S. D. Ngo, J. R. Davie, E. Seto, R. N. Eisenman, D. W. Rose, C. K. Glass, and M. G. Rosenfeld. A complex containing N-CoR, mSin3, and histone deacetylase mediates transcriptional repression. *Nature* 387:43–48, 1997.

Henkel, T., T. Machleidt, I. Alkalay, M. Kronke, Y. Ben-Neriah, and P. A. Bauerle. Rapid proteolysis of IκB-α is necessary for activation of transcription factor NF-κB. *Nature* 365:182–185, 1993.

Henthorn, P., M. Kiledjian, and T. Kadesch. Two distinct transcription factors that bind the immunoglobulin enhancer μE5/κE2 motif. *Science* 247:467–470, 1990.

Herr, W., R. A. Sturm, R. G. Clerc, L. M. Corcoran, D. Baltimore, P. A. Sharp, H. A. Ingraham, M. G. Rosenfeld, M. Finney, G. Ruvkin, and H. R. Horvitz. The POU domain: a large conserved region in the mammalian Pit-1, oct-1, oct-2 and Caenorhabditis elegans unc-86 gene products. *Genes Dev.* 2:1513–1516, 1988.

Hiebert, S. W., S. P. Chellappan, J. M. Horowitz, and J. R. Nevins. The interaction of RB with E2F coincides with an inhibition of the transcriptional activity of E2F. *Genes Dev.* 6:177–185, 1992.

Hirose, K., M. Morita, M. Ema, J. Mimura, H. Hamada, H. Fujii, Y. Saijo, O. Gotoh, K. Sogawa, and Y. Fujii-Kuriyama. cDNA cloning and tissue-specific expression of a novel basic helix-loop-helix/PAS factor (Arnt2) with close sequence similarity to the aryl hydrocarbon receptor nuclear translocator (Arnt). *Mol. Cell. Biol.* 16: 1706–1713, 1996.

Hirschhorn, J. N., S. A. Brown, C. D. Clark, and F. Winston. Evidence that SNF2/ SWI2 and SNF5 activate transcription in yeast by altering chromatin structure. *Genes Dev.* 6:2288–2298, 1992.

Hoey, T., R. O. J. Weinzierl, G. Gill, J.-L. Chen, B. D. Dynlacht, and R. Tjian. Molecular cloning and functional analysis of Drosophila TAF110 reveal properties expected of coactivators. *Cell* 72:247–260, 1993.

Hoffman, E. C., H. Reyes, F.-F. Chu, F. Sander, L. H. Conley, B. A. Brooks, and O. Hankinson. Cloning of a factor required for activity of the Ah (dioxin) receptor. *Science* 252:954–958, 1991.

Hoffmann, A., C.-M. Chiang, T. Oelgeschlager, X. Xie, S. K. Burley, Y. Nakatani, and R. G. Roeder. A histone octamer-like structure within TFIID. *Nature* 380: 356–359, 1996.

Hope, I. A., S. Mahadevan, and K. Struhl. Structural and functional characterization of the short acidic transcriptional activation region of yeast GCN4 protein. *Nature* 333:635–640, 1988.

Horiuchi, J., N. Silverman, G. A. Marcus, and L. Guarente. ADA3, a putative transcriptional adaptor, consists of two separable domains and interacts with ADA2 and GCN5 in a trimeric complex. *Mol. Cell. Biol.* 15:1203–1209, 1995.

Horlein, A. J., A. M. Naar, T. Heinzel, J. Torchia, B. Gloss, R. Kurokawa, A. Ryan, Y. Kamei, M. Soderstrom, C. K. Glass, and M. G. Rosenfeld. Ligand-independent repression by the thyroid hormone receptor mediated by a nuclear receptor co-repressor. *Nature* 377:397–404, 1995.

Hu, J.-S., E. N. Olson, and R. E. Kingston. HEB, a helix-loop-helix protein related to E2A and ITF2 that can modulate the DNA-binding ability of myogenic regulatory factors. *Mol. Cell. Biol.* 12:1031–1042, 1992.

Hunter, T., and M. Karin. The regulation of transcription by phosphorylation. *Cell* 70:375–387, 1992.

Hurlin, P. J., C. Queva, P. J. Koskinen, E. Steingrimsson, D. E. Ayer, N. G. Copeland, N. A. Jenkins, and R. N. Eisenman. Mad3 and Mad4: novel Max-interacting transcriptional repressors that suppress c-myc dependent transformation and are expressed during neural and epidermal differentiation. *EMBO J.* 14:5646–5659, 1995.

Isaac, D. D., and D. J. Andrew. Tubulogenesis in Drosophila: a requirement for the trachealess gene product. *Genes Dev.* 10:103–117, 1996.

Ishibashi, M., K. Moriyoshi, Y. Sasai, K. Shiota, S. Nakanishi, and R. Kageyama. Persistent expression of helix-loop-helix factor HES-1 prevents mammalian neural differentiation in the central nervous system. *EMBO J.* 13:1799–1805, 1994.

Jabs, E. W., U. Muller, X. Li, L. Ma, W. Luo, I. S. Haworth, I. Klisak, R. Sparkes, M. L. Warman, J. B. Mulliken, M. L. Snead, and R. Maxson. A mutation in

the homeodomain of the human MSX2 gene in a family affected with autosomal dominant craniosynostosis. *Cell* 75:443–450, 1993.

Jacq, X., C. Brou, Y. Lutz, I. Davidson, P. Chambon, and L. Tora. Human $TAF_{II}30$
is present in a distinct TFIID complex and is required for transcriptional
activation by the estrogen receptor. *Cell* 79:107–117, 1994.

Jain, J., P. G. McCaffrey, Z. Miner, T. K. Kerppola, J. N. Lambert, G. L. Verdine,
T. Curran, and A. Rao. The T-cell transcription factor $NFAT_p$ is a substrate
for calcineurin and interacts with Fos and Jun. *Nature* 365:352–355,
1993.

Janknecht, R., and T. Hunter. Transcriptional control: versatile molecular glue.
Curr. Biol. 6:951–954, 1996.

Jen, Y., H. Weintraub, and R. Benezra. Overexpression of Id protein inhibits the
muscle differentiation program: in vivo association of Id with E2A proteins.
Genes Dev. 6:1466–1479, 1992.

Jiang, B.-H., E. Rue, G. L. Wang, R. Roe, and G. L. Semenza. Dimerization, DNA
binding, and transactivation properties of hypoxia-inducible factor 1. *J. Biol.
Chem.* 271:17771–17778, 1996.

Kadesch, T. Helix-loop-helix proteins in the regulation of immunoglobulin gene
transcription. *Immunol. Today* 13:31–36, 1992.

Kamei, Y., L. Xu, T. Heinzel, J. Torchia, R. Kurokawa, B. Gloss, S.-C. Lin, R. A.
Heyman, D. W. Rose, C. K. Glass, and M. G. Rosenfeld. A CBP integrator
complex mediates transcriptional activation and AP-1 inhibition by nuclear
receptors. *Cell* 85:403–414, 1996.

Karin, M., and T. Hunter, T. Transcriptional control by protein phosphorylation:
signal transmission from the cell surface to the nucleus. *Curr. Biol.* 5:747–
757, 1995.

Kasten, M. M., D. E. Ayer, and D. J. Stillman. SIN3–dependent transcriptional
repression by interaction with the Mad1 DNA-binding protein. *Mol. Cell.
Biol.* 16:4215–4221, 1996.

Keegan, L., G. Gill, and M. Ptashne. Separation of DNA binding from the tran-
scription-activating function of a eukaryotic regulatory protein. *Science* 231:
699–704, 1986.

Khavari, P. A., C. L. Peterson, J. W. Tamkun, D. B. Mendel, and G. R. Crabtree.
BRG1 contains a conserved domain of the SWI2/SNF2 family necessary for
normal mitotic growth and transcription. *Nature* 366:170–174, 1993.

Kibel, A., O. Iliopoulos, J. A. DeCaprio, and W. G. Kaelin, Jr. Binding of the von
Hippel-Lindau tumor suppressor protein to Elongin B and C. *Science* 269:
1444–1446, 1995.

Kim, Y.-J., S. Bjorklund, Y. Li, M. H. Sayre, and R. D. Kornberg. A multiprotein
mediator of transcriptional activation and its interaction with the C-terminal
repeat domain of RNA polymerase II. *Cell* 77:599–608, 1994.

Kingston, R. E., C. A. Bunker, and A. N. Imbalzano. Repression and activation
by multiprotein complexes that alter chromatin structure. *Genes Dev.* 10:905–
920, 1996.

Klambt, C., E. Knust, K. Tietze, and J. A. Campos-Ortega. Closely related transcripts encoded by the neurogenic gene complex Enhancer of split of Drosophila melanogaster. *EMBO J.* 8:203–210, 1989.

Klemm, R., J. Goodrich, S. Zhou, and R. Tjian. Molecular cloning and expression
of the 32-kDa subunit of human TFIID reveals interactions with VP16 and

TFIIB that mediate transcriptional activation. *Proc. Natl. Acad. Sci. U. S. A.* 92:5788–5792, 1995.

Knust, E., H. Schrons, F. Grawe, and J. A. Campos-Ortega. Seven genes of the Enhancer of split complex of Drosophila melanogaster encode helix-loop-helix proteins. *Genetics* 132:505–518, 1992.

Korinek, V., N. Barker, P. J. Morin, D. van Wichen, R. de Weger, K. W. Kinzler, B. Vogelstein, and H. Clevers. Constitutive transactivation by a β-catenin-Tcf complex in APC$^{-/-}$ colon carcinoma. *Science* 275:1784–1787, 1997.

Kouzarides, T., and E. Ziff. The role of the leucine zipper in the fos-jun interaction. *Nature* 336:646–651, 1988.

Kretzner, L., E. M. Blackwood, and R. N. Eisenman. Myc and Max proteins possess distinct transcriptional activities. *Nature* 359:426–429, 1992.

Krude, T., and S. C. R. Elgin. Chromatin: pushing nucleosomes around. *Curr. Biol.* 6:511–515, 1996.

Kruger, W., C. L. Peterson, A. Sil, C. Coburn, G. Arents, E. N. Moudrianakis, and I. Herskowitz. Amino acid substitutions in the structured domains of histones H3 and H4 partially relieve the requirement of the yeast SWI/SNF complex for transcription. *Genes Dev.* 9:2770–2779, 1995.

Krumm, A., and M. Groudine. Tumor suppression and transcription elongation: the dire consequences of changing partners. *Science* 269:1400–1401, 1995.

Kumar, S., A. B. Rabson, and C. Gelinas. The RXXRXRXXC motif conserved in all Rel/κB proteins is essential for the DNA-binding activity and redox regulation of the v-Rel oncoprotein. *Mol. Cell. Biol.* 12:3094–3106, 1992.

Kwok, R. P. S., J. R. Lundblad, J. C. Chrivia, J. P. Richards, H. P. Bachinger, R. G. Brennan, S. G. E. Roberts, M. R. Green, and R. H. Goodman. Nuclear protein CBP is a coactivator for the transcription factor CREB. *Nature* 370: 223–226, 1994.

Kwon, H., A. N. Imbalzano, P. A. Khavari, R. E. Kingston, and M. R. Green. Nucleosome disruption and enhancement of activator binding by a human SWI/SNF complex. *Nature* 370:477–481, 1994.

Laherty, C. D., W.-M. Yang, J.-M. Sun, J. R. Davie, E. Seto, and R. N. Eisenman. Histone deacetylases associated with the mSin3 corepressor mediate Mad transcriptional repression. *Cell* 89:349–356, 1997.

Landschulz, W. H., P. F. Johnson, and S. L. McKnight. The leucine zipper: a hypothetical structure common to a new class of DNA binding proteins. *Science* 240:1759–1764, 1988.

Larner, A. C., M. David, G. M. Feldman, K. Igarashi, R. H. Hackett, D. S. A. Webb, D. M. Sweitzer, E. F. Petricoin III, and D. S. Finbloom. Tyrosine phosphorylation of DNA binding proteins by multiple cytokines.*Science* 261: 1730–1733, 1993.

Laudet, V., D. Stehelin, and H. Clevers. Ancestry and diversity of the HMG box superfamily. *Nucleic Acids Res* 21:2493–2501, 1993.

Lee, S., D. Y. T. Chen, J. S. Humphrey, J. R. Gnarra, W. M. Linehan, and R. D. Klausner. Nuclear/cytoplasmic localization of the von Hippel-Lindau tumor suppressor gene product is determined by cell density. *Proc. Natl. Acad. Sci. U. S. A.* 93:1770–1775, 1996.

Leuther, K. K., J. M. Salmeron, and S. A. Johnston. Genetic evidence that an activation domain of GAL4 does not require acidity and may form a β sheet. *Cell* 72:575–585, 1993.

Levy, D. E., D. S. Kessler, R. Pine, N. Reich, and J.E. Darnell, Jr. Interferon-induced nuclear factors that bind a shared promoter element correlate with positive and negative control. *Genes Dev.* 2:383–393, 1988.

Levy, D. E., D. S. Kessler, R. Pine, and J. E. Darnell, Jr. Cytoplasmic activation of ISGF3, the positive regulator of interferon-α-stimulated transcription, reconstituted in vitro. *Genes Dev.* 3:1362–1371, 1989.

Li, T., M. R. Stark, A. D. Johnson, and C. Wolberger. Crystal structure of the MATa1/MATα2 homeodomain heterodimer bound to DNA. *Science* 270: 262–269, 1995.

Lin, Y.-C., K. Brown, and U. Siebenlist. Activation of NF-κB requires proteolysis of the inhibitor IκB-α: signal-induced phosphorylation of IκB-α alone does not release active NF-κB. *Proc. Natl. Acad. Sci. U. S. A.* 92:552–556, 1995.

Lin, Y.-S., and M. R. Green. Mechanism of action of an acidic transcriptional activator in vitro. *Cell* 64:971–981, 1991.

Lindebro, M. C., L. Poellinger, and M. L. Whitelaw. Protein-protein interaction via PAS domains: role of the PAS domain in positive and negative regulation of the bHLH/PAS dioxin receptor-Arnt transcription factor complex. *EMBO J.* 14:3528–3539, 1995.

Liu, X., C. W. Miller, P. H. Koeffler, and A. J. Berk. The p53 activation domain binds the TATA box-binding protein in holo-TFIID and a neighboring p53 domain inhibits transcription. *Mol. Cell. Biol.* 13:3291–3300, 1993.

Lu, H., and A. J. Levine. Human TAF$_{II}$31 protein is a transcriptional coactivator of the p53 protein. *Proc. Natl. Acad. Sci. U. S. A.* 92:5154–5158, 1995.

Lundblad, J. R., R. P. S. Kwok, M. E. Laurance, M. L. Harter, and R. H. Goodman. Adenoviral E1A-associated protein p300 as a functional homologue of the transcriptional co-activator CBP. *Nature* 374:85–88, 1995.

Luo, Y., H. Fujii, T. Gerster, and R. G. Roeder. A novel B cell-derived coactivator potentiates the activator of immunoglobulin promoters by octamer-binding transcription factors. *Cell* 71:231–241, 1992.

Luo, Y., and R. G. Roeder. Cloning, functional characterization, and mechanism of action of the B-cell-specific transcriptional coactivator OCA-B. *Mol. Cell. Biol.* 15:4115–4124, 1995.

Ma, J., and M. Ptashne. A new class of yeast transcriptional activators. *Cell* 51: 113–119, 1987.

Madden, S. L., D.M. Cook, J. F. Morris, A. Gashler, V. P. Sukhatme, and F. J. Rauscher III. Transcriptional repression mediated by the WT1 Wilms tumor gene product. *Science* 253:1550–1553, 1991.

Mangelsdorf, D. J., C. Thummel, M. Beato, P. Herrlich, G. Schutz, K. Umesono, B. Blumberg, P. Kastner, M. Mark, P. Chambon, and R. M. Evans. The nuclear receptor superfamily: the second decade. *Cell* 83:835–839, 1995.

Marais, R., J. Wynne, and R. Treisman. The SRF accessory factor Elk-1 contains a growth factor-regulated transcriptional activation domain. *Cell* 73:381–393, 1993.

Marcus, G. A., J. Horiuchi, N. Silverman, and L. Guarente. ADA/SPT20 links the ADA and SPT genes, which are involved in yeast transcription. *Mol. Cell. Biol.* 16:3197–3205, 1996.

Marcus, G. A., N. Silverman, S. Berger, J. Horiuchi, and L. Guarente. Functional similarity and physical association between GCN5 and ADA2—putative transcriptional adaptors. *EMBO J.* 13:4807–4815, 1994.

Martin, D. I. K., and S. H. Orkin. Transcriptional activation and DNA binding by the erythroid factor GF-1/NF-E1/Eryf1. *Genes Dev* 4:1886–1898, 1990.

Martin, D. W., R. M. Munoz, M. A. Subler, and S. Deb. p53 binds to the TATA-binding protein-TATA complex. *J. Biol. Chem.* 268:13062–13067, 1993.

McGinnis, W., and R. Krumlauf. Homeobox genes and axial patterning. *Cell* 66: 283–302, 1992.

McPherson, C. E., E.-Y. Shim, D. S. Friedman, and K. S. Zaret. An active tissue-specific enhancer and bound transcription factors existing in a precisely positioned nucleosomal array. *Cell* 75:387–398, 1993.

Mendel, D. B., P. A. Khavari, P. B. Conley, M. K. Graves, L. P. Hansen, A. Admon, and G. R. Crabtree. Characterization of a cofactor that regulates dimerization of a mammalian homeodomain protein. *Science* 254:1762–1767, 1991.

Mermod, N., E. A. O'Neill, T. J. Kelly, and R. Tjian. The proline-rich transcriptional activator of CTF/NF-1 is distinct from the replication and DNA-binding domain. *Cell* 58:741–753, 1989.

Mitchell, P. J., and R. Tjian. Transcriptional regulation in mammalian cells by sequence-specific DNA binding proteins. *Science* 245:371–378, 1989.

Mizzen, C. A., X.-J. Yang, T. Kokubo, J. E. Brownell, A. J. Bannister, T. Owen-Hughes, J. Workman, L. Wang, S. L. Berger, T. Kouzarides, Y. Nakatani, and C. D. Allis. The $TAF_{II}250$ subunit of TFIID has histone acetyltransferase activity. *Cell* 87:1261–1270, 1996.

Molenaar, M., M. van de Wetering, M. Oosterwegel, J. Peterson-Maduro, S. Godsave, V. Korinek, J. Roose, O. Destree, and H. Clevers. XTcf-3 transcription factor mediates β-catenin-induced axis formation in Xenopus embryos. *Cell* 86:391–399, 1996.

Monica, K., N. Galili, J. Nourse, D. Saltman, and M. L. Cleary. PBX2 and PBX3, new homeobox genes with extensive homology to the human proto-oncogene PBX1. *Mol. Cell. Biol.* 11:6149–6157, 1991.

Moore, K. Insight into the microphthalmia gene. *Trends Genet.* 11:442–448, 1995.

Moqtaderi, Z., Y. Bai, D. Poon, P. A. Weil, and K. Struhl. TBP-associated factors are not generally required for transcriptional activation in yeast. *Nature* 383: 188–191, 1996.

Moran, E. DNA tumor virus transforming proteins and the cell cycle. *Curr. Opin. Genet. Dev.* 3:63–70, 1993.

Morin, P. J., A. B. Sparks, V. Korinek, N. Barker, H. Clevers, B. Vogelstein, and K. W. Kinzler. Activation of β-catenin-Tcf signalling in colon cancer by mutations in β-catenin or APC. *Science* 275:1787–1790, 1997.

Muchardt, C., and M. Yaniv. A human homologue of Saccharomyces cerevisiae SNF2/SWI2 and Drosophila brm genes potentiates transcriptional activation by the glucocorticoid receptor. *EMBO J.* 12:4279–4290, 1993.

Muller, M. M., S. Ruppert., W. Schaffner, and P. Matthias. A cloned octamer transcription factor stimulates transcription from lymphoid-specific promoters in non-B cells. *Nature* 336:544–551, 1988.

Mumberg, D., F. C. Lucibello, M. Schuermann, and R. Muller. Alternative splicing of fosB transcripts results in differentially expressed mRNAs encoding functionally antagonistic proteins. *Genes Dev.* 5:1212–1223, 1991.

Murre, C., P. S. McCaw, and D. Baltimore. A new DNA binding and dimerization motif in immunoglobulin enhancer binding, daughterless, Myo D, and myc proteins. *Cell* 56:777–784, 1989a.

Murre, C., P. S. McCaw, H. Vaessin, M. Caudy, L. Y. Jan, Y. N. Jan, C. V. Cabrera, J. N. Buskin, S. D. Hauschka, and A. I. Et. Interactions between heterologous helix-loop-helix proteins generate complexes that bind specifically to a common DNA sequence. *Cell* 58:537–544, 1989b.

Nagy, L., H.-Y. Kao, D. Chakravarti, R. J. Lin, C. A. Hassig, D. E. Ayer, S. L. Schreiber, and R. M. Evans. Nuclear receptor repression mediated by a complex containing SMRT, mSin3A, and histone deacetylase. *Cell* 89:373–380, 1997.

Nakabeppu, Y., and D. Nathans. A naturally occurring truncated form of FosB that inhibits Fos/Jun transcriptional activity. *Cell* 64:751–759, 1991.

Nakatani, Y., S. Bagby, and M. Ikura. The histone folds in transcription factor TFIID. *J. Biol. Chem.* 271:6575–6578, 1996.

Nambu, J. R., J. O. Lewis, K. A. Wharton, and S. T. Crews. The Drosophila single-minded gene encodes a helix-loop-helix protein that acts as a master regulator of CNS midline development. *Cell* 67:1157–1167, 1991.

Nigg, E. A., H. Hilz, H. M. Eppenberger, and F. Dutly. Rapid and reversible translocation of the catalytic subunit of cAMP-dependent protein kinase type II from the Golgi complex to the nucleus. *EMBO J.* 4:2801–2806, 1985.

Nonet, M. L., and R. A. Young. Intragenic and extragenic suppressors of mutations in the heptapeptide repeat domain of Saccharomyces cerevisiae RNA polymerase II. *Genetics* 123:715–724, 1989.

Ogryzko, V. V., R. L. Schlitz, V. Russanova, B. H. Howard, and Y. Nakatani. The transcriptional coactivators P300 and CBP are histone acetyltransferases. *Cell* 87:953–959, 1996.

Ohsako, S., J. Hyer, G. Panganiban, I. Oliver, and M. Caudy. Hairy functions as a DNA-binding helix-loop-helix repressor of Drosophila sensory organ formation. *Genes Dev.* 8:2743–2755, 1994.

Okabe, I., L. C. Bailey, O. Attree, S. Srinivasan, J. M. Perkel, B. C. Laurent, M. Carlson, D. L. Nelson, and R. L. Nussbaum. Cloning of human and bovine homologs of SNF2/SWI2, a global activator of transcription in yeast S. cerevisiae. *Nucleic Acids Res.* 20:4649–4655, 1992.

Onate, S., S. Y. Tsai, M.-J. Tsai, and B. W. O'Malley. Sequence and characterization of a coactivator for the steroid hormone receptor superfamily. *Science* 270:1354–1357, 1995.

Orkin, S. H. GATA-binding transcription factors in hematopoietic cells. *Blood* 80:575–581, 1992.

Owen-Hughes, T., R. T. Utley, J. Cote, C. L. Peterson, and J. L. Workman. Persistent site-specific remodeling of a nucleosome array by transient action of the SWI/SNF complex. *Science* 273:513–516, 1996.

Palombella, V. J., O. J. Rando, A. L. Goldberg, and T. Maniatis. The ubiquitin-proteasome pathway is required for processing the NF-κB1 precursor protein and the activation of NF-κB. *Cell* 78:773–785, 1994.

Papavassiliou, A. G. Transcription factors. *N. Engl. J. Med.* 332:45–47, 1995.

Parker, D., K. Ferreri, T. Nakajima, V. J. LaMorte, R. Evans, S. C. Koerber, C. Hoeger, and M. R. Montminy. Phosphorylation of CREB at Ser-133 induces complex formation with CREB-binding protein via a direct mechanism. *Mol. Cell. Biol.* 16:694–703, 1996.

Paroush, Z., R. Finley, T. Kidd, S. M. Wainwright, P. Ingham, R. Brent, and D. Ish-Horowicz. Groucho is required for Drosophila neurogenesis, segmentation, and sex determination and interacts directly with hairy-related bHLH proteins. *Cell* 79:805–815, 1994.

Pavletich, N. P., and C. O. Pabo. Zinc finger-DNA recognition: crystal structure of a Zif268-DNA complex at 2.1 A. *Science* 252:809–817, 1991.

Peifer, M., and E. Wieschaus. Mutations in the Drosophila gene extradenticle affect the way specific homeodomain proteins regulate segmental identity. *Genes Dev.* 4:1209–1223, 1990.

Pina, B., S. Berger, G. A. Marcus, N. Silverman, J. Agapite, and L. Guarente. ADA3: a gene, identified by resistance to GAL4–VP16, with properties similar to and different from those of ADA2. *Mol. Cell. Biol.* 13:5981–5989, 1993.

Pina, B., U. Burggemeier, and M. Beato. Nucleosome positioning modulates accessibility of regulatory proteins to the mouse mammary tumor virus promoter. *Cell* 60:719–731, 1990.

Pollenz, R. S., C. A. Sattler, and A. Poland. The aryl hydrocarbon receptor and aryl hydrocarbon receptor nuclear translocator protein show distinct subcellular localizations in Hepa 1c1c7 cells by immunofluorescence microscopy. *Mol. Pharmacol.* 45:428–438, 1994.

Pratt, W. B. The role of heat shock proteins in regulating the function, folding, and trafficking of the glucocorticoid receptor. *J. Biol. Chem.* 268:21455–21458, 1993.

Ptashne, M. How eukaryotic transcriptional activators work. *Nature* 335:683–689, 1988.

Rauskolb, C., M. Peifer, and E. Wieschaus. extradenticle, a regulator of homeotic gene activity, is a homolog of the homeobox-containing human proto-oncogene pbx1. *Cell* 1101–1112, 1993.

Regier, J. L., F. Shen, and S. J. Triezenberg. Pattern of aromatic and hydrophobic amino acids critical for one of two subdomains of the VP16 transcriptional activator. *Proc. Natl. Acad. Sci. U.S.A.* 90:883–887, 1993.

Reisz-Porszasz, S., M. R. Probst, B. N. Fukunaga, and O. Hankinson. Identification of functional domains of the aryl hydrocarbon receptor nuclear translocator protein (ARNT). *Mol. Cell. Biol.* 14:6075–6086, 1994.

Reyes, H., S. Reisz-Porszasz, and O. Hankinson. Identification of the Ah receptor nuclear translocator protein (Arnt) as a component of the DNA binding form of the Ah receptor. *Science* 256:1193–1195, 1992.

Rochette-Egly, C., S. Adam, M. Rossignol, J.-M. Egly, and P. Chambon. Stimulation of RARα activation function AF-1 through binding to the general transcription factor TFIIH and phosphorylation by CDK7. *Cell* 90:97–107, 1997.

Roman, C., L. Cohn, and K. Calame. A dominant negative form of transcription activator mTFE3 created by differential splicing. *Science* 254:94–97, 1991.

Rubinfeld, B., I. Albert, E. Porfiri, C. Fiol, S. Munemitsu, and P. Polakis. Binding of GSK3β to the APC-β-catenin complex and regulation of complex assembly. *Science* 272:1023–1026, 1996.

Rubinfeld, B., P. Robbins, M. El-Gamil, I. Albert, E. Porfiri, and P. Polakis. Stabilization of β-catenin by genetic defects in melanoma cell lines. *Science* 275:1790–1792, 1997.

Rudnicki, M. A., and R. Jaenisch. The MyoD family of transcription factors and skeletal myogenesis. *Bioessays* 17:203–209, 1995.

Ruff-Jamison, S., K. Chen, and S. Cohen. Induction by EGF and interferon-γ of tyrosine phosphorylated DNA binding proteins in mouse liver nuclei. *Science* 261:1733–1736, 1993.

Sadowski, H., K. Shuai, J. E. Darnell, Jr., and M. Z. Gilman. A common nuclear signal transduction pathway activated by growth factor and cytokine receptors. *Science* 261:1739–1744, 1993.

Sadowski, I., J. Ma, S. J. Triezenberg, and M. Ptashne. GAL4-VP16 is an unusually potent transcriptional activator. *Nature* 335:563–564, 1988.

Sasai, Y., R. Kageyama, Y. Tagawa, R. Shigemoto, and S. Nakanishi. Two mammalian helix-loop-helix factors structurally related to Drosophila hairy and Enhancer of split. *Genes Dev.* 6:2620–2634, 1992.

Satokata, I., and R. Maas. Msx1 deficient mice exhibit cleft palate and abnormalities of craniofacial and tooth development. *Nat. Genet.* 6:348–355, 1994.

Sauer, F., S. K. Hansen, and R. Tjian. DNA template and activator-coactivator requirements for transcriptional synergism by Drosophila bicoid. *Science* 270:1825–1828, 1995a.

Sauer, F., S. K. Hansen, and R. Tjian. Multiple TAF$_{II}$s directing synergistic activation of transcription. *Science* 270:1783–1788, 1995b.

Sauer, F., D. A. Wassarman, G. M. Rubin, and R. Tjian. TAF$_{II}$s mediate activation of transcription in the Drosophila embryo. *Cell* 87:1271–1284, 1996.

Schindler, C., X.-Y. Fu, T. Improta, R. Aebersold, and J. E Darnell, Jr. Proteins of transcription factor ISGF-3: one gene encodes the 91- and 84-kDa ISGF-3 proteins that are activated by interferon a. *Proc. Natl. Acad. Sci. U.S.A.* 89:7836–7839, 1992a.

Schindler, C., K. Shuai, V. R. Prezioso, and J. E. Darnell, Jr. Interferon-dependent tyrosine phosphorylation of a latent cytoplasmic transcription factor. *Science* 257:809–812, 1992b.

Schreiber-Agus, N., L. Chin, K. Chen, R. Torres, G. Rao, P. Guida, A. I. Skoultchi, and R. A. DePinho. An amino-terminal domain of Mxi1 mediates anti-Myc oncogenic activity and interacts wtih a homolog of the yeast transcriptional repressor SIN3. *Cell* 80:777–786, 1995.

Scott, M.P. Vertebrate homeobox gene nomenclature. *Cell* 71:551–553, 1992.

Semenza, G. L., G. L. Wang, and R. Kundu. DNA binding and transcriptional properties of wild-type and mutant forms of the homeodomain protein MSX2. *Biochem. Biophys. Res. Comm.* 209:257–262, 1995.

Sen, C. K., and L. Packer. Antioxidant and redox regulation of gene transcription. *FASEB J.* 10:709–720, 1996.

Seto, E., A. Usheva, G. P. Zambetti, J. Momand, N. Horikoshi, R. Weinmann, A. J. Levine, and T. Shenk. Wild-type p53 binds to the TATA-binding protein and represses transcription. *Proc. Natl. Acad. Sci. U. S. A.* 89:12028–12032, 1992.

Shashikant, C. S., M. F. Utset, S. M. Violette, T. L. Wise, P. Einat, J. W. Pendleton, K. Schughart, and F. H. Ruddle. Homeobox genes in mouse development. *Crit. Rev. Eukaryotic Gene Expression* 1:207–245, 1991.

Shaw, P. E., H. Schroter, and A. Nordheim. The ability of a ternary complex to form over the serum response element correlates with serum induciblility of the human c-fos promoter. *Cell* 56:563–572, 1989.

Shibasaki, F., E. R. Price, D. Milan, and F. McKeon. Role of kinases and the phosphatase calcineurin in the nuclear shuttling of transcription factor NF-AT4. *Nature* 382:370–373, 1996.

Shuai, K., C. Schindler, V. R. Prezioso, and J. E. Darnell, Jr. Activation of trancription by IFN-γ: tyrosine phosphorylation of a 91-kD DNA binding protein. *Science* 258:1808–1812, 1992.

Sigler, P. B. Acid blobs and negative noodles. *Nature* 333:210–212, 1988.

Silvennoinen, O., C. Schindler, J. Schlessinger, and D. E. Levy. Ras-independent growth factor signaling by transcription factor tyrosine phosphorylation. *Science* 261:1736–1739, 1993.

Smeal, T., B. Binetruy, D. A. Mercola, M. Birrer, and M. Karin. Oncogenic and transcriptional cooperation with Ha-Ras requires phosphorylation of c-Jun on serines 63 and 73. *Nature* 354:494–496, 1991.

Sogawa, K., R. Nakano, A. Kobayashi, Y. Kikuchi, N. Ohe, N. Matsushita, and Y. Fujii-Kuriyama. Possible function of the Ah receptor nuclear translocator (Arnt) homodimer in transcriptional regulation. *Proc. Natl. Acad. Sci. U.S.A.* 92:1936–1940, 1995.

Spencer, T. E., G. Jenster, M. M. Burcin, C. D. Allis, J. Zhou, C. A. Mizzen, N. J. McKenna, S. A. Onate, S. Y. Tsai, M.-J. Tsai, and B. W. O'Malley. Steroid receptor coactivator-1 is a histone acetyltransferase. *Nature* 389:194–198, 1997.

Stahl, N., T. J. Farruggella, T. G. Boulton, Z. Zhong, J. E. Darnell, Jr., and G. D. Yancopoulos. Choice of STATs and other substrates specified by modular tyrosine-based motifs in cytokine receptors. *Science* 267:1349–1353, 1995.

Staudt, L. M., and M. J. Lenardo. Immunoglobulin gene transcription. *Annu. Rev. Immunol.* 9:373–398, 1991.

Staudt, L. M., H. Singh, R. Sen, T. Wirth, P. A. Sharp, and D. Baltimore. A lymphoid-specific protein binding to the octamer motif of immunoglobulin genes. *Nature* 323:640–643, 1986.

Strubin, M., J. W. Newell, and P. Matthias. OBF-1, a novel B cell-specific coactivator that stimulates immunoglobulin promoter activity through association with octamer-binding proteins. *Cell* 80:497–506, 1995.

Struhl, K. Yeast transcriptional regulatory mechanisms. *Annu. Rev. Genet.* 29:651–674, 1995.

Sturm, R. A., G. Das, and W. Herr. The ubiquitous octamer-binding protein Oct-1 contains a POU domain with a homeo box subdomain. *Genes Dev.* 2:1582–1599, 1988.

Sun, S.-C., J. Elwood, C. Beruad, and W. C. Greene. Human T-cell leukemia type I virus Tax activation of NF-κB/Rel involves phosphorylation and degradation of IκBα and RelA (p65)-mediated induction of the c-rel gene. *Mol. Cell. Biol.* 14:7377–7384, 1994.

Swanson, H. I., W. K. Chan, and C. A. Bradfield. DNA binding specificities and pairing rules of the Ah receptor, ARNT, and SIM proteins. *J. Biol. Chem.* 270:26292–26302, 1995.

Takebayashi, K., C. Akazawa, S. Nakanishi, and R. Kageyama. Structure and promoter analysis of the gene encoding the mouse helix-loop-helix factor HES-5. *J. Biol. Chem.* 270:1342–1349, 1995.

Tanaka, M. Modulation of promoter occupancy by cooperative DNA binding and activation-domain function is a major determinant of transcriptional regulation by activators in vivo. *Proc. Natl. Acad. Sci. U. S. A.* 93:4311–4315, 1996.

Tapscott, S. J., R. L. Davis, M. J. Thayer, P.-F. Cheng, H. Weintraub, and A. Lassar. MyoD: a nuclear phosphoprotein requiring a Myc homology region to convert fibroblasts to myoblasts. *Science* 242:405–411, 1988.

Taunton, J., C. A. Hassig, and S. L. Schreiber. A mammalian histone deacetylase related to the yeast transcriptional regulator Rpd3p. *Science* 272:408–411, 1996.

Thanos, D., and T. Maniatis. NF-κB: a lesson in family values. *Cell* 80:529–532, 1995.

Theill, L. E., J.-L. Castrillo, D. Wu, and M. Karin. Dissection of functional domains of the pituitary-specific transcription factor GHF-1. *Nature* 342:945–948, 1989.

Thut, C., J. L. Chen, R. Klemm, and R. Tjian. p53 transcriptional activation mediated by coactivators TAF$_{II}$40 and TAF$_{II}$60. *Science* 267:100–104, 1995.

Traenckner, E. B.-M., H. L. Pahl, T. Henkel, K. N. Schmidt, S. Wilk, and P. A. Bauerle. Phosphorylation of human IκBa on serines 32 and 36 controls IκB-α proteolysis and NF-κB activation in response to diverse stimuli. *EMBO J.* 14:2876–2883, 1995.

Traenckner, E. B.-M., S. Wilk, and P. A. Bauerle. A proteasome inhibitor prevents activation of NF-κB and stabilizes a newly phosphorylated form of IκB-a that is still bound to NF-κB. *EMBO J.* 13:5433–5441, 1994.

Travis, A., A. Amsterdam, C. Belancger, and R. Grosschedl. LEF-1, a gene encoding a lymphoid-specific protein with an HMG domain, regulates T-cell receptor alpha enhancer function. *Genes Dev.* 5:880–894, 1991.

Treisman, R. The SRE: a growth factor responsive transcriptional regulator. *Sem. Cancer Biol.* 1:47–58, 1990.

Triezenberg, S. J. Structure and function of transcriptional activation domains. *Curr. Opin. Genet. Dev.* 5:190–196, 1995.

Triezenberg, S. J., R. C. Kingsbury, and S. L. McKnight. Functional dissection of VP16, the trans-activator of herpes simplex virus immediate early gene expression. *Genes Dev.* 2:718–729, 1988.

Trouche, D., and T. Kouzarides. E2F1 and E1A$_{12S}$ have a homologous activation domain regulated by RB and CBP. *Proc. Natl. Acad. Sci. U.S.A.* 93:1439–1442, 1996.

Tsang, A. P., J. E. Visvader, C. A. Turner, Y. Fujiwara, C. Yu, M. J. Weiss, M. Crossley, and S. H. Orkin. FOG, a multitype zinc finger protein, acts as a cofactor for transcription factor GATA-1 in erythroid and megakaryocytic differentiation. *Cell* 90:109–119, 1997.

Tsukiyama, T., C. Daniel, J. Tamkun, and C. Wu. ISWI, a member of the SWI2/SNF2 ATPase family, encodes the 140 kDa subunit of the nucleosome remodeling factor. *Cell* 83:1021–1026, 1995.

Tsukiyama, T., and C. Wu. Purification and properties of an ATP-dependent nucleosome remodeling factor. *Cell* 83:1011–1020, 1995.

van Dijk, M. A., and C. Murre. extradenticle raises the DNA binding specificity of homeotic selector gene products. *Cell* 78:617–624, 1994.

Van Hoy, M., K. K. Leuther, T. Kodadek, and S. A. Johnston. The acidic activation domains of the GCN4 and GAL4 proteins are not α helical but form β sheets. *Cell* 72:587–594, 1993.

Velazquez, L., M. Fellous, G. R. Stark, and S. Pellegrini. A protein tyrosine kinase in the interferon α/β signaling pathway. *Cell* 70:313–322, 1992.

Verrijzer, C. P., and R. Tjian. TAFs mediate transcriptional activation and promoter selectivity. *Trends Biochem. Sci.* 21:338–342, 1996.

Vinson, C. R., P. B. Sigler, S. L. McKnight. Scissors-grip model for DNA recognition by a family of leucine zipper proteins. *Science* 246:911–916, 1989.

Visvader, J. E., M. Crossley, J. Hill, S. H. Orkin, and J. M. Davis. The C-terminal zinc finger of GATA-1 or GATA-2 is sufficient to induce megakaryocytic differentiation of an early myeloid cell line. *Mol. Cell. Biol.* 15:634–641, 1995.

Walker, S. S., J. C. Reese, L. M. Apone, and M. R. Green. Transcription activation in cells lacking $TAF_{II}s$. *Nature* 383:185–188, 1996.

Wang, G. L., B.-H. Jiang, E. A. Rue, and G. L. Semenza. Hypoxia-inducible factor 1 is a basic-helix-loop-helix-PAS heterodimer regulated by cellular O_2 tension. *Proc. Natl. Acad. Sci. U.S.A.* 92:5510–5514, 1995.

Wang, L., C. Mizzen, C. Ying, R. Candau, N. Barlev, J. Brownell, C. D. Allis, and S. L. Berger. Histone acetyltransferase activity is conserved between yeast and human GCN5 and is required for complementation of growth and transcriptional activation. *Mol. Cell. Biol.* 17:519–527, 1997.

Wang, W., J. Cote, Y. Xue, S. Zhou, P. A. Khavar, S. R. Biggar, C. Muchardt, G. V. Kalpana, S. P. Goff, M. Yaniv, J. L. Workman, and G. R. Crabtree. Purification and biochemical heterogeneity of the mammalian SWI/SNF complex. *EMBO J.* 15:5370–5382, 1996.

Wang, W., Y. Xue, S. Zhou, A. Kuo, B. R. Cairns, and G. R. Crabtree. Diversity and specialization of mammalian SWI/SNF complexes. *Genes Dev.* 10:2117–2130, 1996b.

Waterman, M. L., W. H. Fischer, and K. A. Jones. A thymus-specific member of the HMG protein family regulates the human T cell receptor alpha enhancer. *Genes Dev.* 5:656–669, 1991.

Weintraub, H. The MyoD family and myogenesis: redundancy, networks, and thresholds. *Cell* 75:1241–1244, 1993.

Weintraub, H., V. J. Dwarki, I. Verma, R. Davis, S. Hollenberg, L. Snider, A. Lassar, and S. J. Tapscott. Muscle-specific transcriptional activation by MyoD. *Genes Dev.* 5:1377–1386, 1991.

Weintraub, S. J., K. N. B. Chow, R. X. Luo, S. H. Zhang, S. He, and D. C. Dean. Mechanism of active transcriptional repression by the retinoblastoma protein. *Nature* 375:812–815, 1995.

Weintraub, S. J., C. A. Prater, and D. C. Dean. Retinoblastoma protein switches the E2F site from positive to negative element. *Nature* 358:259–261, 1992.

Whitelaw, M. L., J. McGuire, D. Picard, J.-A. Gustafsson, and L. Poellinger. Heat shock protein hsp90 regulates dioxin receptor function in vivo. *Proc. Natl. Acad. Sci. U.S.A.* 92:4437–4441, 1995.

Wilk, R., I. Weizman, and B.-Z. Shilo. *tracheless* encodes a bHLH-PAS protein that is an inducer of tracheal cell fates in *Drosophila*. *Genes Dev.* 10: 93–102, 1996.

Wilson, C. J., D. M. Chao, A. N. Imbalzano, G. R. Schnitzler, R. E. Kingston, and R. A. Young. RNA polymerase II holoenzyme contains SWI/SNF regulators involved in chromatin remodeling. *Cell* 84:235–244, 1996.

Winston, F., and M. Carlson. Yeast SNF/SWI transcriptional activators and the SPT/SIN chromatin connection. *Trends Genet.* 8:387–391, 1992.

Wolffe, A. Histone deacetylase: a regulator of transcription. *Science* 272:371–372, 1996.

Wolffe, A. P., and D. Pruss. Targeting chromatin disruption: transcription regulators that acetylate histones. *Cell* 86:817–819, 1996.

Xanthoudakis, S., and T. Curran. Identification and characterization of Ref-1, a nuclear protein that facilitates AP-1 DNA-binding activity. *EMBO J.* 11:653–665, 1992.

Xiao, H., A. Pearsdon, B. Coulombe, R. Truant, S. Zhang, J. L. Regier, S. J. Triezenberg, D. Reinberg, O. Flores, C. J. Ingles, and J. Greenblatt. Binding of basal transcription factor TFIIH to the acidic activation domains of VP16 and p53. *Mol. Cell. Biol.* 14:7013–7024, 1994.

Xie, X., T. Kokubo, S. L. Cohen, U. A. Mirza, A. Hoffmann, B .T. Chait, R. G. Roeder, Y. Nakatani, and R. G. Roeder. Structural similarity between TAFs and the heterotetrameric core of the histone octamer. *Nature* 380:316–322, 1996.

Yang, X.-J., V. V. Ogryzko, J. Nishikawa, B. H. Howard, and Y. Nakatani. A p300/CBP-associated factor that competes with the adenoviral oncoprotein E1A. *Nature* 382:319–324, 1996.

Yankulov, K., J. Blau, T. Purton, S. Roberts, and D. L. Bentley. Transcriptional elongation by RNA polymerase II is stimulated by transactivators. *Cell* 77:749–759, 1994.

Yen, J., R. M. Wisdom, I. Tratner, and I. M. Verma. An alternative spliced form of FosB is a negative regulator of transcriptional activation and transformation by Fos proteins. *Proc. Natl. Acad. Sci. U. S. A.* 88:5077–5081, 1991.

Zervos, A. S. , J. Gyuris, and R. Brent. Mxi1, a protein that specifically interacts with Max to bind Myc-Max recognition sites. *Cell* 72:223–232, 1993.

Zhang, H., K. M. Catron, and C. Abate-Shen. A role for the Msx-1 homeodomain in transcriptional regulation: residues in the N-terminal arm mediate TATA binding protein interaction and transcriptional repression. *Proc. Natl. Acad. Sci. U.S.A.* 93:1764–1769, 1996.

Zhang, Y., R. Iratni, H. Erdjument-Bromage, P. Tempst, and D. Reinberg. Histone deacetylases and SAP-18, a novel polypeptide, are components of a human Sin3 complex. *Cell* 89:357–364, 1997.

Zhang, X., J. Blenis, H.-C. Li, C. Schindler, and S. Chen-Kiang. Requirement of serine phosphorylation for formation of STAT-promoter complexes. *Science* 267:1990–1994, 1995.

Zhao, G., T. Xia, J. Song, R. A. Jensen. Pseudomonas aeruginosa possesses homologues of mammalian phenylalanine hydroxylase and 4 alpha-carbinolamine dehydratase/DCoH as part of a three-component gene cluster. *Proc. Natl. Acad. Sci. U. S. A.* 91:1366–1370, 1994.

Zhong, Z., Z. Wen, and J. E. Darnell, Jr. Stat3: a STAT family member activated by tyrosine phosphorylation in response to epidermal growth factor and interleukin-6. *Science* 264:95–98, 1994.

Zhuang, Y., C. G. Kim, S. Bartelmez, P. Cheng, M. Groudine, and H. Weintraub. Helix-loop-helix transcription factors E12 and E47 are not essential for skeletal or cardiac myogenesis, erythropoiesis, chondrogenesis, or neurogenesis. *Proc. Natl. Acad. Sci. U.S.A.* 89:12132–12136, 1992.

Transcriptional
Pathophysiology

Part **II**

Mutations in *CIS*-Acting Transcriptional Regulatory Elements   4

This and subsequent chapters of Part Two will focus on human diseases that are caused by abnormal structure and/or function of the *cis*-acting DNA sequences or *trans*-acting protein factors that represent the two major components of transcriptional systems. Part Two will differ from Part One by the introduction of clinical data into the discussion. In order to provide a resource for further exploration, the description of each clinical condition will include the relevant catalogue (MIM) number in the Online Mendelian Inheritance in Man (OMIM™) database, which can be accessed at the National Center for Biotechnology Information, National Library of Medicine, via the World Wide Web (http://www.ncbi.nlm.nih.gov/Omim). A less up-to-date hard copy of MIM is also available (McKusick, 1994).

The discussion of transcriptional pathophysiology begins with a description of the less common mechanism by which transcription is deranged, mutations within *cis*-acting DNA sequences that represent transcription factor binding sites. Binding site mutations may represent a less common cause of transcriptional derangement because of the cooperative nature of DNA binding in which protein-protein interactions between factors binding at adjacent sites (either directly or via interactions with common coactivators) may stabilize DNA binding. Under these circumstances a point mutation might decrease the affinity of a transcription factor for its cognate nucleotide sequence so that the factor could no longer bind to the isolated DNA sequence in vitro, yet might still be capable of binding in vivo. This hypothesis is not easily tested, because there is no simple means of ascertaining presumably rare mutations in the absence of a phenotype. However, there are a limited number of cases in which single nucleotide substitutions have a sufficiently disruptive effect on transcription factor binding to result in disease, and several illustrative examples are provided below. Larger deletions of long-range-acting chromatin domain elements that affect expression of globin genes are also discussed. In addition, the effect of a specific trinucleotide repeat expansion on DNA methylation and transcription of the *FMR1* gene is described. Finally, the effect of promoter DNA sequence polymorphisms on gene transcription and predisposition to what would otherwise be considered a nongenetic disorder is described.

β-Thalassemia Due to Mutations in the β-globin Gene Promoter

The first mutations in *cis*-acting transcriptional regulatory elements were identified by analysis of the β-globin genes of patients with β thalassemia (MIM 141900), an inherited anemia due to deficient production of β-globin protein by erythroid cells (reviewed by Orkin and Kazazian, 1984). In contrast to frameshift, nonsense, and splice junction mutations which resulted in a complete lack of β-globin mRNA synthesis from the mutant gene (null allele) and a severe clinical phenotype in the homozygous state, the effect of promoter mutations were clinically mild and were detected only in patients who were compound heterozygotes for a promoter mutation and a null allele. The motif 5'-ACACCC-3' is present at nucleotides -92 to -86 relative to the β-globin gene transcription initiation site and mutations at positions -92, -90, -88, -87, and -86 have been identified in patients with β thalassemia (reviewed by Cooper et al., 1995). Although ubiquitously expressed factors have been shown to bind to the CACCC motif, binding of the erythroid Kruppel-like factor (EKLF) plays an essential role in activation of the β globin promoter through this site, and mice lacking EKLF die *in utero* of severe β thalassemia (Miller and Bieker, 1993; Nuez et al., 1995; Perkins et al., 1995).

In addition to the CACCC box mutations that affect the binding of the sequence-specific transcription factor EKLF, mutations at -31, -30, -29, and -28 within the TATA box of the β-globin promoter have also been identified in β-thalassemia alleles (reviewed by Cooper et al., 1995). These mutations also have mild clinical effects and result in decreased transcription of the affected allele, presumably due to inefficient binding of the general transcription factor TFIID (see Chapter 1) to the mutant DNA sequence.

Hereditary Persistence of Fetal Hemoglobin Due to Mutations in the γ-Globin Gene Promoter

As described in Chapter 2, the β-globin gene cluster contains the embryonic ε, fetal Gγ and Aγ, and adult δ and β globin genes (see Fig. 2.6). In

the erythroid cells of individuals with hereditary persistence of fetal hemoglobin (HPFH; MIM 141749), γ-globin gene expression persists in
adult life rather than being repressed after birth. In several patients with
HPFH, mutations have been identified within the promoter of the ^{G}γ- or
^{A}γ-globin gene at positions -114, -175, and -202 relative to the transcription initiation site (reviewed by Cooper et al., 1995). The molecular basis
for the increased γ globin gene transcription that results from these mutations has not been fully elucidated but appears to involve decreased
binding of transcriptional repressors (such as the ubiquitous factor OTF-
1) and/or increased binding of transcriptional activators (such as the
erythroid-specific factor GATA-1) to the mutant DNA sequence (Martin
et al., 1989). The-202 mutation resulted in the creation of a new binding
site for a factor, the stage selector protein, that may normally mediate
preferential activation of γ- over β-globin gene transcription in fetal erythroid cells, suggesting that the presence of this binding site at an abnormal location may result in constitutive γ-globin gene transcription
(Jane et al., 1993). Thus, in contrast to the other mutations described in
this chapter, HPFH may be due to gain-of-function mutations in *cis*-
acting transcriptional regulatory elements.

Thalassemia Due to Deletion of the Locus Control Region of the α- or β-Globin Gene Cluster

γδβ Thalassemia Due to Deletion of the Locus Control Region of the β-Globin Gene Cluster

As described in Chapter 2, the *cis*-acting locus control region (LCR) plays
an essential role in the erythroid-specific expression of all genes in the
β-globin gene cluster (see Fig. 2.6). A family was identified in which
DNA sequences located from 9.5 to 39 kb 5' to the ε-globin gene, a region
that encompassed the LCR, were deleted (Driscoll et al., 1989). Deletion
of the LCR completely eliminated expression of the ε-, ^{G}γ-, ^{A}γ-, δ-, and
β-globin genes in *cis*, despite the fact that these genes, as well as their
promoter and enhancer elements, remained intact. The entire β-globin
gene cluster normally exists in the nuclei of erythroid precursor cells as
an open chromatin domain that is sensitive to DNase I digestion, indicating an alteration of higher-order nucleosome packing. Deletion of the
LCR affected chromatin structure of DNA sequences extending approximately 100 kb 5' and 3' to the β-globin gene (Forrester et al., 1990),
preventing the formation of this open chromatin structure that is probably a prerequisite for gene expression. In addition, the wild-type locus
replicated early in S phase in mitotic erythroid progenitor cells whereas

the mutant locus replicated late in S phase in the absence of the LCR (Forrester et al., 1990).

α-Thalassemia Due to Deletion of the Locus Control Region of the α-globin Gene Cluster

Patients with α-thalassemia were identified in which the α-globin gene cluster was intact but sequences 5' to the cluster were deleted (Hatton et al., 1990; Liebhaber et al., 1990; Wilkie et al., 1990). The subsequent identification of the α-globin LCR within the region encompassed by the deletion (Jarman et al., 1991) provided a molecular understanding for the absence of α-globin gene expression in *cis* to the deletion.

Loss of Duffy Blood Group Antigen Due to Mutations in the *DARC* Gene Promoter

The *DARC* gene encodes the Duffy antigen receptor for chemokines, a seven-transmembrane-domain receptor for proinflammatory cytokines that also serves as the receptor for the malarial parasite *Plasmodium vivax* (Chauduri et al., 1994; Neote et al., 1994). Red cells lacking Duffy antigen are resistant to invasion by *P. vivax* and the Duffy negative (−) phenotype is present at high frequency in West Africa where malaria is endemic (Miller et al., 1976). In addition to expression in erythroid precursors, the *DARC* gene is widely expressed throughout the body within endothelial cells of postcapillary venules (Hadley et al., 1994). Comparison of the DNA sequence of the *DARC* gene from Duffy postitive (+) and (−) individuals revealed a T-to-C transition at nucleotide -46 relative to the transcription initiation site (Tournamille et al., 1995). This point mutation occurred within the context of the sequence 5'-TTATCT-3', which on the antisense strand is a perfect match to the consensus sequence (5'-(A/T)GATA(A/G)-3') for binding by the erythroid-specific transcription factor GATA-1, which was shown to bind to an oligonucleotide containing the wild-type, but not the mutant, sequence. In addition, the wild-type, but not the mutant, promoter was active in directing reporter gene expression in an erythroid cell line (Tournamille et al., 1995). Remarkably, DARC mRNA is expressed in endothelial cells of Duffy (−) individuals (Peiper et al., 1995), indicating that the mutation selectively eliminates *DARC* gene expression in erythroid cells as predicted by the erythroid-specific expression of GATA-1. Thus, while complete loss of *DARC* expression might not be compatible with normal development and/or postnatal physiology, the selective loss of expression in erythroid cells provides a means of acquiring resistance to a life-threatening disease.

Coagulation Disorders Due to Promoter Mutations in the *F9* and *F7* Genes

Developmentally Limited Factor IX Deficiency: Hemophilia B Leyden

Mutations in the X-linked gene encoding factor IX (*F9*) result in hemophilia B (MIM 306900). A variant form, hemophilia B Leyden, has been described in which affected males have less than 1% of normal factor IX activity until puberty, when levels spontaneously rise to approximately 60% of normal activity (Briet et al., 1982). All Leyden patients studied have a mutation within 20 bp of the *F9* gene transcription initiation site (Fig. 4.1): T→A (−20), G→A (−6), G→C (−6), A→T (−5), T→A (+6), T→C (+8), A→G (+13), A→C (+13), and del A (+13) (Crossley and Brownlee, 1990; Crossley et al., 1990, 1992; Freedenberg and Black, 1991; Hirosawa et al., 1990; Picketts et al., 1992, 1993; Reijnen et al., 1992; Reitsma et al., 1988, 1989; Royle et al., 1991). The mutations affecting nt +13 disrupt the binding site for C/EBP, a bZIP factor that activates transcription of many liver-specific genes including *F9* (Crossley and Brownlee, 1990). The −20 mutation disrupts binding of hepatocyte nuclear factor 4 (HNF-4), another transcriptional activator of many liver-specific genes (Reijnen et al., 1992). The *F9* gene promoter sequence between −38 and −22 (Fig. 4.1) is similar to the consensus sequence for androgen receptor binding sites (5'-AGNACANNNTGTNCT-3'), and transcription of reporter plasmids containing four copies of the *F9* promoter sequence

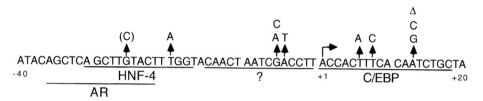

FIGURE 4-1. Point mutations in the *F9* gene promoter associated with hemophilia B Leyden. The nucleotide sequence surrounding the transcription initiation site (bent arrow at +1) is shown. Vertical arrow, a nucleotide substitution or deletion (Δ) found in genomic DNA of an individual with hemophilia B Leyden. (C), Brandenburg mutation. Underscore, binding sites for AR, C/EBP, HNF-4, and an undetermined factor (?).

between -42 and -17 linked to the herpes simplex virus thymidine kinase promoter was activated by androgen receptor (in the presence of 5α-dihydrotestosterone) in cotransfection assays (Crossley et al., 1992).

The androgen receptor shares with all steroid hormone receptors the fact that it is a zinc finger transcription factor that binds to DNA and activates transcription only in the presence of its ligand, 5α-dihydrotestosterone, the production of which increases in males at the time of puberty. Thus, binding of the androgen receptor in postpubertal males may compensate for the lack of C/EBP or HNF-4 binding to activate transcription of the $F9$ gene. This hypothesis was supported by analysis of the Brandenburg mutation at -26, which was found in the DNA of an affected male who showed no improvement at puberty. This mutation disrupts binding of both HNF-4 and the androgen receptor because the binding sites for these two factors (-22 to -38 and -15 to -27, respectively) overlap (Crossley et al., 1992).

An alternative explanation for the recovery of patients with hemophilia B Leyden has been proposed based on the observation that C/EBP binds at a site approximately 200 nucleotides (nt) 5' to the $F9$ transcription initiation site and that this binding is enhanced 20-fold by the presence of DBP, a related bZIP factor that is first expressed in rat liver at approximately one month of age, suggesting that in humans DBP may be expressed at puberty (Picketts et al., 1993). These two proposed mechanisms are not mutually exclusive, and the developmentally regulated expression of the androgen receptor and DBP may both play a role in the recovery of $F9$ transcription after puberty.

Factor VII Deficiency

Recently, severe factor VII deficiency (MIM 227500) has also been associated with a mutation that disrupts the binding of HNF-4 to a site in the promoter of the gene encoding factor VII (Arbini et al., 1997). The mutation changes the sequence 5'-ACTTTG-3' to 5'-ACGTTG-3', which is similar to the mutation of 5'-ACTTTG-3' to 5'-ACTTAG-3' that is associated with hemophilia B Leyden (Fig. 4.1). The mutation disrupts HNF-4 binding, decreases transcription directed by the promoter and eliminates transcriptional activation by cotransfected HNF-4 in transiently transfected reporter gene assays (Arbini et al., 1997). Because the $F7$ gene is not located on the X chromosome and its promoter does not contain the same unusual arrangement of AR, HNF-4, and C/EBP binding sites that are found in the $F9$ gene, there are no reported cases of males with puberty-limited factor VII deficiency. However, the fact that mutations in HNF-4 binding sites in both the $F7$ and $F9$ promoters have drastic effects on gene transcription suggest that this transcription factor plays a key role in coordinating the synthesis of coagulation factors within hepatocytes.

Fragile X Mental Retardation Syndrome

The fragile X (Martin-Bell) syndrome (MIM 309550) is an X-linked disorder characterized by mental retardation, dysmorphic facial features, and postpubertal macroorchidism (enlarged testicles) (reviewed by Nussbaum and Ledbetter, 1989). The disorder affects approximately 1 in 1000 to 1500 males (Gustavson et al., 1986; Webb et al., 1986). Approximately four fifths of hemizygous males are mentally retarded and one third of heterozygous females are mildly mentally impaired (Sherman et al., 1985). It is thus the most common hereditable cause of mental retardation. The clinical syndrome is associated with a dynamic cytogenetic abnormality, a fragile site on chromosome Xq27 that can be induced by culturing cells from affected males in medium that is either deficient in folate or contains the folate inhibitor methotrexate (Sutherland, 1977).

The DNA encompassing the fragile site was cloned and the gene responsible for the fragile X syndrome, *FMR1*, was identified and shown to contain a CGG repeat sequence (Heitz et al., 1991; Kremer et al., 1991; Oberle et al., 1991; Verkerk et al., 1991; Yu et al., 1991). The number of copies of the CGG repeat was directly related to phenotype: in normal individuals, the number of repeats was polymorphic, varying between 6 and 54 copies; in unaffected male and female carriers, a premutation consisting of expansion of the repeat length, ranging in size from 50 to 200 repeats, was present; and in affected males, repeat length was invariably greater than 200 copies (Fu et al., 1991). Expansion of premutations to full mutations occurs only during female meiosis (Fig. 4.2) and the risk of expansion increases with repeat number (Fu et al., 1991; Oberle et al., 1991). However, mitotic instability of repeat length has also been detected in males with the full mutation (Fu et al., 1991).

FMR1 is expressed in many tissues, with highest levels of mRNA detected in brain and testes (reviewed by Caskey et al., 1992). Cells from fragile X males have greatly reduced amounts of *FMR1* mRNA (Pieretti et al., 1991). The CGG repeat is located in the 5'-untranslated region of the *FMR1* gene, which contains a CpG island that encompasses the 5'-flanking region and first exon. CpG dinucleotides are underrepresented in mammalian DNA and are substrates for methylation by cytosine methyltransferase. CpG islands, which can be detected by the presence of multiple BssH II (5'-GCGCGC-3'), Eag I/Xma III (5'-CGGCCG-3'), Sac II (5'-CCGCGG-3'), and Not I (5'-GCGGCCGC-3') restriction sites, are of-

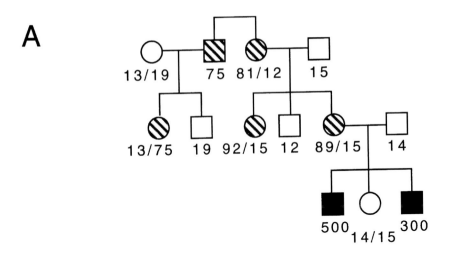

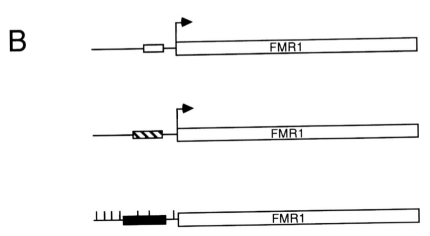

FIGURE 4-2. Fragile X syndrome. (A) Inheritance pattern. Pedigree shows a family in which fragile X mental retardation syndrome was diagnosed in two brothers in the third generation (filled boxes). CGG repeat number was determined for all family members and revealed the presence of five individuals (hatched symbols) carrying premutations with repeat expansion to 75–92 copies. Note the progressive increase in repeat length of premutation, but not wild-type, alleles when transmitted from the mother but not when transmitted from the father. (B) Molecular pathophysiology. Repeat expansion in premutation allele (hatched box) has no effect on transcription of the *FMR1* gene. However, expansion to full mutation (filled box) results in cytosine methylation (tick marks) of CpG sequences in the 5'-flanking sequence and transcriptional silencing of the *FMR1* gene.

ten found at the 5' ends of ubiquitously expressed genes and their methylation is associated with transcriptional inactivation. It appears that CGG repeat amplification exerts its effect on *FMR1* gene expression by facilitating the methylation of cytosine residues in the CpG island that is associated with concomitant transcriptional inactivation (Bell et al., 1991; Pieretti et al., 1991; Vincent et al., 1991). The mild mental impairment in carrier females may be due to partial methylation induced by partial repeat expansion or may reflect mitotic expansion of the premutation to full mutation within a limited number of cells during development. Thus, the fragile X mutation represents a defect in transcriptional control in which a *cis*-acting regulatory element is not itself mutated but is instead adversely affected by a mutation within flanking DNA sequences.

Mutations Affecting Transcription as Disease Modifiers

Most genes contain multiple binding sites for transcription factors and these factors rely on both protein-protein and protein-DNA interactions to bind to DNA. Most single nucleotide substitutions in *cis*-acting transcriptional regulatory elements are thus unlikely to have a significant effect on the level of gene transcription. In the case of Hemophilia B Leyden and Duffy Blood Group Antigen, single transcription factor binding sites play sufficiently major roles in mediating the transcription of the *F9* and *DARC* genes, respectively, that mutations in these sites result in decreased gene expression sufficient to result in a clinical phenotype. In the case of HPFH, point mutations either eliminate repressor or establish activator binding sites that result in γ-globin gene transcription at a time when the gene is normally not expressed. Mutations in *cis*-acting sequences may have more subtle effects on gene transcription that in isolation might not be sufficient to result in a disease phenotype but which in combination with other genetic or environmental factors could contribute significantly to multifactorial disease pathogenesis. Conversely, such mutations may function to ameliorate an otherwise severe disorder. For example, the relative severity of sickle cell anemia is inversely related to the levels of hemoglobin F, and pharmacologic induction of γ-globin gene transcription by hydroxyurea administration has been shown to ameliorate sickling episodes in some patients (Steinberg et al., 1997). Individuals with mild sickle cell disease carry an allele for high Hb F that is located on the X chromosome and is therefore unlinked to the γ-globin gene, suggesting the involvement of a *trans*-acting factor (Chang et al., 1997). Cancer, coronary artery disease, and stroke are multifactorial in nature, and mutations affecting gene transcription probably contribute to the genetic component of these common human diseases.

Susceptibility to Cerebral Malaria Associated with a Polymorphism in the Tumor Necrosis Factor-α Gene Promoter

An example of these types of potential interactions occurs in the case of malaria, a common life-threatening illness in the Mediterranean area and Africa. Alleles for sickle cell anemia, thalassemia, and Duffy blood group all occur at high frequency in malarial areas because erythrocytes from sickle and thalassemia heterozygotes and Duffy (−) homozygotes are resistant to invasion by the *Plasmodium* parasite. Thus, not all individuals exposed to the parasite develop malaria. Only a fraction of those individuals who do develop malaria progress to cerebral malaria, which can result in death or severe neurologic sequelae. Among children with cerebral malaria, levels of the cytokine tumor necrosis factor–α (TNF-α) are higher than in those with uncomplicated malaria, and TNF-α levels are highest in those children who die or develop neurologic sequelae from cerebral malaria (McGuire et al., 1994). In this condition, the parasites bind to the cerebral vasculature by recognizing endothelial cell adhesion molecules, the expression of which is stimulated by TNF-α. In addition, TNF-α stimulates production of nitric oxide, which has been implicated in the pathogenesis of cerebral malaria. A polymorphism was detected at nt −308 in the *TNF-α* gene promoter. The *TNF1* and *TNF2* alleles contained G and A, respectively, at this position, and were present with frequencies of 0.84 and 0.16 in the Gambian population studied. Whereas *TNF2* homozygotes represented only 1.2% of non-malaria patients and 1.8% of patients with uncomplicated malaria or malaria complicated by severe anemia, there was a significantly higher frequency of *TNF2* homozygotes among patients with cerebral malaria (4.5%) and especially among those who died or developed sequelae (8.1%) (McGuire et al., 1994). Transcriptional studies of the *TNF-α* promoter linked to a reporter gene demonstrated higher levels of expression when the promoter contained the *TNF2* as compared to the *TNF1* allele. These data suggest that a point mutation within the *TNF-α* promoter represents a genetic predisposition to the development of cerebral malaria.

References

Arbini, A. A., E. S. Pollak, J. K. Bayleran, K. A. High, and K. A. Bauer. Severe factor VII deficiency due to a mutation disrupting a hepatocyte nuclear factor 4 binding site in the factor VII promoter. *Blood* 89:176–182, 1997.

Bell, M. V., M. C. Hirst, Y. Nakahori, R. N. Mackinnon, A. Roche, T. J. Flint, P. A. Jacobs, N. Tommerup, L. Tranebjaerg, U. Froster-Iskenius, B. Kerr, G. Turner, R. H. Lindenbaum, R. Winter, M. Pembrey, S. Thibodeau, and K. E. Davies. Physical mapping across the fragile X: hypermethylation and clinical expression of the fragile X syndrome. *Cell* 64:861–866, 1991.

Briet, E., R. M. Bertina, N. H. van Tilburg, and J. J. Veltkamp. Hemophilia B Leyden: a sex linked hereditary disorder that improves after puberty. *N. Engl. J. Med.* 306:788–790, 1982.

Caskey, C. T., A. Pizzuti, Y.-H. Fu, R. G. Fenwick, Jr., and D. L. Nelson. Triplet repeat mutations in human disease. *Science* 256:784–789, 1992.

Chang, Y. P., M. Maier-Redelsperger, K. D. Smith, L. Contu, R. Ducroco, M. de Montalembert, M. Belloy, J. Elion, G. J. Dover, and R. Girot. The relative importance of the X-linked FCP locus and beta-globin haplotypes in determining haemoglobin F levels: a study of SS patients homozygous for beta S haplotypes. *Br. J. Haematol.* 96:806–814, 1997.

Chauduri, A., V. Zbrzezna, J. Polyakova, A. O. Pogo, J. Hesselgesser, and R. Horuk. Expression of the Duffy antigen in K562 cells: Evidence that it is the human erythrocyte chemokine receptor. *J. Biol. Chem.* 269:7835–7838, 1994.

Cooper, D. N., M. Krawczak, and S. E. Antonarakis. The nature and mechanisms of human gene mutation. In C. R. Scriver, A. L. Beaudet, W. S. Sly, and D. Valle, eds. *The Metabolic and Molecular Bases of Inherited Disease*, 7th ed. New York: McGraw-Hill, 1995.

Crossley, M., and G. G. Brownlee. Disruption of a C/EBP binding site in the factor IX promoter is associated with hemophilia B. *Nature* 345:444–446, 1990.

Crossley, M., M. Ludwig, K. M. Stowell, P. De Vos, K. Olek, and G. G. Brownlee. Recovery from hemophilia B Leyden: an androgen responsive element in the factor IX promoter. *Science* 257:377–379, 1992.

Crossley, M., P. R. Winship, D. E. G. Austen, C. R. Rizza, and G. G. Brownlee. A less severe form of hemophilia B Leyden. *Nucleic Acids Res.* 18:4633, 1990.

Driscoll, M. C., C. S. Dobkin, and B. P. Alter. γδβ-thalassemia due to a de novo mutation deleting the 5' β-globin gene activation-region hypersensitive sites. *Proc. Natl. Acad. Sci. U.S.A.* 86:7470–7474, 1989.

Forrester, W. C., E. Epner, M. C. Driscoll, T. Enver, M. Brice, T. Papayannopoulou, and M. Groudine. A deletion of the human β-globin locus activator region (LAR) causes a major alteration in chromatin structure and replication across the entire β-globin locus. *Genes Dev.* 4:1637–1649, 1990.

Freedenberg, D. L., and B. Black. Altered developmental control of the factor IX gene: a new T to A mutation at position +6 of the FIX gene resulting in hemophilia B Leyden. *Thromb. Haemost.* 65:964, 1991.

Fu, Y.-H., D. P. A. Kuhl, A. Pizzuti, M. Pieretti, J. S. Sutcliffe, S. Richards, A. J. M. H. Verkerk, J. J. A. Holden, R .G. Fenwick, Jr., S. T. Warren, B.A. Oostra, D. L. Nelson, and C. T. Caskey. Variation of the CGG repeat at the fragile X site results in genetic instability: resolution of the Sherman paradox. *Cell* 67:1047–1058, 1991.

Gustavson, K. H., H. K. Blomquist, and G. Holmgren. Prevalence of the fragile-X syndrome in mentally retarded boys in a Swedish county. *Am. J. Med. Genet.* 23:581–587, 1986.

Hadley, T. J., Z. H. Lu, K. Wasniowska, A. W. Martin, S. C. Peiper, J. Hesselgesser, and R. Horuk. Postcapillary venule endothelial cells in kidney express a multispecific chemokine receptor that is structurally and functionally identical to the erythroid isoform, which is the Duffy blood group antigen. *J. Clin. Invest.* 94:985–991, 1994.

Hatton, C., A. O. M. Wilkie, H. C. Drysdale, W. G. Wood, M. A. Vickers, J. Sharpe, H. Ayyub, I.-M. Pretorius, V. J. Buckle, and D. R. Higgs. Alpha thalassemia caused by a large (62 kb) deletion upstream of the human α globin gene cluster. *Blood* 76:221–227, 1990.

Heitz, D., F. Rousseau, D. Dvys, S. Saccone, H. Abderrahim, D. Le Paslier, D. Cohen, A. Vincent, D. Toniolo, G. Della Valle, S. Johnson, D. Schlessinger, I. Oberle, and J. L. Mandel. Isolation of sequences that span the fragile X and identification of a fragile X-related CpG island. *Science* 251:1236–1239, 1991.

Hirosawa, S., J. B. Fahner, J. P. Salier, C. T. Wu, E. W. Lorrien, and K. Kurachi. Structural and functional basis of the developmental regulation of human cogulation factor IX gene. *Proc. Natl. Acad. Sci. U.S.A.* 87:4421–4425, 1990.

Jane, S. M., D. L. Gumucio, P. A. Ney, J. M. Cunningham, and A. W. Nienhuis. Methylation-enhanced binding of Sp1 to the stage selector element of the human γ-globin gene promoter may regulate developmental specificity of expression. *Mol. Cell. Biol.* 13:3272–3281, 1993.

Jarman, A. P., W. G. Wood, J. A. Sharpe, G. Gourdon, H. Ayyub, and D. R. Higgs. Characterization of the major regulatory element upstream of the human α-globin gene cluster. *Mol. Cell. Biol.* 11:4679–4689, 1991.

Kremer, E. J., M. Pritchard, M. Lynch, S. Yu, K. Homan, E. Baker, S. T. Warren, D. Schlessinger, G. R. Sutherland, and R. I. Richards. Mapping of DNA instability at the Fragile X to a trinucleotide repeat p(CGG)n. *Science* 252:1711–1714, 1991.

Liebhaber, S. A., E.-U. Griese, I. Weiss, F. E. Cash, H. Ayyub, D. R. Higgs, and J. Horst. Inactivation of human α-globin gene expression by a de novo deletion located upstream of the α-globin gene cluster. *Proc. Natl. Acad. Sci. U.S.A.* 87:9431–9435, 1990.

Martin, D. I. K., S.-F. Tsai, and S. H. Orkin. Increased γ-globin expression in a nondeletion HPFH mediated by an erythroid-specific DNA-binding factor. *Nature* 338:435–438, 1989.

McGuire, W., A. V. S. Hill, C. E. M. Allsopp, B. M. Greenwood, and D. Kwiatkowski. Variation in the TNF-α promoter region associated with susceptibility to cerebral malaria. *Nature* 371:508–511, 1994.

McKusick, V.A. *Mendelian Inheritance in Man. Catalogs of Human Genes and Genetic Disorders,* 11th edition. Baltimore: Johns Hopkins University Press, 1994.

Miller, I. J., and J. J. Bieker. A novel, erythroid cell-specific murine transcription factor that binds to the CACCC element and is related to the Kruppel family of nuclear proteins. *Mol. Cell. Biol.* 13:2776–2786, 1993.

Miller, L. H., S. J. Mason, D. F. Clyde, and M. H. McGinnis. The resistance factor to Plasmodium vivax in blacks: the Duffy blood group phenotype, FyFy. *N. Engl. J. Med.* 295:302–305, 1976.

Neote, K., J. Y. Mak, L. F. Kolakowski, and T. J. Schall. Functional and biochemical analysis of the cloned Duffy antigen: identity with the red blood cell chemokine receptor. *Blood* 84:44–52, 1994.

Nuez, B., D. Michalovich, A. Bygrave, R. Ploemacher, and F. Grosveld. Defective haematopoiesis in fetal liver resulting from inactivation of the EKLF gene. *Nature* 375:316–318, 1995.

Nussbaum, R. L., and D. H. Ledbetter. The fragile X syndrome. In *Metabolic Basis of Inherited Disease*, C. R. Scriver, A. L. Beaudet, W. S. Sly, D. Valle, Eds. New York: McGraw-Hill, pp. 327–341, 1989.

Oberle, I., F. Rousseau, D. Heitz, C. Kretz, D. Devys, A. Hanauer, J. Boue, M. F. Bertheas, and J. L. Mandel. Instability of a 550-base pair DNA segment and abnormal methylation in fragile X syndrome. *Science* 252:1097–1102, 1991.

Orkin, S. H., and H. H. Kazazian, Jr. The mutation and polymorphism of the human β-globin gene and its surrounding DNA. *Annu. Rev. Genet.* 18:131–171, 1984.

Peiper, S. C., Z. X. Wang, K. Neote, A. W. Martin, H. J. Showell, M. J. Conklyn, K. Ogborne, T. J. Hadley, Z. H. Lu, J. Hesselgesser, et al. The Duffy antigen/receptor for chemokines (DARC) is expressed in endothelial cells of Duffy negative individuals who lack the erythrocyte receptor. *J. Exp. Med.* 181:1311–1317, 1995.

Perkins, A. C., A. H. Sharpe, and S. H. Orkin. Lethal β-thalassemia in mice lacking the erythroid CACCC-transcription factor EKLF. *Nature* 375:318–322, 1995.

Picketts, D. J., C. D'Souza, P. J. Bridge, and D. Lillicrap. An A to T transversion at position −5 of the factor IX promoter results in hemophilia B. *Genomics* 12:161–163, 1992.

Picketts, D. J., D. P. Lillicrap, and C. R. Muller. Synergy between transcription factors DBP and C/EBP compensates for a haemophilia B Leyden factor IX mutation. *Nat. Genet.* 3:175–179, 1993.

Pieretti, M., F. Zhang, Y.-H. Fu, S. T. Warren, B. A. Oostra, C. T. Caskey, and D. L. Nelson. Absence of expression of the FMR-1 gene in fragile X syndrome. *Cell* 66:817–822, 1991.

Reijnen, M. J., F. M. Sladek, R. M. Bertina, and P. H. Reitsma. Disruption of a binding site for hepatic nuclear factor 4 results in hemophilia B Leyden. *Proc. Natl. Acad. Sci. U.S.A.* 89:6300–6303, 1992.

Reitsma, P. H., R. M. Bertina, J. K. Ploos van Amste, A. Riemans, and E. Briet. The putative factor IX promoter in hemophilia B Leyden. *Blood* 72:1074–1076, 1988.

Reitsma, P. H., T. Mandalaki, C. K. Kasper, R. M. Bertina, and E. Briet. Two novel point mutations correlate with an altered developmental expression of blood coagulation factor IX (hemophilia B Leyden phenotype). *Blood* 73:743–746, 1989.

Royle, G., N. S. Van De Water, E. Berry, P. A. Ockelford, and P. J. Browett. Haemophilia B Leyden arising de novo by point mutation in the putative factor IX promoter region. *Br. J. Haematol.* 77:191–194, 1991.

Sherman, S. L., P. A. Jacobs, N. E. Morton, U. Froster-Iskenius, P. N. Howard-Peebles, K. B. Nielsen, M. W. Partington, G. R. Sutherland, G. Turner, and M. Watson. Further segregation analysis of the fragile X syndrome with special reference to transmitting males. *Hum. Genet.* 69:289–299, 1985.

Steinberg, M. H., Z. H. Lu, F. B. Barton, M. L. Terrin, S. Charache, and G. J. Dover. Fetal hemoglobin in sickle cell anemia: determinants of response to hydroxyurea: multicenter study of hydroxyurea. *Blood* 89:1078–1088, 1997.

Sutherland, G. R. Fragile sites on human chromosomes: demonstration of their dependence on the type of tissue culture medium. *Science* 197:265–266, 1977.

Tournamille, C., Y. Colin, J. P. Cartron, and C. Le Van Kim. Disruption of a GATA motif in the Duffy gene promoter abolishes erythroid gene expression in Duffy-negative individuals. *Nat. Genet.* 10:224–228, 1995.

Verkerk, A. J. M. H., M. Piearetti, J. S. Sutcliffe, Y.-H. Fu, D. P. A. Kuhl, A. Pizzuti, O. Reiner, S. Richards, M. F. Victoria, F. Zhang, B. E. Eussen, G. J. B. van Ommen, L. A. J. Blonden, G. J. Riggins, J. L. Chastain, C. B. Kunst, H. Galjaard, C. T. Caskey, D. L. Nelson, B. A. Oostra, and S. T. Warren. Identification of a gene (FMR-1) containing a CGG repeat coincident with a breakpoint cluster region exhibiting length variation in fragile X syndrome. *Cell* 65:905–914, 1991.

Vincent, A., D. Heitz, C. Petit, C. Kretz, I. Oberle, and J. L. Mandel. Abnormal pattern detected in fragile X patients by pulsed-field gel electrophoresis. *Nature* 349:624–626, 1991.

Webb, T. P., S. Bundey, A. Thak, and J. Todd. The frequency of the fragile X chromosome among schoolchildren in Coventry. *J. Med. Genet.* 23:396–399, 1986.

Wilkie, A. O. M., J. Lamb, P. C. Harris, R. D. Finney, and D. R. Higgs. A truncated human chromosome 16 associated with α thalassemia is stabilized by addition of telomeric repeat (TTAGGG)$_n$. *Nature* 346:868–871, 1990.

Yu, S., M. Pritchard, E. Kremer, M. Lynch, J. Nancarrow, E Baker, K. Holman, J. C. Mulley, S. T. Warren, D. Schlessnger, G. R. Sutherland, and R. I. Richards. Fragile X genotype characterized by an unstable region of DNA. *Science* 252:1179–1181, 1991.

Mutations in Genes Encoding   5
Transcription Factors:
The Nuclear Receptor
Superfamily

In Chapters 5 through 14, mutations that affect the structure and/or function of specific transcription factors and result in human disease will be described. As in the previous chapter, the intent is not to catalogue all known mutations but rather to provide examples that illustrate principles of molecular pathophysiology that will be applicable to the ever-expanding list of such conditions that is being reported in the molecular biology and clinical literature. In contrast to the mutations in *cis*-acting elements, the mutations in *trans*-acting factors affect the structure of the protein product of a gene. In the text, gene symbols will be indicated by italicized letters (all capitalized for human genes, first letter only for mouse genes), whereas the protein product of a gene will be indicated by unitalicized capital letters (for both human and mouse proteins). Missense mutations result in substitution of one amino acid for another and will be designated in the text using the single-letter code for amino acids (see Table 5.1). For example, the mutation C23S (due to a TGT → AGT transversion) would result in substitution of serine for cysteine at residue 23 of the protein. Nonsense mutations result in premature termination of translation, which is designated by an X. Thus, the mutation C23X (due to a TGT → TGA transversion) would result in translation of a truncated polypeptide containing only 22 amino acid residues.

Both dominant and recessive disease phenotypes will be described. Phenotypes that demonstrate recessive inheritance are due to loss-of-function mutations. In contrast, several different molecular mechanisms underlie diseases with dominant inheritance, in which the inheritance of a single mutant allele is sufficient to cause disease despite the presence of a wild-type allele. First, heterozygosity for a loss-of-function mutation that results in 50% of normal levels of functioning protein may not be sufficient for normal transcriptional regulation. This mechanism is referred to as

TABLE 5.1. Amino acid codes

Amino Acid	Single-Letter Code	Triple-Letter Code
alanine	A	Ala
arginine	R	Arg
asparagine	N	Asn
aspartic acid	D	Asp
cysteine	C	Cys
glutamic acid	E	Glu
glutamine	Q	Gln
glycine	G	Gly
histidine	H	His
isoleucine	I	Ile
leucine	L	Leu
lysine	K	Lys
methionine	M	Met
phenylalanine	F	Phe
proline	P	Pro
serine	S	Ser
threonine	T	Thr
tryptophan	W	Trp
tyrosine	Y	Tyr
valine	V	Val
termination	X	Ter

haploinsufficiency or gene dosage, because individuals homozygous for the mutant allele (~0% of wild-type protein activity) generally manifest a more severe phenotype than those heterozygous for the mutant allele (~50% of wild-type protein activity). Second, a missense mutation may result in the synthesis of a mutant protein that not only is inactive but also interferes with the activity of the wild-type protein, the so-called dominant-negative mechanism. This mechanism often involves transcription factors that must dimerize in order to bind to DNA and activate transcription. Third, a mutation may result in the synthesis of a mutant protein that has a novel property. In this case, the presence or absence of the wild-type protein is irrelevant. Gain-of-function mutants are much less common than loss-of-function and dominant-negative mutants.

The survey of mutations in *trans*-acting factors will begin in this chapter with a description of one of the largest categories of transcription factors, the nuclear receptor superfamily. Members of this group of proteins have been described in both invertebrates and vertebrates. In mammals, they have been shown to play essential roles in embryonic development and postnatal physiology. Mutations within genes encoding these proteins are responsible for a large number of congenital disorders.

Classification and Structure of Nuclear Receptors

The nuclear receptor superfamily represents an extensive group of zinc finger transcription factors (reviewed by Mangelsdorf and Evans, 1995; Mangelsdorf et al., 1995). Most proteins within this superfamily contain three essential domains: (1) The DNA-binding domain consists of two highly conserved zinc fingers (Berg, 1989; Klug and Schwabe, 1995). (2) The ligand-binding domain regulates transcriptional activity of the protein by stimulating nuclear localization, dimerization, DNA binding, and/or transactivation functions of the protein on ligand binding. Heptad amino acid repeats within the ligand-binding domain are specifically involved in ligand-induced dimerization. (3) One or more transactivation domains are present, the function of which may or may not be modulated by ligand binding. The general structure of members of the steroid hormone receptor subfamily of nuclear receptors is shown in Figure 5.1.

The nuclear receptor superfamily can be divided into two large groups of factors, those that are known to bind specific small organic ligands and orphan receptors for which a ligand may exist (based on

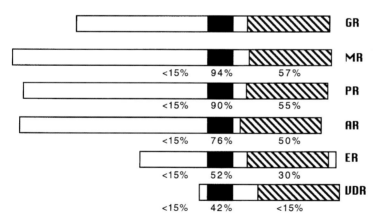

FIGURE 5-1. General structure of steroid hormone receptors. The glucocorticoid (GR), mineralocorticoid (MR), progesterone (PR), androgen (AR), estrogen (ER), and vitamin D (VDR) receptors are shown with DNA-binding (solid box) and ligand-binding (hatched box) domains indicated. Sequence similarity between receptors is restricted to these two domains. The steroid hormone receptors, which homodimerize, show greater similarity when compared with each other than when compared with the VDR, which is a member of the subfamily that heterodimerizes with retinoid x receptors (RXRs) (percent identity with GR is shown to the amino-terminal, DNA-binding, and ligand-binding domains). (Adapted from Chrousos et al., 1993.)

TABLE 5.2. Organization of the mammalian nuclear receptor superfamily

1. Nuclear receptors (with known ligands)
    a. Steroid hormone receptors [class I]
        i. Androgen receptor (5α-dihydrotestosterone)
        ii. Estrogen receptor (estradiol)
        iii. Glucocorticoid receptor (cortisol)
        iv. Mineralocorticoid receptor (aldosterone)
        v. Progesterone receptor (progesterone)
    b. Non-steroid-hormone receptors [class II]
        i. Retinoic acid receptors α, β, γ (all *trans*-retinoic acid)
        ii. Retinoid X receptors α, β, γ (9-*cis*-retinoic acid)
        iii. Thyroid hormone receptors α, β (3,5,3'-L-triiodothyronine)
        iv. Vitamin D receptor (1,25-dihydroxyvitamin D_3)
        v. Peroxisome proliferator-activated receptors α, β, γ (eicosanoids)
        vi. Farnesoid X-activated receptor (farnesoids)
2. Orphan nuclear receptors
    a. Homodimeric receptors [class III]
        i. COUP α, β, γ
        ii. HNF-4
    b. Monomeric receptors [class IV]
        i. NGFI-B
        ii. Retinoid-related orphan receptors α, β, γ
        iii. Steroidogenic factor 1
    c. Truncated receptors [Class V]
        i. DAX-1

similarity of structure within the ligand-binding domain) but has not been identified (Table 5.2). In addition, the ligand-binding receptors can be subdivided into those that bind steroid hormones and form homodimers (androgen, estrogen, glucocorticoid, mineralocorticoid, and progesterone receptors [class I]) and those that form heterodimers with the retinoid X receptor (RXR) (e.g., *trans*-retinoic acid, thyroid hormone, and vitamin D receptors [class II]). Finally, the orphan receptors can be subdivided into those that form homodimers (e.g., hepatocyte nuclear factor 4 [class III]), those that bind DNA as a monomer (e.g., steroidogenic factor-1 [class IV]), and truncated receptors that contain a ligand-binding domain but lack the conserved zinc finger DNA-binding domain (e.g., DAX-1 [class V]).

DNA-Binding Specificity

The class I steroid hormone receptors all bind to inverted repeat DNA sequences. The androgen, glucocorticoid, mineralocorticoid, and progesterone receptors all bind to sites containing the consensus sequence 5'-

AGAACA-3' as an inverted repeat with half-sites separated by three nucleotides (IR-3), whereas the estrogen receptor binds to the half-site sequence 5'-RGGTCA-3' (R = A or G) in an IR-3 configuration. In contrast, many of the class II nuclear receptors that form heterodimers with RXR and class III orphan receptors recognize the half-site sequence 5'-RGKTCA-3' (K = G or T) as a direct repeat separated by one to five nucleotides, whereas the class IV orphan receptors recognize a single copy of this sequence, usually with a requirement for specific flanking nucleotides.

The binding site sequences described above clearly do not provide adequate information to insure recognition of specific sites by specific nuclear receptors. One mechanism by which specific binding is achieved for class II receptors involves the number of nucleotides separating the direct repeats. The vitamin D, thyroid hormone, and retinoic acid receptors (as RXR heterodimers) were shown to bind preferentially to 5'-AGGTCA-3' half-site direct repeats separated by three, four, and five nucleotides, respectively (Naar et al., 1991; Umesono et al., 1991). The binding at these sites appears to be highly organized; in all cases studied, the RXR subunit has been shown to bind to the 5' half-site whereas the specific subunit (retinoic acid, thyroid hormone, or vitamin D receptor) contacts the 3' half-site (Kurokawa et al., 1993, 1994; Perlmann et al., 1993; Zechel et al., 1994). Subsequently, direct repeats separated by one nucleotide were shown to be preferentially bound by RXR homodimers and RXR-peroxisome proliferator-activated receptor heterodimers whereas direct repeats separated by two nucleotides were also recognized by RXR–retinoic acid receptor heterodimers (reviewed by Mangelsdorf et al., 1994). Although these binding site preferences are by no means absolute, they represent one factor that contributes to binding site selection. Other factors include the specific nucleotide composition of the repeats as well as interstitial and flanking sequences (Mader et al., 1993). In addition, as for other transcription factors, the presence of adjacent transcription factor binding sites may also influence binding.

Nuclear Hormone Receptor Pathophysiology

The estrogen, glucocorticoid, and thyroid hormone receptors represent the first mammalian transcription factors for which cDNA sequences were isolated just over a decade ago (Green et al., 1986; Hollenberg et al., 1985; Jansson et al., 1983; Sap et al., 1986; Weinberger et al., 1986). Even before the identification of the steroid hormone receptors, a variety of clinical conditions were characterized by endocrinologists that shared in common the property of hormone resistance, in which affected individuals had normal circulating levels of the hormone in question but showed no evidence of normal developmental or physiologic effects of the hormone and supplemental hormone administration was often ineffective in ameliorating the disease symptoms. Subsequently, mutations have been identified within genes encoding the androgen, estrogen, glucocorticoid, thyroid hormone, and vitamin D receptors as described in detail below. A comprehensive database containing current information on mutations in the androgen, glucocorticoid, mineralocorticoid, vitamin D, and thyroid hormone receptors has recently been established: the Nuclear Receptor Resource; the project's home page can be reached via the Internet at http://nrr.georgetown.edu/nrr.html (Martinez et al., 1997).

Androgen Receptor

Androgen Insensitivity Syndromes

The pubertal development of male secondary sexual characteristics is mediated by the binding of the biologically active androgens testosterone and 5α-dihydrotestosterone to the androgen receptor present within target tissues (reviewed by Wilson et al., 1981a,b, 1995). The identification of mutations at the X-linked androgen receptor (*AR*) locus in males with defects in sexual differentiation has demonstrated the essential role of the AR in this process. In addition, important genotype-phenotype and protein structure-function relationships have been revealed by molecular analysis of these patients (Bevan et al., 1996; Brinkmann et al., 1995; Klocker et al., 1992; Lobaccaro et al., 1996; Lubahn et al., 1990; McPhaul et al., 1991, 1992; Marcelli et al., 1990a,b, 1991; Ris-Stalpers et al., 1991, 1994; Sai et al., 1990; Zoppi et al., 1992; and references therein). More mutations have been identified in the AR than in any other transcription factor, due to the ascertainment of mutations in the hemizygous state.

The most severe phenotype is testicular feminization, or more properly, complete androgen insensitivity syndrome (AIS; MIM 300068), in which affected individuals with a 46,XY chromosome constitution manifest female secondary sexual characteristics. In contrast, 46,XY individuals with partial AIS demonstrate a broad spectrum of incomplete virilization ranging from apparently overvirilized female secondary sexual characteristics such as clitoromegaly or labial fusion to undervirilized male secondary sexual development with findings such as azoospermia, cryptorchidism, gynecomastia, hypogonadism, hypospadias, and/or microphallus. Some patients with partial AIS have been assigned an alternative eponymic designation, Reifenstein syndrome (MIM 312300).

The clinical heterogeneity has been associated with heterogeneity in the ligand-binding properties of the AR assayed in fibroblasts cultured from affected individuals. Four categories of binding of dihydrotestosterone (DHT) to AR have been defined: (1) no DHT-AR binding; (2) decreased DHT-AR binding; (3) qualitatively abnormal binding, such as increased thermal lability and increased hormone-receptor dissociation kinetics; and (4) normal DHT-AR binding. The first three categories involve mutations affecting the ligand-binding domain (Table 5.3), whereas the last category includes mutations affecting the structure of the two zinc fingers of the DNA-binding domain (Fig. 5.2).

There is no correlation between the AR domain that is affected by mutation and the clinical phenotype. Rather, the degree to which the mutation disrupts AR biological activity, either at the level of hormone binding, DNA binding, or transactivation, may determine the clinical severity. For example, the nonsense mutations W794X and W717X (Marcelli et al., 1990b; Sai et al., 1990) cause premature translation termination within the hormone-binding domain and the truncated receptor showed no detectable binding of DHT, resulting in complete AIS. In contrast, the missense mutation A594T, involving an amino acid substitution in the second zinc finger of the DNA-binding domain, resulted in an AR that

TABLE 5.3. Androgen receptor mutations responsible for complete (C) or partial (P) androgen insensitivity syndrome

Hormone-Binding Domain				
Abnormal Binding	No Binding	Decreased Binding	Normal Binding	DNA-binding Domain
L726S (P)	W717X (C)	R853H (C)	Q798E (P)	C550Y (C)
M742I (P)	W739R (C)	R853H (P)		G559V (P)
A746D (P)	F762L (C)			G559W (P)
Y761C (P)	R772C (C)			A564D (C)
P764S (C)	W794X (C)			C567R (C)
M780I (P)	R829Q (C)			C567F (C)
R838C (P)	Y832C (C)			V572F (C)
R840C (P)	R838H (P)			Del F573/F574 (C)
R852K (P)	R853C (C)			K581X (C)
R855H (P)	V864E (C)			A587T (P)
V864M (P)	P902H (C)			S588G (P)
I869M (P)				C592F (C)
V901M (P)				R589Q (P)
				R599K (P)
				R606H (C)
				Del R606 (C)
				L607R (P)
				R608P (C)

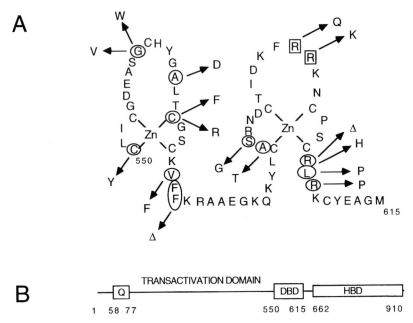

FIGURE 5-2. Mutations in the androgen receptor (AR) DNA-binding domain. (A) Amino acid residues 550–615, constituting the zinc (Zn) finger DNA-binding domain (DBD) of the AR are shown with arrows indicating missense mutations identified in patients with complete or partial androgen insensitivity syndrome (AIS) (circle) or partial AIS and breast cancer (square). Δ, deletion of amino acid(s). (B) Structure of the approximately 917–amino-acid AR (with variability depending on the length of the amino-terminal polyglutamine tract), showing the location of the DBD, hormone-binding domain (HBD), and transactivation domain including the polymorphic polyglutamine stretch (Q), which is expanded in patients with spinal and bulbar muscular atrophy. Note that the numbering of amino acid residues in the AR varies among different publications due to the presence of polymorphic homopolymeric stretches within the protein. In the 910-amino-acid protein shown, the polyglutamine and polyglycine runs are 20 and 16 residues long, respectively.

bound DHT normally but activated transcription at one third of the normal level (compared to the wild-type AR) and was associated with the clinical phenotype of partial AIS/Reifenstein syndrome (Klocker et al., 1992). Thus, a mutation that had a milder effect on AR transcriptional activity was associated with a less severe clinical phenotype. Another mutation that affected DNA binding involved a 6-kb deletion in intron 2 that disrupted pre-mRNA splicing so that greater than 90% of the processed mRNA lacked exon 2 sequences encoding the second zinc finger of the DNA-binding domain (Ris-Stalpers et al., 1994). Despite the apparent severity of the defect, this mutation was identified in a patient diagnosed with the Reifenstein syndrome. Because the mutant protein was functionally inactive in transcription assays but did not interfere with the activity of coexpressed wild-type protein, these results indicate that approximately 10% of normal levels of wild-type AR protein are insufficient for normal male secondary sexual development.

Some of the missense mutations associated with partial AIS have been identified in more than one patient and assays of receptor activity in these patients have given different results. For example, the R838H mutation was associated with a qualitative defect in DHT binding in one patient, whereas in another patient it was associated with an apparently complete lack of DHT binding (McPhaul et al., 1992). The latter patient did not manifest complete AIS, suggesting that the mutant receptor could still bind DHT and/or testosterone in vivo. A second example involves two individuals carrying an R853H mutation, one with complete and the other with incomplete AIS (McPhaul et al., 1992). These observations indicate that other genetic differences, either linked or unlinked to the *AR* locus, may affect receptor function and influence the severity of the clinical phenotype.

Another missense mutation associated with partial AIS that provides insight into the functional activity of the AR is Q798E, which, despite its location in the ligand-binding domain, demonstrated normal androgen binding activity (Bevan et al., 1996). However, the mutant AR did show decreased transcriptional activity in androgen-treated cells, suggesting either that the mutation affected some aspect of binding not assayed or that it affected some other aspect of AR function, such as dimerization or transactivation. Both ligand-activated homodimerization and transactivation functions have been attributed to the AR ligand-binding domain but have not been localized to specific amino acid residues. Further analysis of the molecular pathophysiology of the Q798E mutation may therefore further our understanding of the complex structural and functional changes of the AR that occur as a result of androgen binding.

The analysis of *AR* mutations in patients with AIS indicates that missense mutations within the ligand- or DNA-binding domain within the carboxyl-terminal half of the protein are sufficient to result in disease. In contrast, no mutations affecting the amino-terminal half of the AR, which contains the transactivation domain(s), have been shown to result in AIS. These results are consistent with the observation that in contrast to the highly ordered structure of the DNA- and ligand-binding domains, transactivation domains demonstrate a much less ordered structure in solution. As a result, there may be fewer crucial residues that are absolutely required to maintain a particular tertiary structure necessary for domain function. Experimental evidence from the analysis of a variety of transcription factors is consistent with this hypothesis because single missense mutations usually result at most in a minor decrease in transactivation function. In contrast, substitution of the cysteine residues required for the formation of the zinc fingers (e.g., C550Y, C567F, C567R and C592F in Fig. 5.2) result in complete loss of DNA-binding activity and of biological function. A comprehensive current compilation of all known *AR* mutations can be obtained through the Androgen Receptor Mutations Database World Wide Web Server, which can be accessed on the Internet at http://www.mcgill.ca/androgendb/ (Gottlieb et al., 1997).

Male Breast Cancer

The incidence of breast cancer in males is 100-fold lower than in females (Crichlow and Galt, 1990) and usually occurs in association with androgen deficiency (Thomas et al., 1992). Two pedigrees have been described in which affected males manifested partial AIS and breast cancer. *AR* missense mutations were identified that affected contiguous arginine residues in the second zinc finger of the androgen receptor (Fig. 5.2) (Lobaccaro et al., 1993a,b; Wooster et al., 1992). Thus, these mutations, as in the case of other mutations affecting the zinc fingers, inhibit androgen receptor from directing the normal program of male sexual differentiation. However, unlike other mutations, these two mutations in some way also result in an increased risk of breast cancer, perhaps by either promoting or failing to inhibit cellular proliferation. Androgens have been shown to inhibit the proliferation of MFM-223 breast cancer cells (Hackenberg and Schulz, 1996), and it would be interesting to compare the antiproliferative effects of wild-type, AIS, and AIS/cancer *AR* alleles in these cells. These mutations are analogous to mutations in sequences encoding the zinc fingers of the WT1 transcription factor that result in both abnormal genitourinary development and predisposition to Wilms tumor (Baird et al., 1992; Bruening et al., 1992; Pelletier et al., 1991), as will be described in detail in Chapter 6. In addition to germline *AR* mutations that predispose to breast cancer, somatic mutations in the *AR* gene are also associated with prostate cancer (reviewed by Brinkmann et al., 1995).

Spinal and Bulbar Muscular Atrophy (Kennedy Disease)

X-linked spinal and bulbar muscular atrophy (MIM 313200) was first reported in nine males from two unrelated pedigrees (Kennedy et al.,

1968). The clinical hallmarks of this condition are X-linked inheritance and onset of neuromuscular symptoms in the third to fifth decade with involvement of the facial and bulbar muscles, wasting of the proximal limb muscles, fasciculations of perioral muscles, and intention tremor (Warner et al., 1992). Remarkably, gynecomastia was reported as the first clinical sign of disease. Furthermore, in one group of patients the onset of neuromuscular symptoms was coincident with disturbances of sexual function, which in some patients included sterility (Hausmanowa-Petrusewicz et al., 1983). The molecular basis for this phenotype was identified as an expansion of a CAG trinucleotide repeat, normally present in 11 to 31 copies and coding for a polyglutamine tract at the amino-terminal end of the androgen receptor beginning at codon 58, so that the *AR* gene of affected males contains 40 to 52 copies of the trinucleotide repeat (LaSpada et al., 1991).

Expansion of the AR polyglutamine tract has been associated with decreased ligand binding affinity (MacLean et al., 1995) and with decreased transactivation function (Brinkmann et al., 1995; Chamberlain et al., 1994; Mhatre et al., 1993). However, because *AR* mutations that result in complete or partial AIS (without neuromuscular disease) can also affect ligand binding or transactivation, the mechanism by which the polyglutamine expansion results in selective toxicity to motor neurons remains undetermined but is likely to involve a gain-of-function effect. Because several other neurodegenerative disorders are associated with the expansion of trinucleotide repeats within genes that do not encode transcription factors, the pathophysiologic effect of the mutation may be independent of transcription.

Prostate Cancer

Prostate cancer is the most common malignancy in humans. Primary prostate cancers are believed to consist of a heterogeneous collection of cells: androgen-dependent cells, which require androgens for proliferation and survival; androgen-sensitive cells, which undergo cell cycle arrest but do not die when androgens are withdrawn; and androgen-independent cells (reviewed by Scher and Fossa, 1995). Death from prostate cancer is generally associated with increased tumor cell proliferation in the absence of androgens. *AR* gene mutations have been detected in prostate cancer. These are somatic (non-heritable) mutations that are present in the tumor and not in the patient's germline DNA. Amplification of the *AR* gene was detected in 30% of recurrent tumors after androgen deprivation therapy, whereas tumor biopsies from the same patients before therapy showed no evidence of *AR* amplification (Visakorpi et al., 1995). These results provide a mechanism by which androgen-sensitive tumor cells can continue to proliferate in the presence of low concentrations of androgen. Somatic point mutations in the *AR* gene have been reported in prostate cancer (Newmark et al., 1992). Some of these mutations may allow ligand-independent transcriptional activity, as described for the estrogen receptor in breast cancer (see below), thus providing a molecular basis for androgen-independent proliferation of prostate cancer cells.

Estrogen Receptor

Estrogen Insensitivity Syndrome

Unlike the X-linked *AR*, the *ER* gene has been mapped to chromosome 6q24-q27, and in contrast to the multitude of mutations involving the androgen receptor, only a single patient has been described with disease attributable to a mutation affecting the estrogen receptor (Smith et al., 1994). The 28-year-old male patient was extremely tall (204 cm) and his linear growth had continued despite otherwise normal masculine pubertal changes. Radiographically, the long-bone epiphyseal growth plates were unfused, the bone age was 15 years, and generalized osteopenia was noted. Serum concentrations of luteinizing hormone, follicle-stimulating hormone, estrone, and estradiol were increased whereas testosterone levels were normal. Other evidence of hormonal imbalance included glucose intolerance, hyperinsulinism, acanthosis nigricans, and reduced sperm viability. Parenteral high-dose estrogen administration for 6 months had no effect on bone density nor did it affect secondary sexual characteristics. DNA analysis revealed homozygosity for a R157X nonsense mutation that predicts the synthesis of a truncated estrogen receptor lacking both the DNA- and hormone-binding domains and is therefore likely to represent a null (complete loss-of-function) allele. His parents were second cousins, were both heterozygous for the mutant allele, and were clinically unaffected. Taken together these data provide important insights into the function of the estrogen receptor. First, estrogen receptor function is not required for normal male development. Second, males and females with a single functioning estrogen receptor gene also develop normally. Third, estrogen is required for epiphyseal fusion and normal bone mineralization in postpubertal males. Fourth, estrogen regulates gonadotropin levels in males and may play a role in sperm viability.

Breast Cancer

In stage I breast cancer, absence of ER expression is the most important risk factor for disease relapse and mortality (Clark and McGuire, 1988). Many ER-positive breast cancer patients who receive hormonal therapy eventually become unresponsive despite continued ER expression, suggesting the occurrence of somatic mutations in the *ER* gene that result in ligand-independent ER transcriptional activity (Fuqua et al., 1993). Analysis of mutant ER proteins generated by in vitro mutagenesis revealed that the mutation Y537S resulted in transcriptional activity in the absence of estradiol equivalent to that of the wild-type ER in the presence of estradiol, indicating that Tyr-537 plays an important role in ligand regulation of ER transcriptional activity (Weis et al., 1996).

Glucocorticoid Receptor

Glucocorticoid resistance syndromes (MIM 138040) are characterized by elevated serum levels of cortisol in the absence of clinical signs of glucocorticoid excess (Chrousos et al., 1982, 1993). Plasma ACTH levels are elevated, cannot be suppressed by exogenous cortisol, and stimulate secretion of mineralocorticoids and androgens that interact with their cognate receptors in target tissues to activate genetic programs that result in hypertension and hypokalemic alkalosis as well as virilization in females. In one sibship, the severely affected proband was found to be homozygous for a D641V substitution in the hormone-binding domain of the glucocorticoid receptor (Hurley et al., 1991). The proband's mildly affected brother and son were heterozygous for the mutation. The mutant glucocorticoid receptor (GR) was unable to activate transcription of a reporter gene containing a glucocorticoid response element in the presence of up to 1 µM dexamethasone, whereas the wild-type GR maximally transactivated the reporter gene at a concentration of 1 nM. The effect of the mutant protein on wild-type GR function was not investigated. The pedigree analysis is therefore consistent with either a gene dosage (loss-of-function) or mild dominant-negative effect in the heterozygous state. In another family, affected individuals were heterozygous for a 4-bp deletion at a splice junction that resulted in complete loss-of-function of the mutant allele, suggesting that a 50% decrease in normal GR levels is sufficient to cause glucocorticoid resistance (Karl et al., 1993).

Thyroid Hormone Receptors

The thyroid hormone receptors TRα and TRβ are encoded by two unlinked genes, *THRA* (*THR1*) and *THRB* (*THR2*), respectively (Jansson et al., 1983; Sap et al., 1986; Weinberger et al., 1986; reviewed by Lazar and Chin, 1990). Unlike the AR, ER, and GR, which form homodimers, the TRs form heterodimers with retinoid X receptors (RXRs). Thyroid hormone resistance syndromes (MIM 188570) are characterized by increased levels of triiodothyronine and thyroid-stimulating hormone, clinical hypothyroidism, and unresponsiveness to thyroid hormone administration in pharmacologic doses (reviewed by Weiss and Refetoff, 1992; Refetoff, 1994). Remarkably, in almost all cases the underlying molecular pathophysiology is heterozygosity for a missense mutation in the hormone-binding domain of TRβ (Table 5.4), either between amino acids 316 and 345 or 438 and 453 (Kitajima et al., 1995; Parrilla et al., 1991; Tsukaguchi et al., 1995; Weiss and Refetoff, 1992; and references therein). This clustering strongly resembles the findings for the X-linked *AR* gene described above in which 90% of mutations affecting the hormone-binding domain were clustered between amino acids 726–772 and 826–864 (McPhaul et al., 1992). However, in the case of the autosomal *THRB* gene, a functional copy remains active in affected individuals, suggesting that the mutant TRβ has a dominant-negative effect (Parrilla et al., 1991; Weiss and Refetoff, 1992). A gene dosage effect is not operative, because heterozygous deletion of *THRB* does not result in disease and patients homozygous for *THRB* deletions are responsive to pharmacologic doses of thyroid hormone, unlike individuals heterozygous for hormone-binding-domain missense mutations (Weiss and Refetoff, 1992). In transfection assays, expression of mutant TRβ encoded by DNA cloned from affected individuals has been shown to repress the transactivation func-

TABLE 5.4. Thyroid hormone receptor β mutations
responsible for thyroid hormone resistance

Hormone-Binding Domain	DNA-Binding Domain
R316H	None
A317T	
R320H, R320C	
G332R	
T337Δ	
R338W	
Q340H	
G345R, G345N, G345V	
H435L, H435Q	
R438H	
M442V	
F451I	
P453T, P453H, P453S	

tion of both wild-type TRβ and TRα (Krishna et al., 1991; Ozata et al., 1995; Sakurai et al., 1990). The mechanism by which this occurs is unknown. The dominant-negative effect may be mediated by mutant TRβ-RXR heterodimers functioning as a repressor rather than an activator and/or may involve heterodimerization of wild-type and mutant TRβ (Zhu et al., 1996). In mice, homozygous inactivation of the *Thrb* gene encoding TRβ results in thyroid hormone resistance, indicating that some TRβ functions cannot be assumed by TRα (Forrest et al., 1996).

Vitamin D Receptor

Adequate intake and proper metabolism of vitamin D is required for normal bone and calcium homeostasis. After absorption from the gastrointestinal tract, vitamin D is subjected to two separate hydroxylation reactions to form the biologically active molecule 1, 25-dihydroxycholecalciferol (1, 25-dihydroxyvitamin D_3). All known biological effects of vitamin D are mediated by the binding of 1, 25-dihydroxyvitamin D_3 to the vitamin D receptor.

Type II Hereditary Vitamin D–Resistant Rickets

Hereditary vitamin D–resistant rickets (MIM 277440) is characterized by the clinically and radiographically demonstrable osseous deformities known as rickets, hypocalcemia, and secondary hyperparathyroidism, despite adequate vitamin D intake. Type I vitamin D–resistant rickets is due to inadequate production of 1, 25-dihydroxyvitamin D_3 due to deficiency of the enzyme 1α-hydroxylase (reviewed by Hewison and O'Riordan, 1994). In contrast, in type II vitamin D–resistant rickets, there is end organ resistance to 1, 25-dihydroxyvitamin D_3, a steroid hormone whose effects are mediated by the vitamin D receptor (VDR).

As in the case of the AR mutations in patients with androgen insensitivity syndrome, missense and nonsense mutations in the DNA binding domain (Fig. 5.3) and the hormone binding domain (Table 5.5) of the VDR have been identified in patients with type II vitamin D–resistant rickets (Hughes et al., 1988; Kristjansson et al., 1993; Malloy et al., 1997; Ritchie et al., 1989; Saijo et al., 1991; Sone et al., 1990). The autosomal recessive inheritance suggests that these mutations represent simple loss-of-function alleles. Thus, diseases involving mutations in genes encoding nuclear receptors demonstrate the three classical modes of mendelian inheritance: autosomal recessive (vitamin D–resistant rickets), autosomal dominant (thyroid hormone resistance syndromes), and X-linked recessive (androgen insensitivity syndromes).

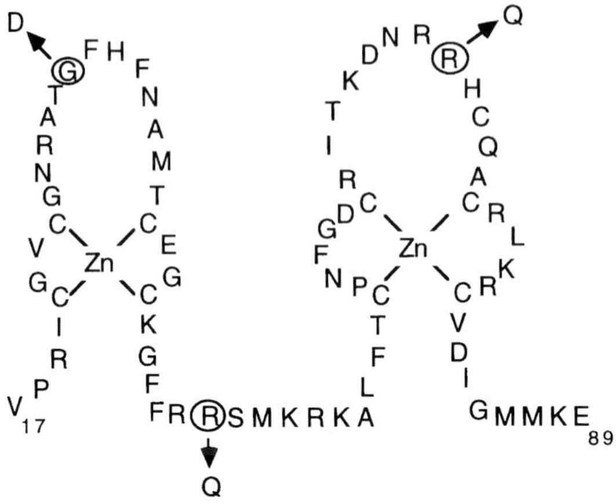

FIGURE 5-3. Mutations in the vitamin D receptor DNA-binding domain. Amino acid residues 17–89, spanning the zinc (Zn) finger DNA-binding domain, are shown.

As in the case of the AR, structure-function correlations have been made based on the analysis of *VDR* mutations that cause vitamin D–resistant rickets. The *VDR (Y292X)* allele encodes a truncated VDR that lacks amino acids 292–424 within the hormone binding domain and therefore cannot bind vitamin D or activate transcription (Ritchie et al., 1989). In contrast, the R271L missense mutation within the hormone binding domain decreases the affinity of the VDR for its ligand. In transfection assays, the mutant VDR activated transcription to wild-type levels but only in the presence of 1 µM vitamin D_3 as opposed to 1 nM required by the wild-type VDR (Kristjansson et al., 1993). Mutations in the DNA-binding domain do not affect ligand binding but have the same end result of eliminating transcriptional activation mediated by binding of the vitamin D_3-VDR-RXR complex to target DNA sequences. The

TABLE 5.5. Vitamin D receptor mutations responsible for type II vitamin D–resistant rickets

DNA-Binding Domain	Hormone-Binding Domain
G30D	Q149X
R47Q	R271L
R70Q	Y292X
	H305Q

H305Q mutation in the ligand-binding domain was shown to cause an eightfold decrease in the affinity of the VDR for $1,25(OH)_2D_3$ (Malloy et al., 1997). Treatment of the patient with cholecalciferol at a dosage that maintained the serum concentration of $1,25(OH)_2D_3$ 20–25-fold higher than normal levels was successful in eliminating hypercalcemia. Thus, the affinity defect of the receptor could be overcome by increasing the concentration of the ligand. Once the receptor-ligand complex formed, its ability to activate transcription was apparently normal. This study demonstrates that knowledge of the molecular defect is important because the finding of a missense mutation in the ligand-binding domain (of VDR as well as other nuclear hormone receptors) indicates the potential for successful pharmacologic therapy.

It also appears that mutations at loci other than *VDR* can affect VDR function and cause type II vitamin D–resistant rickets. In cells from one patient, binding of 1, 25-dihydroxyvitamin D_3 by the VDR appeared normal, but the hormone-receptor complex did not translocate to the nucleus (Hewison et al., 1993). Analysis of the *VDR* coding sequence failed to reveal a mutation, suggesting a defect in a protein with which VDR must interact in order to enter the nucleus and bind to DNA.

Osteoporosis

Loss of bone density (osteoporosis) occurs at high frequency in the elderly population, especially among females, with risk increasing as a function of age. Predisposition to the development of osteoporosis also segregates as a multifactorial trait indicating the contribution of both genetic and environmental factors (reviewed by Eisman, 1996). Given the important role of vitamin D in bone metabolism, the effect of genetic variation at the *VDR* locus on bone density was investigated. In order to eliminate the confounding effect of age, dizygotic twins were examined for bone density and genotyped using restriction fragment length polymorphisms (RFLPs) in the *VDR* gene (Morrison et al., 1994). The within-pair difference in bone density was significantly less in female twins that shared the same genotype relative to twins that were discordant for *VDR* genotype. The genotype associated with lower bone density in the twins was overrepresented in a second group of postmenopausal women with bone densities more than two standard deviations below the mean for premenopausal women, providing further evidence in support of the hypothesis that genetic variation at the *VDR* locus contributes to the predisposition to osteoporosis (Morrison et al., 1994).

These results were not replicated in subsequent studies by other investigators, but there are many potential confounding factors in this type of analysis, including activity level, age, calcium and vitamin intake, and other dietary factors (reviewed by Eisman, 1996). Taken together, the evidence at present suggests that genetic differences at the *VDR* locus may represent one factor that determines the risk of developing osteoporosis. Several other polymorphisms were in linkage disequilibrium with the RFLPs used for genotyping, including nucleotide differences in the 3'-untranslated region of the *VDR* gene that may affect VDR expression by increasing the mRNA stability (Morrison et al., 1994).

Prostate Cancer

Whereas osteoporosis is a major cause of morbidity and mortality among elderly females, prostate cancer is a major killer of older men. In the United States, mortality rates for prostate cancer are higher in the north than in the south, correlating inversely with exposure to ultraviolet radiation (Hanchette and Schwartz, 1992). Vitamin D is synthesized in the skin in response to UV irradiation, and higher serum 1, 25-dihydroxyvitamin D_3 levels are associated with a decreased risk of developing prostate cancer (Corder et al., 1993). To investigate whether genetic differences at the *VDR* locus contribute to the risk of developing prostate cancer, patients and controls were genotyped for the same RFLP (identified by the restriction endonuclease Taq I) utilized in the osteoporosis study. Men homozygous for the *t/t* genotype had one third the risk of developing prostate cancer as men with the *T/t* or *T/T* genotype (Taylor et al., 1996). Data from the osteoporosis study (Morrison et al., 1994) indicated that serum 1, 25-dihydroxyvitamin D_3 levels were significantly higher ($P = 0.0008$) in *t/t* individuals (134 ± 42 pM) compared with *T/t* or *T/T* individuals (104 ± 30 pM and 99 ± 40 pM, respectively).

Thus, genetic variation at the *VDR* locus may contribute significantly to two major causes of morbidity and mortality in the adult population. In each case, relatively subtle differences in *VDR* expression may interact with environmental and other genetic factors to determine an individual's risk of developing disease. Identifying such contributing genetic factors to common human diseases represents one of the greatest challenges for the field of medical genetics in the next century.

DAX-1

X-Linked Adrenal Hypoplasia Congenita

Both autosomal recessive and X-linked recessive forms of adrenal hypoplasia congenita (AHC) have been described in which normal adrenal

gland development is disturbed, resulting in profound hormonal deficiencies. X-linked adrenal hypoplasia congenita (MIM 300200) is characterized by glandular dysplasia, absence of the permanent zone of the
adrenal cortex, congenital adrenal insufficiency (deficient production of
glucocorticoids, mineralocorticoids, and androgens that is unresponsive
to administration of adrenocorticotropic hormone), and hypogonadotropic hypogonadism. Patients with X-linked adrenal hypoplasia congenita were found to have loss-of-function mutations in the *DAX1* gene
located at Xp21 that included frameshift and nonsense mutations as well
as whole gene deletions (Zanaria et al., 1994). In addition, a missense
mutation and a single amino-acid deletion, both in the putative ligand-
binding domain, were identified in two patients (Muscatelli et al, 1994).
DAX-1 mRNA and protein expression in adult tissues appeared to be
restricted to the adrenal gland and testis.

Sequence analysis revealed that *DAX1* encoded a 470-amino-acid
protein which at its carboxyl terminus (amino acids 253–470) showed
similarity to the ligand binding domain of nuclear receptor superfamily
members, especially the retinoid X receptor (RXR) subfamily (Fig. 5.4).
In contrast, the amino-terminal half of DAX-1 was unrelated to nuclear
receptors and instead contained four incomplete direct repeats of a 65–
67 amino acid sequence. Despite the lack of the zinc fingers that are
required for DNA binding by nuclear receptors, DAX-1 could compete
with retinoic acid receptor α (RARα) or RXRβ for binding to a retinoic
acid response element (RARE). However, whereas expression of RARα
or RXRβ resulted in transcriptional activation of a reporter gene containing a RARE, coexpression of DAX-1 repressed the transcription mediated

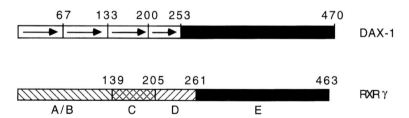

FIGURE 5-4. Structure of DAX-1. The 470-amino-acid residue DAX-1 protein is
shown schematically with the putative ligand-binding domain indicated by black
box and the four incomplete direct repeats indicated by the arrows. DAX-1 shares
26% amino-acid identity with the ligand-binding domain (E) of mouse RARγ.
The other domains of RARγ, including the zinc finger DNA-binding domain (C),
which are conserved in all other members of the nuclear receptor superfamily,
are not present in DAX-1. (Adapted from Zanaria et al., 1994.)

by RARα or RXRβ (Zanaria et al., 1994). Further studies will be required to determine whether these findings are relevant to the function of DAX-1 in vivo.

Dosage-Sensitive Sex Reversal

Several 46,XY individuals with sex reversal were shown to carry duplications of a region of the short arm of the X chromosome. The minimal duplication was a 160-kb region of Xp21, which was designated the *DSS* (dosage sensitive sex-reversal) locus (Bardoni et al., 1994). Although duplication of this locus caused sex reversal, its deletion had no effect on gonadal development. *DAX1* was mapped within the *DSS* critical region (Zanaria et al., 1994). During mouse embryogenesis, *Dax1* was expressed at the earliest stages of gonadal and adrenal development and expression was downregulated at the time of testicular differentiation but persisted in developing ovaries (Swain et al., 1996). The *Dax1* expression pattern in the developing gonads is consistent with a role in sex determination, suggesting that duplication of *DAX1* may in fact result in sex reversal. (The role of DAX-1 in sex determination is further considered in Chapter 10.) Furthermore, the expression of *Dax1* in the developing adrenals and hypothalamus (Swain et al., 1996) is consistent with the adrenal hypoplasia and hypogonadotropic hypogonadism associated with loss-of-function mutations in *DAX1* described above.

SF-1

Steroidogenic factor 1 (SF-1) was identified as a transcriptional regulator of genes encoding steroidogenic enzymes in cells of the adrenal cortex and shown to be the mammalian homologue of the *Drosophila* orphan nuclear receptor fushi tarazu factor 1 (Ftz-F1) (Honda et al., 1993; Lala et al., 1992; Rice et al., 1991). SF-1 expression was demonstrated in all primary steroidogenic tissues including adrenal cortex, testicular Leydig cells, and ovarian corpus luteum, theca, and granulosa cells (Ikeda et al., 1993). SF-1 expression was also detected in the urogenital ridge of mouse embryos at E9, the earliest stage of gonadogenesis, as well as in fetal Sertoli cells of the testis (Ikeda et al., 1994). Mice that were homozygous for a targeted disruption of the *Ftz-F1* (*Sf-1*) gene lacked adrenal glands and gonads and developed oviducts, uterus, and vagina regardless of their genetic sex (Luo et al., 1994). In these knockout mice, the ventromedial nucleus of the hypothalamus, which has been implicated in the neural control of reproductive behaviors, also did not develop properly (Ikeda et al., 1995), resulting in loss of pituitary gonadotropin production (Ingraham et al., 1994). Thus, like DAX-1, SF-1 appears to act at multiple levels of the reproductive axis and to play a key role in the development of the adrenals, gonads, and hypothalamus. Spontaneous mutations in the human or mouse gene encoding SF-1 have not yet been described.

RORα

Given the growing number of nuclear receptor superfamily members, the list of diseases due to mutations in these genes will also continue to grow rapidly. For example, RORα is an orphan (class IV) nuclear receptor that binds to DNA as a monomer and activates transcription in the absence of any known ligand (Giguere et al., 1994). Positional cloning of the gene responsible for the autosomal recessive *staggerer* phenotype in mice revealed a 122-bp frameshift deletion in the mRNA encoding RORα that is predicted to prevent synthesis of a functional protein (Hamilton et al., 1996). The *staggerer* phenotype is characterized by cerebellar ataxia due to a cell-autonomous defect in Purkinje cell development, and RORα mRNA was detected in Purkinje cell precursors of wild-type mice. Autosomal recessive, autosomal dominant, and X-linked recessive forms of hereditary cerebellar ataxia have been described in humans (a total of 154 MIM entries). One or more of these conditions may be caused by mutations in the human gene encoding RORα.

References

Baird, P. N., A. Santos, N. Groves, L. Jadresic, and J. K. Cowell. Constitutional mutations in the WT1 gene in patients with Denys-Drash syndrome. *Hum. Mol. Genet.* 1:301–305, 1992.

Bardoni, B., E. Zanaria, S. Guioli, G. Floridia, K. C. Worley, and G. Tonini. A dosage sensitive locus at chromosome Xp21 is involved in male to female sex reversal. *Nat. Genet.* 7:497–501, 1994.

Berg, J. M. DNA binding specificity of steroid receptors. *Cell* 57:1065–1068, 1989.

Bevan, C. L., B. B. Brown, H. R. Davies, B. A. J. Evans, I. A. Hughes, and M. N. Patterson. Functional analysis of six androgen receptor mutations identified in patients with partial androgen insensitivity syndrome. *Hum. Mol. Genet.* 5:265–273, 1996.

Brinkmann, A. O., G. Jenster, C. Ris-Stalpers, J. A. G. M. van der Korput, H. T. Bruggenwirth, A. L. M. Boehmer, and J. Trapman. Androgen receptor mutations. *J. Steroid Biochem. Mol. Biol.* 53:443–448, 1995.

Bruening, W., N. Bardessy, B. L. Silverman, R. A. Cohn, G. A. Machin, A. J. Aronson, D. Housman, and J. Pelletier. Germline intronic and exonic mutations in the Wilms' tumor gene (WT1) affecting urogenital development. *Nat. Genet.* 1:144–148, 1992.

Chamberlain, N. L., E. D. Driver, and R. L. Miesfeld. The length and location of CAG trinucleotide repeats in the androgen receptor N-terminal domain affect transactivation function. *Nucleic Acids Res.* 22:3181–3186, 1994.

Chrousos, G. P., S. Detera-Wadleigh, and M. Karl. Syndromes of glucocorticoid resistance. *Ann. Intern. Med.* 119:1113–1124, 1993.

Chrousos, G. P., A. Vingerhoeds, D. Brandon, C. Eil, M. Pugeat, M. DeVroede, D. L. Loriaux, and M. B. Lipsett. Primary cortisol resistance in man. *J. Clin. Invest.* 69:1261–1269, 1982.

Clark, G. M., and W. L. McGuire. Steroid receptors and other prognostic factors in primary breast cancer. *Semin. Oncol.* 15(suppl 1):20–25, 1988.

Corder, E. H., H. A. Guess, B. S. Hulka, G. D. Friedman, M. Sadler, R. T. Vollmer, B. Lobaugh, M. K. Drezner, J. H. Vogelman, and N. Orentreich. Vitamin D and prostate cancer: a prediagnostic study with stored sera. *Cancer Epidemiol. Biomarkers Prev.* 2:467–472, 1993.

Crichlow, R. W., and S. W. Galt. Male breast cancer. *Surg. Clin. North Am.* 70: 1165–1177, 1990.

Eisman, J. A. Vitamin D receptor gene variants: implications for therapy. *Curr. Opin. Genet. Devel.* 6:361–365, 1996.

Forrest, D., E. Hanebuth, R. J. Smeyne, N. Everds, C. L. Stewart, J. M. Wehner, and T. Curran. Recessive resistance to thyroid hormone in mice lacking thyroid hormone receptor β: evidence for tissue-specific modulation of receptor function. *EMBO J.* 15:3006–3015, 1996.

Fuqua, S. A., G. C. Chamness, and W. L. McGuire. Estrogen receptor mutations in breast cancer. *J. Cell. Biochem.* 51:135–139, 1993.

Giguere, V., M. Tini, G. Flock, E. S. Ong, R. M. Evans, and G Otulakowski. Isoform-specific amino-terminal domains dictate DNA-binding properties of RORα, a novel family of orphan nuclear receptors. *Genes Dev.* 8:538–553, 1994.

Gottlieb, B., M. Trifiro, R. Lumbroso, and L. Pinsky. The androgen receptor gene mutations database. *Nucleic Acids Res.* 25:158–162, 1997.

Green, S., P. Walter, V. Kumar, A. Krust, J.-M. Bornert, P. Argos, and P. Chambon. Human oestrogen receptor cDNA: sequence, expression and homology to v-erb-A. *Nature* 320:134–139, 1986.

Hackenberg, R., and K. D. Schulz. Androgen receptor mediated growth control of breast cancer and endometrial cancer modulated by antiandrogen- and androgen-like steroids. *J. Steroid Biochem. Mol. Biol.* 56:113–137, 1996

Hamilton, B. A., W. N. Frankel, A. W. Kerrebrock, T. L. Hawkins, W. FitzHugh, K. Kusumi, L. B. Russell, K. L. Mueller, V. van Berkel, B. W. Birren, L. Kruglyak, and E. S. Lander. Disruption of the nuclear hormone receptor RORα in staggerer mice. *Nature* 379:736–739, 1996.

Hanchette, C. L., and G. G. Schwartz. Geographic patterns of prostate cancer mortality: evidence for a protective effect of ultraviolet radiation. *Cancer* 70: 2861–2869, 1992.

Hausmanowa-Petrusewicz, I., J. Borkowska, and Z. Janczewski. X-linked adult form of spinal muscular atrophy. *J. Neurol.* 229:175–188, 1983.

Hewison, M., and J. L. O'Riordan. Hormone-nuclear receptor interactions in health and disease: vitamin D resistance. *Baillieres Clin. Endocrinol. Metab.* 8: 305–315, 1994.

Hewison, M., A. R. Rut, K. Kristjansson, R. E. Walker, M. J. Dillon, M. R. Hughes, and J. L. O'Riordan. Tissue resistance to 1,25-dihydroxyvitamin D without a mutation of the vitamin D receptor gene. *Clin. Endocrinol.* 39:663–670, 1993.

Hollenberg, S. M., C. Weinberger, E. S. Ong, G. Cerelli, A. E. Oro, R. Lebo, E. B. Thompson, M. G. Rosenfeld, and R. M. Evans. Primary structure and expression of a functional glucocorticoid receptor cDNA. *Nature* 318:635–641, 1985.

Honda, S.-I., K.-I. Morohashi, M. Nomura, H. Takeya, M. Kitajima, and T. Omura. Ad4BP-regulating steroidogenic P-450 gene is a member of the steroid hormone receptor superfamily. *J. Biol. Chem.* 268:7492–7502, 1993.

Hughes, M. R., P. J. Malloy, D. G. Kieback, R. A. Kesterson, J. W. Pike, D. Feldman, and B. W. O'Malley. Point mutations in the human vitamin D receptor gene associated with hypocalcemic rickets. *Science* 242:1702–1705, 1988.

Hurley, D. M., D. Accili, C. A. Stratakis, M. Karl, N. Vamvakopoulos, E. Rorer, K. Constantine, S. I. Taylor, and G. P. Chrousos. Point mutation causing a single amino acid substitution in the hormone binding domain of the glucocorticoid receptor in familial glucocorticoid resistance. *J. Clin. Invest.* 87: 680–686, 1991.

Ikeda, Y., D. S. Lala, X. Luo, E. Kim, M.-P. Moisan, and K. L. Parker. Characterization of the mouse FTZ-F1 gene, which encodes a key regulator of steroid hydroxylases. *Mol. Endocrinol.* 8:852–860, 1993.

Ikeda, Y., X. Luo, R. Abbud, J. H. Nilson, and K. L. Parker. The nuclear receptor steroidogenic factor 1 is essential for the formation of the ventromedial hypothalamic nucleus. *Mol. Endocrinol.* 9:478–486, 1995.

Ikeda, Y., W. H. Shen, H. A. Ingraham, and K. L. Parker. Developmental expression of mouse steroidogenic factor-1, an essential regulator of the steroid hydroxylases. *Mol. Endocrinol.* 8:654–662, 1994.

Ingraham, H. A., D. S. Lala, Y. Ikeda, X. Luo, W. H. Shen, M. W. Nachtigal, R. Abbud, J. H. Nilson, and K. L. Parker. The nuclear receptor steroidogenic factor 1 acts at multiple levels of the reproductive axis. *Genes Dev.* 8:2302–2312, 1994.

Jansson, M., L. Philipson, and B. Vennstrom. Isolation and characterization of multiple human genes homologous to the oncogenes of avian erythroblastosis virus. *EMBO J.* 2: 561–565, 1983.

Karl, M., S. W. Lamberts, S. D. Detera-Wadleigh, I. J. Encio, C. A. Stratakis, D. M. Hurley, D. Accili, and G. P. Chrousos. Familial glucocorticoid resistance caused by a splice site deletion in the human glucocorticoid receptor gene. *J. Clin. Endocrinol. Metab.* 76:683–689, 1993.

Kennedy, W. R., M. Alter, and J. H. Sung. Progressive proximal spinal and bulbar muscular atrophy of late onset: a sex-linked recessive trait. *Neurology* 18:671–680, 1968.

Kitajima, K., T. Nagaya, and J. L. Jameson. Dominant negative and DNA-binding properties of mutant thyroid hormone receptors that are defective in homodimerization but not heterodimerization. *Thyroid* 5:343–353, 1995.

Klocker, H., F. Kaspar, J. Eberle, S. Uberreiter, C. Radmayr, and G. Bartsch. Point mutation in the DNA binding domain of the androgen receptor in two families with Reifenstein syndrome. *Am. J. Hum. Genet.* 50:1318–1327, 1992.

Klug, A., and J. W. R. Schwabe. Zinc fingers. *FASEB J.* 9:597–604, 1995.

Krishna, V. K. K., T. Nagaya, L. D. Madison, S. Datta, A. Rentoumis, and J. L. Jameson. Thyroid hormone resistance syndrome: inhibition of normal receptor function by mutant thyroid hormone receptors. *J. Clin. Invest.* 87:1977–1984, 1991.

Kristjansson, K., A. R. Rut, M. Hervison, J. L. H. O'Riordan, and M. R. Hughes. Two mutations in the hormone binding domain of the vitamin D receptor cause tissue resistance to 1, 25 dihydroxyvitamin D_3. *J. Clin. Invest.* 92:12–16, 1993.

Kurokawa, R., J. DiRenzo, M. Boehm, J. Sugarman, B. Gloss, M. G. Rosenfeld, R. A. Heyman, and C. K. Glass. Regulation of retinoid signalling by receptor polarity and allosteric control of ligand binding. *Nature* 371:528–531, 1994.

Kurokawa, R., V. C. Yu, A. Naar, S. Kyakumoto, Z. Han, S Silverman, M. G. Rosenfeld, and C. K. Glass. Differential orientations of the DNA-binding domain and carboxy-terminal dimerization interface regulate binding site selection by nuclear receptor heterodimers. *Genes Dev.* 7:1423–1435, 1993.

Lala, D. S., D. A. Rice, and K. L. Parker. Steroidogenic factor 1, a key regulator of steroidogenic enzyme expression, is the mouse homolog of fushi tarazu factor 1. *Mol. Endocrinol.* 6:1249–1258, 1992.

LaSpada, A. R., E. Wilson, D. B. Lubahn, and K. H. Fishbeck. Androgen receptor gene mutations in X-linked spinal and bulbar muscular atrophy. *Nature* 352: 77–79, 1991.

Lazar, M. A., and W. W. Chin. Nuclear thyroid hormone receptors. *J. Clin. Invest.* 86: 1777–1782, 1990.

Lobaccaro, J.-M., S. Lumbroso, C. Belon, F. Galtier-Dereure, J. Bringer, T. Lesimple, J.-F. Heron, H. Pujol, and C. Sultan. Male breast cancer and the androgen receptor gene. *Nat. Genet.* 5:109–110, 1993a.

Lobaccaro, J.-M., S. Lumbroso, C. Belon, F. Galtier-Dereure, J. Bringer, T. Lesimple, M. Namer, B. F. Cutuli, H. Pujol, and C. Sultan. Androgen receptor gene mutation in male breast cancer. *Hum. Mol. Genet.* 2:1799–1802, 1993b.

Lobaccaro, J.- M., N. Poujol, L. Chiche, S. Lumbroso, T. R. Brown, and C. Sultan. Molecular modeling and in vitro investigations of the human androgen receptor DNA-binding domain: application for the study of two mutations. *Mol. Cell. Endocrinol.* 116:137–147, 1996.

Lubahn, D. B., T. R. Brown, J. A. Simental, H. N. Higgs, C. J. Migeon, E. M. Wilson, and J. S. French. Sequence of the intron/exon junctions of the coding region of the human androgen receptor gene and identification of a point mutation in a family with complete androgen insensitivity. *Proc. Natl. Acad. Sci. U.S.A.* 86:9534–9538, 1990.

Luo, X., Y. Ikeda, and K. L. Parker. A cell-specific nuclear receptor is essential for adrenal and gonadal development and sexual differentiation. *Cell* 77: 481–490, 1994.

MacLean, H. E., W. T. Choi, G. Rekaris, G. L. Warne, and J. D. Zajac. Abnormal androgen receptor binding affinity in subjects with Kennedy's disease (spinal and bulbar muscular atrophy). *J. Clin. Endocrinol. Metab.* 80:508–516, 1995.

Mader, S., P. Leroy, J.-Y. Chen, and P. Chambon. Multiple parameters control the selectivity of nuclear receptors for their response elements: selectivity and promiscuity in response element recognition by retinoic acid receptors and retinoid X receptors. *J. Biol. Chem.* 268:591–600, 1993.

Malloy, P. J., T. R. Eccleshall, C. Gross, L. Van Maldergem, R Bouillon, and D. Feldman. Hereditary vitamin D resistant rickets caused by a novel mutation in the vitamin D receptor that results in decreased affinity for hormone and cellular responsiveness. *J. Clin. Invest.* 99:297–304, 1997.

Mangelsdorf, D. J., and R. M. Evans. The RXR heterodimers and orphan receptors. *Cell* 83:841–850, 1995.

Mangelsdorf, D. J., C. Thummel, M. Beato, P. Herrlich, G. Schutz, K. Umesono,

B. Blumberg, P. Kastner, M. Mark, P. Chambon, and R. M. Evans. The nuclear receptor superfamily: the second decade. *Cell* 83:835–839, 1995.

Mangelsdorf, D. J., K. Umesono, and R. M. Evans. The retinoid receptors. In *The Retinoids: Biology, Chemistry, and Medicine*, M. B. Sporn, A. B. Roberts, and D. S. Goodman eds. New York: Raven Press, pp. 319–349, 1994.

Marcelli, M., W. D. Tilley, C. M. Wilson, J. E. Griffin, J. D. Wilson, and M. J. McPhaul. Definition of the human androgen receptor gene structure permits the identification of mutations that cause androgen resistance: premature termination of the receptor protein at amino acid residue 588 causes complete androgen resistance. *Mol. Endocrinol.* 4:1105–1116, 1990a.

Marcelli, M., W. D. Tilley, C. M. Wilson, J. E. Griffin, C. M. Wilson, J. D. Wilson, and M. J. McPhaul. A single nucleotide substitution introduces a premature termination codon into the androgen receptor gene of a patient with receptor-negative androgen resistance. *J. Clin. Invest.* 85:1522–1528, 1990b.

Marcelli, M., S. Zoppi, P. B. Grino, J. E. Griffin, J. D. Wilson, and M. J. McPhaul. A mutation in the DNA-binding domain of the androgen receptor gene causes complete testicular feminization in a patient with receptor-positive androgen resistance. *J. Clin. Invest.* 87:1123–1126, 1991.

Martinez, E., D. D. Moore, E. Keller, D. Pearce, V. Robinson, P. N. MacDonald, S. S. Simons Jr., E. Sanchez, and M. Danielsen. The nuclear receptor resource project. *Nucleic Acids Res.* 25:163–165, 1997.

McPhaul, M. J., M. Marcelli, W. D. Tilley, J. E. Griffin, R. F. Isidoro-Guiteres, and J. D. Wilson. Molecular basis of androgen resistance in a family with a qualitative abnormality of the AR and responsive to high-dose androgen therapy. *J. Clin. Invest.* 87:1413–1416, 1991.

McPhaul, M. J., M. Marcelli, S. Zoppi, C. M. Wilson, J. E. Griffin, and J. D. Wilson. Mutations in the ligand-binding domain of the androgen receptor gene cluster in two regions of the gene. *J. Clin. Invest.* 90:2097–2101, 1992.

Mhatre, A. N., M. A. Trifiro, M. Kaufman, P. Kazemi-Esfarjani, D. Figlewicz, G. Rouleau, and L. Pinsky. Reduced transcriptional regulatory competence of the androgen receptor in X-linked spinal and bulbar muscular atrophy. *Nat. Genet.* 5:184–188, 1993.

Morrison, N. A., J. C. Qi, A. Tokita, P. J. Kelly, L. Crofts, T. V. Nguyen, P. N. Sambrook, and J. A. Eisman. Prediction of bone density from vitamin D receptor alleles. *Nature* 367:284–287, 1994.

Muscatelli, F., T. M. Strom, A. P. Walker, E. Zanaria, D. Recan, A. Meindl, B. Bardoni, S. Guioli, G. Zehetner, W. Rabl, H. P. Schwartz, J.-C. Kaplan, G. Camerino, T. Meitinger, and A. P. Monaco. Mutations in the DAX-1 gene give rise to both X-linked adrenal hypoplasia congenita and hypogonadotropic hypogonadism. *Nature* 372:672–676, 1994.

Naar, A. M., J.-M. Boutin, S. M. Lipkin, V. C. Yu, J. M. Holloway, C. K. Glass, and M. G. Rosenfeld. The orientation and spacing of core DNA-binding motifs dictate selective transcriptional responses to three nuclear receptors. *Cell* 65:1267–1279, 1991.

Newmark, J. R., D. O. Hardy, D. C. Tonb, B. S. Carter, J. I. Epstein, W. B. Isaacs, T. R. Brown, and E. R. Barrack. Androgen receptor gene mutations in human prostate cancer. *Proc. Natl. Acad. Sci. U. S. A.* 89:6319–6323, 1992.

Ozata, M., S. Suzuki, T. Takeda, D. G. Malkin, T. Miyamoto, R. T. Liu, N. Suzuki, J. D. Silverberg, D. Daneman, and L. J. DeGroot. Functional analysis of a proline to serine mutation in codon 453 of the thyroid hormone receptor beta 1 gene. *J. Clin. Endocrinol. Metab.* 80:3239–3245, 1995.

Parrilla, R., A. J. Mixson, J. A. McPherson, J. H. McClaskey, and B. D. Weintraub. Characterization of seven novel mutations of the c-erbAβ gene in unrelated kindreds with generalized thyroid hormone resistance. *J. Clin. Invest.* 88: 2123–2130, 1991.

Pelletier, J., W. Bruening, C. E. Kashtan, S. M. Mauer, J. C. Manivel, J. E. Striegel, D. C. Houghton, C. Junien, R. Habib, L. Fouser, R. N. Fine, B. L. Silverman, D. A. Haber, and D. Housman. Germline mutations in the Wilms' tumor suppressor gene are associated with abnormal urogenital development in Denys-Drash syndrome. *Cell* 67:437–447, 1991.

Perlmann, T., P. N. Rangarajan, K. Umesono, and R. M. Evans. Determinants for selective RAR and TR recognition of direct repeat HREs. *Genes Dev.* 7:1411–1422, 1993.

Refetoff, S. Resistance to thyroid hormone: an historical overview. *Thyroid* 4:345–349, 1994.

Rice, D. A., A. R. Mouw, A. M. Bogerd, and K. L. Parker. A shared promoter element regulates the expression of three steroidogenic enzymes. *Mol. Endocrinol.* 5:1552–1561, 1991.

Ris-Stalpers, C., M. A. Trifiro, G. G. J. M. Kuiper, G. Jenster, G. Romalo, T. Sai, H. C. J. van Rooij, M. Kaufman, R. L. Rosenfield, and A. O. Brinkmann. Substitution of aspartic acid-686 by histidine or asparagine in the human androgen receptor leads to a functionally inactive protein with altered hormone-binding characteristics. *Mol. Endocrinol.* 5:1562–1569, 1991.

Ris-Stalpers, C., M. C. T. Verleun-Mooijman, T .J. P. de Blaeij, H. J. Degenhart, J. Trapman, and A. O. Brinkmann. Differential splicing of human androgen receptor pre-mRNA in X-linked Reifenstein syndrome, because of a deletion involving a putative branch site. *Am. J. Hum. Genet.* 54:609–617, 1994.

Ritchie, H. H., M. R. Hughes, E. T. Thompson, P. J. Malloy, Z. Hochberg, D. Feldman, J. W. Pike, and B. W. O'Malley. An ochre mutation in the vitamin D receptor gene causes hereditary 1, 25-dihydroxyvitamin D_3-resistant rickets in three families. *Proc. Natl. Acad. Sci. U.S.A.* 86:9783–9787, 1989.

Sai, T., S. Seino, C. Chang, M. Trifiro, L. Pinsky, A. Mhatre, M. Kaufman, B. Lambert, J. Trapman, A. O. Brinkmann, R. L. Rosenfield, and S. Liao. An exonic point mutation of the androgen receptor gene in a family with complete androgen insensitivity. *Am. J. Hum. Genet.* 46:1095–1100, 1990.

Saijo, T., M. Ito, E. Takeda, A. H. M. Mahbubul Huq, E. Naito, I. Yokota, T. Sone, J. W. Pike, and V. Kuroda. A unique mutation in the vitamin D receptor gene in three Japanese patients with vitamin D-dependent rickets type II: utility of single-strand conformation polymorphism analysis for heterozygous carrier detection. *Am. J. Hum. Genet.* 49:668–673, 1991.

Sakurai, A., T. Miyamoto, S. Refetoff, and L. DeGroot. Dominant negative transcriptional regulation by a mutant thyroid hormone receptor-β in a family with generalized resistance to thyroid hormone. *Mol. Endocrinol.* 4:1988–1994, 1990.

Sap, J., A. Munoz, K. Damm, Y. Goldberg, J. Ghysdael, A. Leutz, H. Beug, and B. Vennstrom. The c-erb-A protein is a high-affinity receptor for thyroid hormone. *Nature* 324: 635–640, 1986.

Scher, H. I., and S. Fossa. Prostate cancer in the era of prostate-specific antigen. *Curr. Opin. Oncol.* 7:281–291, 1995.

Smith, E. P., J. Boyd, G. R. Frank, H. Takahashi, R. M. Cohen, B. Specker, T. C. Williams, D. B. Lubahn, and K. S. Korach. Estrogen resistance caused by a mutation in the estrogen-receptor gene in a man. *N. Engl. J. Med.* 331:1056–1061, 1994.

Sone, T., S. J. Marx, U. A. Liberman, and J. W. Pike. A unique point mutation in the human vitamin D receptor gene confers hereditary resistance to 1, 25 dihydroxyvitamin D$_3$. *Mol. Endocrinol.* 4:623–631, 1990.

Swain, A., E. Zanaria, A. Hacker, R. Lovell-Badge, and G. Camerino. Mouse Dax1 expression is consistent with a role in sex determination as well as in adrenal and hypothalamus function. *Nat. Genet.* 12:404–409, 1996.

Taylor, J. A., A. Hirvonen, M. Watson, G. Pittman, J. L. Mohler, and D. A. Bell. Association of prostate cancer with vitamin D receptor gene polymorphism. *Cancer Res.* 56:4108–4110, 1996.

Thomas, D. B., L. M. Jimenez, A. McTiernan, K. Rosenblatt, H. Stalsberg, A. Stemhagen, W. D. Thompson, M. G. Curnen, W. Satariano, D. F. Austin, R. S. Greenberg, C. Key, L. N. Lolonel, and D. W. West. Breast cancer in men: risk factors with hormonal implications. *Am. J. Epidemiol.* 135:734–748, 1992.

Tsukaguchi, H., Y. Yoshimasa, K. Fujimoto, H. Ishii, T. Yamamoto, T. Yoshimasa, T. Yagura, and J. Takamatsu. Three novel mutations of thyroid hormone receptor beta gene in unrelated patients with resistance to thyroid hormone: two mutations of the same codon (H435L and H435Q) produce separate subtypes of resistance. *J. Clin. Endocrinol. Metab.* 80:3613–3616, 1995.

Umesono, K., K. K. Murakami, C. C. Thompson, and R. M. Evans. Direct repeats as selective response elements for the thyroid hormone, retinoic acid, and vitamin D$_3$ receptors. *Cell* 65:1255–1266, 1991.

Visakorpi, T., E. Hyytinen, P. Koivisto, M. Tanner, R. Keinanen, C. Palmberg, A. Palotie, T. Tammela, J. Isola, O. P. Kallioniemi. In vivo amplification of the androgen receptor gene and progression of human prostate cancer. *Nat. Genet.* 9:401–406, 1995.

Warner, C. L., J. E. Griffin, J. D. Wilson, L. D. Jacobs, K. R. Murray, K. H. Fishbeck, D. Dickoff, and R. C. Griggs. X-linked spinomuscular atrophy: a kindred with associated abnormal androgen receptor binding. *Neurology* 42: 2181–2184, 1992.

Weinberger, C., C. C. Thompson, E. S. Ong, R. Lebo, D. J. Gruol, and R. M. Evans. The c-erb-A gene encodes a thyroid hormone receptor. *Nature* 324:641–646, 1986.

Weis, K. E, K. Ekena, J. A. Thomas, G. Lazennec, and B. S. Katzenellenbogen. Constitutively active human estrogen receptors containing amino acid substitutions for tyrosine 537 in the receptor protein. *Mol. Endocrinol.* 10:1388–1398, 1996.

Weiss, R. E., and S. Refetoff. Thyroid hormone resistance. *Annu. Rev. Med.* 93: 363–375, 1992.

Wilson, J. D., F. W. George, and J. E. Griffin. The hormonal control of sexual development. *Science* 211:1278–1284, 1981a.

Wilson, J. D., J. E. Griffin, M. Leshin, and F. W. George. Role of gonadal hormones in development of the sexual phenotypes. *Hum. Genet.* 58:78–84, 1981b.

Wilson, J. D., F. W. George, and M. B. Renfree. The endocrine role in mammalian sexual differentiation. *Recent Prog. Horm. Res.* 50:349–64, 1995.

Wooster, R., J. Mangion, R. Eeles, S. Smith, M. Dowsett, D. Averill, P. Barrett-Lee, D. F. Easton, B. A. J. Ponder, and M. R. Stratton. A germline mutation in the androgen receptor gene in two brothers with breast cancer and Reifenstein syndrome. *Nat. Genet.* 2:132–134, 1992.

Zanaria, E., F. Muscatelli, B. Bardoni, T. M. Strom, S. Guioli, W. Guo, E. Lalli, C. Moser, A. P. Walker, E. R. B. McCabe, T. Meitinger, A. P. Monaco, P. Sassone-Corsi, and G. Camerino. An unusual member of the nuclear hormone receptor superfamily responsible for X-linked adrenal hypoplasia congenita. *Nature* 372:635–641, 1994.

Zechel, C., X.-Q. Shen, J.-Y. Chen, P. Chambon, and H. Gronemeyer. The dimerization interfaces formed between the DNA binding domains of RXR, RAR and TR determine the binding specificity and polarity of the full-length receptors to direct repeats. *EMBO J.* 13:1425–1433, 1994.

Zhu, X. G., C. L. Yu, P. McPhie, R. Wong, and S. Y. Cheng. Understanding the molecular mechanism of dominant negative action of mutant thyroid hormone beta 1–receptors: the important role of the wild-type/mutant receptor heterodimer. *Endocrinology* 137:712–721, 1996.

Zoppi, S., M. Marcelli, J.-P. Deslypere, J. E. Griffin, J. D. Wilson, and M. J. McPhaul. Amino acid substitutions in the DNA-binding domain of the human androgen receptor are a frequent cause of receptor-binding positive androgen resistance. *Mol. Endocrinol.* 6:409–415, 1992.

Other Zinc Finger Proteins: 6
WT1 and GLI3

Although the nuclear receptor superfamily has an impressive and steadily growing number of members, it represents only a small subset of all known zinc finger transcription factors. Among the dozens of other such factors encoded in the human genome, defects in WT1 and GLI3 have been associated with human malformation syndromes and, in the case of WT1, predisposition to tumorigenesis.

WT1

The WAGR Syndrome

Germline deletions of chromosome 11p13 result in the autosomal dominant WAGR syndrome (MIM 194072), which is characterized by predisposition to Wilms tumor, congenital aniridia, genitourinary malformations, and mental retardation (Riccardi et al., 1978). A contiguous gene syndrome was proposed as the basis for the pleiotropic phenotypic manifestations (Schmickel, 1986). The predisposition to Wilms tumor (nephroblastoma) was proposed to be caused by the presence of an inactivating germline mutation (the 11p13 deletion) that was present in all cells of the target organ (the kidney). If tumorigenesis required the inactivation of both alleles of a "tumor suppressor" gene within a single cell, then the likelihood of this occurring would be greatly increased by the presence of the first "hit" within all cells of the target organ (Knudson, 1971). The presence of multifocal, bilateral tumors of earlier onset in patients with WAGR syndrome compared to patients with isolated, nonhereditary Wilms tumor was also consistent with this "two-hit" hypothesis (Knudson and Strong, 1972). A putative Wilms tumor suppressor gene, WT1, was identified within the region of the 11p13 deletion and shown to encode a transcription factor containing four $(Cys)_2$ $(His)_2$ zinc fingers (Call et al., 1990; Gessler et al., 1990; Ton et al., 1991). *WT1* mutations were subsequently identified in Wilms tumors from patients with WAGR syndrome as well as patients with isolated, nonhereditary Wilms tumors (Baird et al., 1992a; Cowell et al., 1991; Davis et al., 1991; Haber et al., 1990; Haber and Housman, 1992; Huff et al., 1991; Little et al., 1992; Ton et al., 1991).

WT1 is expressed in condensing mesenchyme, renal vesicle, and glomerular epithelium of the developing kidney (Pritchard-Jones et al., 1990). The structure of WT1 is similar to another zinc finger transcription factor, EGR1, and both factors bind to the DNA sequence 5'-CGCCCCCGC-3' (Rauscher et al., 1990). EGR1 is a transcriptional activator that accumulates in the nucleus after induction by various mitogenic stimuli, whereas WT1 is a transcriptional repressor (Drummond et al., 1992; Madden et al., 1991; Wang et al., 1992). These results suggest that WT1 may inhibit cellular proliferation by opposing the action of EGR1 and initiate a program of gene expression leading to kidney differentiation. In the absence of WT1, EGR1 action is unopposed, leading to uncontrolled cellular proliferation and tumor formation.

The importance of WT1 for normal development of the kidneys and genitourinary system is further supported by the analysis of patients with Denys-Drash syndrome and mice deficient for Wt1, as described below. Thus, two components of the WAGR phenotype, Wilms tumor and genitourinary malformations, are in fact due to deletion of a single gene, *WT1*. However, the WAGR syndrome does represent a contiguous gene syndrome because loss of WT1 function does not cause aniridia or mental retardation. Aniridia is caused by the deletion of a second gene at 11p13 that also encodes a transcription factor, PAX6, which will be described in Chapter 7.

Denys-Drash Syndrome

WT1 mRNA was detected in the developing genitourinary system (Pelletier et al., 1991c), suggesting that the genitourinary malformations of the WAGR syndrome might also be related to the deletion of *WT1*. This hypothesis was supported by the analysis of DNA from patients with the Denys-Drash syndrome (MIM 194080), an autosomal dominant disorder characterized by renal dysgenesis, with renal failure by age 2 years; bilateral, early-onset Wilms tumor; and genital abnormalities, including male pseudohermaphroditism (ambiguous or female external genitalia), streak (dysplastic) gonads, and predisposition to gonadoblastoma (Drash et al., 1970). Germline missense mutations that result in amino acid substitutions in zinc fingers 1, 2, and 3 of WT1 (Fig. 6.1) have been identified in genomic DNA from patients with the Denys-Drash syndrome (Baird et al., 1992b; Bruening et al., 1992; Little et al., 1993; Pelletier et al., 1991a). These missense mutations result in substitution either of an essential cysteine or histidine residue, such that the basic zinc finger structure cannot form, or of an amino acid that directly contacts the DNA binding site sequence. In addition, nonsense mutations that result in the synthesis of a truncated protein lacking two or more of the zinc fingers have been identified (Baird et al., 1992b; Little et al., 1993). In all cases tested, the mutations reduced or eliminated the binding of WT1 protein to target DNA sequences (Borel et al., 1996; Little et al., 1995).

The genotype-phenotype comparison for the WAGR and Denys-Drash syndromes is instructive. Both syndromes include a predisposition to Wilms tumor, due to an inactivating germline deletion (WAGR) or point mutation (Denys-Drash) involving *WT1*. In the WAGR syndrome, the genitourinary malformations are mild, consisting of hypospadias, in which the urethral orifice is located on the ventral shaft of the penis, and cryptorchidism, in which the testes have not descended into the scrotum (Baird et al., 1992b; Pelletier et al., 1991b; van Heyningen et al., 1990), and are presumably due to a gene dosage effect resulting from a 50% reduction in the levels of WT1 protein. In contrast, the *WT1* point mutations associated with the Denys-Drash syndrome are associated with a more severe disruption of normal genitourinary development, indicating either a dominant negative effect (i.e., the mutant gene product interferes

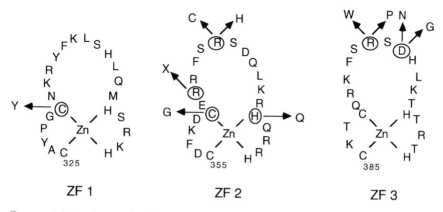

FIGURE 6-1. Amino acid substitutions in the zinc fingers of WT1 associated with Denys-Drash syndrome. The first amino acid of each zinc finger is numbered relative to the initiator methionine. X, introduction of a stop codon.

with the function of the wild-type gene product) or a gain-of-function effect (i.e., the mutant protein has a novel DNA-binding specificity or otherwise acquires biological activity not possessed by the wild-type protein). This conclusion is consistent with the fact that in the WAGR syndrome the mutant allele produces no WT1 protein, whereas in Denys-Drash syndrome the mutant allele always produces a mutant protein in which sequences amino-terminal to the zinc fingers remain intact (Little et al., 1993).

The only mutation associated with Denys-Drash syndrome that does not result in an amino acid substitution in a zinc finger of WT1 is an intervening sequence mutation that eliminates the production of two WT1 isoforms that are normally generated by alternative splicing (Bruening et al., 1992). Of interest, the patient in whom this mutation was identified did not develop Wilms tumor. Of the four WT1 isoforms generated by alternative splicing, isoforms A and B bind to the EGR1 binding site described above and mediate transcriptional repression, whereas isoforms C and D do not bind to the EGR1 site and their function is undefined (Bickmore et al., 1992; Madden et al., 1991; Morris et al., 1991; Rauscher et al., 1990). As a result of alternative splicing, an insertion of three amino acids between the third and fourth zinc fingers is present in isoforms C and D but absent in isoforms A and B. The C and D isoforms are eliminated by the intervening sequence mutation (Bruening et al., 1992). These results suggest that loss of binding of WT1 isoforms C and D to a second recognition site may result in genitourinary malformations.

Wt1 Knockout Mice

The key role played by WT1 in directing normal genitourinary development has also been established by the inactivation of the mouse *Wt1* gene by homologous recombination (Kreidberg et al., 1993). Mice that were heterozygous for the inactivated *Wt1* allele appeared normal and did not develop tumors. Thus, the phenotype associated with the heterozygosity for a null allele at the *WT1* locus in humans was not observed in the mouse strain (C57BL/6) studied. Homozygosity for a null allele at the *WT1* locus has not been reported in humans. Mice homozygous for the *Wt1* null allele died by embryonic day 15 (E15) as a result of cardiac defects. However, in addition, these mice manifested failure of normal renal development with metanephric blastemal cell death and absence of ureteric bud growth (Kreidberg et al., 1993). Gonadal development was arrested at an early stage, a finding similar to the streak gonads associated with Denys-Drash syndrome (Pelletier et al., 1991a).

Although these results suggest differences in the function of WT1 in humans and mice, they also provide strong evidence that WT1 function is essential for normal cardiac, gonadal, and renal development.

GLI3

Greig Syndrome

Greig cephalopolysyndactyly syndrome (MIM 175700) is an autosomal dominant disorder affecting limb and craniofacial development (Greig, 1926; reviewed by Jones, 1988). It is characterized by postaxial polydactyly of the hands, preaxial polydactyly of the feet, macrocephaly with a prominent forehead, hypertelorism, and a broad nasal bridge (Fig. 6.2). The locus for Greig cephalopolysyndactyly syndrome was mapped by the analysis of three familial balanced translocations and two isolated cases with overlapping microdeletions to chromosome 7p13, and all three translocations were found to have breakpoints within or near the

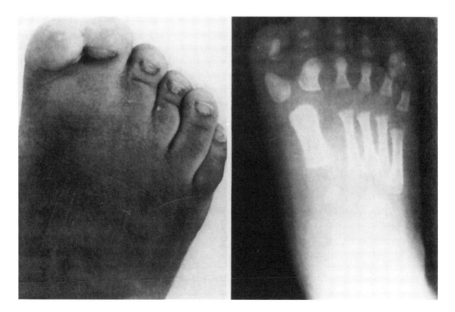

FIGURE 6-2. Malformations in Greig cephalopolysyndactyly syndrome. Preaxial polysyndactyly, manifested by duplication of right great toe. (Reprinted with permission from Duncan et al., 1979. Copyright © 1979 by the American Medical Association.)

GLI3 gene, which spans at least 280 kilobases (Vortkamp et al., 1991, 1995). Two breakpoints interrupted the coding sequence and the third was located 10 kb 3' to the coding sequence. GLI3 encodes a transcription factor that is a member of the GLI-Kruppel family of proteins, which are characterized by the presence of five zinc fingers (Ruppert et al., 1988). Genes encoding the GLI-Kruppel family members *cubitus interruptus* (*ci*) and *tra-1* have been shown to play key roles in *Drosophila* and *Xenopus* development, respectively (Orenic et al., 1990; Zarkower and Hodgkin, 1992). In addition, the GLI3 gene was originally isolated in hybridization experiments that utilized as a probe the GLI gene, which encodes a related zinc finger factor that is amplified in glioblastomas (Ruppert et al., 1990). Thus, a zinc finger transcription factor, GLI3, is implicated in a human malformation syndrome.

extra-toes

Two alleles at the mouse *extra-toes* (*Xt*) locus were characterized as representing partial nonoverlapping intragenic deletions of *Gli3* that result in an autosomal dominant syndrome of craniofacial defects, forelimb postaxial polydactyly, and hindlimb preaxial polydactyly that is remarkably similar to Greig cephalopolysyndactyly syndrome (Hui and Joyner, 1993; Vortkamp et al., 1992). The *Xt* alleles are lethal in the homozygous state and affected animals manifest severe polysyndactyly, with as many as eight digits per foot, severe craniofacial defects, and severe brain malformations such as exencephaly due to a defect in neural tube closure at the midbrain level. *In situ* and blot hybridization experiments demonstrated expression of Gli3 mRNA in the developing brain, craniofacial structures, and limbs of wild-type mouse embryos and a lack of expression in Xt^J/Xt^J homozygotes (Hui and Joyner, 1993). Because both *Xt* alleles studied were intragenic deletions, one of which removed the 5' end of the gene (Vortkamp et al., 1992), and were associated with decreased expression of *Gli3* (Hui and Joyner, 1993; Schimmang et al., 1992), it is likely that a loss-of-function or gene dosage effect is responsible for the pathophysiology of this disorder as well as Greig cephalopolysyndactyly syndrome. The gene dosage effect is most evident with respect to the *Xt* alleles of the mouse, in which it was possible to correlate severity of phenotype with partial and complete loss of *Gli3* expression in heterozygotes and homozygotes, respectively.

Polydactyly Nagoya

Polydactyly Nagoya (Pdn) mice manifest a phenotype that is similar to *Xt* mice due to allelic mutations in the *Gli3* gene (Schimmang et al., 1994).

In these mice, polydactyly has been associated with decreased cell death in the preaxial mesoderm (Naruse and Kameyama, 1984, 1989), whereas arhinencephaly in *Pdn* homozygotes is associated with increased apoptosis in the brain (Keino et al., 1994), suggesting that GLI3 participates in life-or-death decisions during development that are cell-type-specific. Treatment of *Pdn* fetuses *in utero* with cytosine arabinoside, which induces cell death, resulted in decreased frequency of polydactyly (Naruse and Kameyama, 1984, 1986), providing further evidence that the limb defects in *Pdn* mice were due to a reduction in developmentally programmed cell death as a consequence of reduced Gli3 expression.

anterior digit deformity

When exogenous DNA that is microinjected into fertilized mouse eggs integrates into the mouse genome, it may disrupt the expression of an endogenous mouse gene, a process known as insertional mutagenesis. Insertional mutagenesis is estimated to affect perhaps 15% of transgenic mice so that when mice homozygous for the transgene are generated by mating of heterozygotes, a phenotype is evident. One recessive phenotype identified in a homozygous transgenic mouse was *anterior digit deformity* (*add*), characterized by malformations that were restricted to the anterior part of the forelimb and that were caused by transgene integration 5' to *Gli3* coding sequences that resulted in reduced expression of the gene (Pohl et al., 1990; Schimmang et al., 1993; van der Hoeven et al., 1993). Although the relative level of *Gli3* expression in *add* homozygotes compared to wild-type mice has not been determined, it is clear that homozygosity for *add* results in a milder phenotype than what is observed in *Xt* heterozygotes (in which *Gli3* expression is 50% of wild-type levels), suggesting that residual *Gli3* expression in *add* homozygotes is greater than 50% of wild-type levels. However, the possibility that *Gli3* expression levels are affected by the transgene insertion to different degrees in different tissues cannot be excluded. These results provide further evidence that the severity of malformations is proportional to the level of *Gli3* expression.

The precise structures of the human and mouse genes encoding GLI3 have not been completely elucidated, and thus the mechanisms by which the transgene integration 5' to the mouse coding sequences and the translocation 3' to the human coding sequences affect expression have not been determined; these rearrangements may occur either within untranslated sequences or within flanking sequences, and thus could potentially exert their effects at the transcriptional and/or posttranscriptional level. The study of spontaneous mutations in homologous human and mouse genes resulting in analagous malformation syndromes has provided a powerful new approach to understanding both human malformation syndromes and normal mammalian development.

Pallister-Hall Syndrome

The cardinal features of the autosomal-dominant Pallister-Hall syndrome (MIM 146510) include hypothalamic hamartoblastoma, hypopituitarism, imperforate anus, and postaxial polydactyly (Fig. 6.3) (Hall et al., 1980). A genome-wide search for linkage was performed by analyzing DNA from 32 affected and 36 unaffected members of four families, resulting in linkage to the marker D7S691 on chromosome 7p13 with a LOD score of 8.04 at $\theta = 0$ (Kang et al., 1996). Further analysis placed the locus in a 3 Mb region containing the genes encoding GLI3 and inhibin βA. Both of these genes were excellent candidates because *GLI3* mutations were already known to cause polydactyly (see above) and inhibin βA was expressed in the hypothalamus (Kang et al., 1996).

Analysis of the *GLI3* gene in two families with Pallister-Hall syndrome revealed mutations in exon 14 (Kang et al., 1997). In these two families, affected individuals were heterozygous for a single base-pair

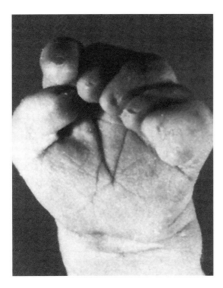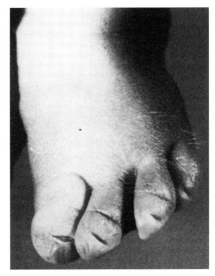

FIGURE 6-3. Limb defects in Pallister-Hall syndrome. Hand and foot of an affected newborn are shown. There are seven digits on the hand and only four digits on the foot. (Reprinted with permission from Hall et al., 1980. Copyright ©1980 by Wiley-Liss Inc., a subsidiary of John Wiley & Sons, Inc.)

deletion. In the two families, the mutant alleles contained deletions (2023delG and 2012delG, respectively) located 11 bp apart that resulted in a frameshift truncation after codon 691 of the 1596–amino-acid coding sequence. The resulting proteins contained the zinc finger DNA-binding domains but lacked the carboxyl-terminal half of the molecule. Thus, whereas Greig syndrome is caused by loss-of-function mutations in *GLI3*, the more severe Pallister-Hall syndrome is caused by mutations that truncate the protein, strongly suggesting a dominant-negative mechanism for pathogenesis of the associated malformations. It is likely that the mutant GLI3 protein can bind to its target sites in genomic DNA but cannot activate transcription and, by competing for DNA binding, prevents the wild-type protein from activating transcription as well. Assuming that the carboxyl-terminal half of GLI3 contains multiple transactivation domains, one can imagine that the more carboxyl-terminal the location of the protein truncation, the less severe the associated malformation phenotype. Thus, patients who do not meet strict criteria for Pallister-Hall syndrome but contain one or more of its cardinal features should be examined for evidence of mutations in *GLI3*. (The principle that more subtle mutations may underlie nonclassical phenotypes is illustrated by the discussion of *PAX2* mutations in Chapter 7.)

Signal Transduction Pathways in Limb Development

During early limb development the proximo-distal (long bones to digits) and anteroposterior (first to fifth digits) axes are established via two specialized morphologic structures. The anterior ectodermal ridge, which extends from anterior to posterior along the distal tip of the limb bud, contains undifferentiated, proliferating mesenchyme cells necessary for continued proximo-distal limb outgrowth. The zone of polarizing activity (ZPA), present in the posterior aspect of the limb bud, determines the anteroposterior axis by the secretion of the SONIC HEDGEHOG (SHH) protein, and transplantation of a ZPA on to the anterior aspect of the limb bud results in mirror image duplications of digits (reviewed by Roberts and Tabin, 1994). Mice lacking SHH expression do not form distal limb structures (Chiang et al., 1996). Binding of SHH to its receptor, PATCHED (PTC), inhibits the ability of PTC to interfere with the function of SMOOTHENED (SMO), a seven-transmembrane signaling protein (Stone et al., 1996). SHH induces expression of *GLI* in the limb bud and the observation that loss-of-function mutations in *PTC* (basal cell nevus syndrome) can result in polysyndactyly suggests that *GLI3* may also be a target of SHH (reviewed by Scott, 1997). Further studies

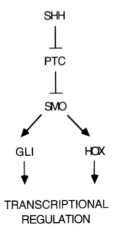

FIGURE 6-4. Genetic interactions in limb development. SHH inhibits PTC, which, in the absence of SHH, inhibits SMO. Signaling via SMO (in the presence of SHH and absence of PTC activity) leads to expression of the GLI and HOX families of transcription factors.

will undoubtedly provide fascinating insights into the relationship between *GLI3* and upstream signaling molecules such as SHH, PTC, and SMO (Fig. 6.4), and possible downstream transcription factors such as those encoded by the *HOX* genes (see Chapter 9). The CUBITUS INTERRUPTUS (CI) protein of *Drosophila melanogaster*, which is homologous to the mammalian GLI proteins, can function as a transcriptional activator or repressor, depending on whether or not proteolytic processing of the primary polypeptide has occurred, a process that is regulated by HEDGEHOG signaling (reviewed by Ruiz i Altaba, 1997). In mammals, transmission of the SHH signal may utilize transcriptional rather than posttranslational mechanisms, as GLI and GLI3 appear to be functionally equivalent to the activating and repressing forms of CI, respectively.

References

Baird, P. N., N. Groves, D. A. Haber, D. E. Housman, and J. K. Cowell. Identification of mutations in the WT1 gene in tumours from patients with the WAGR syndrome. *Oncogene* 7:2141–2149, 1992a.

Baird, P. N., A. Santos, N. Groves, L. Jadresic, and J. K. Cowell. Constitutional mutations in the WT1 gene in patients with Denys-Drash syndrome. *Hum. Mol. Genet.* 1:301–305, 1992b.

Bickmore, W. A., K. Oghene, M. H. Little, A. Seawright, V. van Heyningen, N. D. Hastie. Modulation of DNA binding specificity by alternative splicing of the Wilms tumor wt1 gene transcript. *Science* 257:235–237, 1992.

Borel, F., K. C. Barilla, T. B. Hamilton, M. Iskandar, and P. J. Romaniuk. Effects of Denys-Drash syndrome point mutations on the DNA-binding activity of the Wilms' tumor suppressor protein WT1. *Biochemistry* 35:12070–12076, 1996.

Bruening, W., N. Bardessy, B. L. Silverman, R. A. Cohn, G. A. Machin, A. J. Aronson, D. Housman, and J. Pelletier. Germline intronic and exonic mutations in the Wilms' tumor gene (WT1) affecting urogenital development. *Nat. Genet.* 1:144–148, 1992.

Call, K. M., T. Glaser, C. Y. Ito, A. J. Buckler, J. Pelletier, D. A. Haber, E. A. Rose, A. Kral, H. Yeger, W. H. Lewis, C. Jones, and D. E. Housman. Isolation and characterization of a zinc finger polypeptide gene at the human chromosome 11 Wilms' tumor locus. *Cell* 60:509–520, 1990.

Chiang, C., Y. Litingtung, E. Lee, K. E. Young, J. L. Corden, H. Westphal, and P. A. Beachy. Cyclopia and defective axial patterning in mice lacking Sonic hedgehog gene function. *Nature* 383:407–413, 1996.

Cowell, J. K., R. B. Wadey, D. A. Haber, K. M. Call, D. E. Housman, and J. Pritchard. Structural rearrangements of the WT1 gene in Wilms' tumour cells. *Oncogene* 6:595–599, 1991.

Davis, L. M., B. Zabel, G. Senger, H. J. Ludecke, B. Metzroth, K. Call, D. Housman, U. Claussen, B. Horsthemke, T. B. Shows. A tumor chromosome rearragnement further defines the 11p13 Wilms' tumor locus. *Genomics* 10:588–592, 1991.

Drash, A., F. Sherman, W. H. Hartmann, and R. M. Blizzard. A syndrome of pseudohermaphroditism, Wilms' tumor, hypertension, and degenerative renal disease. *J. Pediatr.* 76:585–593, 1970.

Drummond, I. A., S. L. Madden, N. P. Rohwer, G. I. Bell, V. P. Sukhatme, and F. Rauscher III. Repression of the insulin-like growth factor gene by the Wilms' tumor suppressor gene WT1. *Science* 257:674–678, 1992.

Duncan, P. A., R. M. Klein, P. L. Wilmot, and L. R. Shapiro. Greig cephalopolysyndactyly syndrome. *Am. J. Dis. Child.* 133:818–821, 1979.

Gessler, M., A. Poustka, W. Cavenee, R. L. Neve, S. Orkin, and G. A. P. Bruns. Homozygous deletion in Wilms' tumours of a zinc-finger gene identifed by chromsome jumping. *Nature* 342:774–778, 1990.

Greig, D. M. Oxycephaly. *Edinburgh Med. J.* 33:189–218, 1926.

Haber, D. A., A. J. Buckler, T. Glaser, K. M. Call, J. Pelletier, R. L. Sohn, E. C. Douglass, and D. E. Housman. An internal deletion within an 11p13 zinc finger gene contributes to the development of Wilms tumor. *Cell* 61:1257–1269, 1990.

Haber, D. A., and D. E. Housman. The genetics of Wilms' tumor. *Adv. Cancer Res.* 59:41–68, 1992.

Hall, J. G., P. D. Pallister, S. K. Clarren, J. B. Beckwith, F. W. Wiglesworth, F. C. Fraser, S. Cho, P. J. Benke, and S. D. Reed. Congenital hypothalamic hamartoblastoma, hypopituitarism, imperforate anus, and postaxial polydactyly—a new syndrome? Part I: clinical, causal, and pathogenetic considerations. *Am. J. Med. Genet.* 7: 47–74, 1980.

Huff, V., H. Miwa, D. A. Haber, K. M. Call, D. Housman, L. C. Strong, and G. F. Saunders. Evidence for WT1 as a Wilms' tumor (WT) gene: intragenic germinal deletion in bilateral WT. *Am. J. Hum. Genet.* 48:997–1003, 1991.

Hui, C.-C., and A. L. Joyner. A mouse model of Greig cephalopolysyndactyly syndrome: the extra-toes[J] mutation contains an intragenic deletion of the Gli3 gene. *Nat. Genet.* 3:241–246, 1993.

Jones, K. L. *Smith's Recognizable Patterns of Human Malformation*, 4th ed., Philadelphia: W. B. Saunders Co., 1988.

Kang, S., J. M. Graham, Jr., M. Abbott, A. Schaffer, E. D. Green, M. Rosenberg, J. Allen, C. Clericuzio, T. Grebe, A. Haskins-Olney, and L. G. Biesecker. Autosomal dominant Pallister-Hall syndrome maps to 7p13. *Am. J. Hum. Genet.* 59 (suppl.): A17, 1996.

Kang, S., J. M. Graham, Jr., A. H. Olney, and L. G. Biesecker. GLI3 frameshift mutations cause autosomal dominant Pallister-Hall syndrome. *Nat. Genet.* 15: 266–268, 1997.

Keino, H., S. Masaki, Y. Kawarada, and I. Naruse. Apoptotic degeneration in the arhinencephalic brain of the mouse mutant Pdn/Pdn. *Brain Res. Dev. Brain Res.* 78:161–168, 1994.

Knudson, A. G., Jr. Mutation and cancer: statistical study of retinoblastoma. *Proc. Natl. Acad. Sci. U.S.A.* 68:820–823, 1971.

Knudson, A. G., and L. C. Strong. Mutation and cancer: a model for Wilms tumor of the kidney. *J. Natl. Cancer Inst.* 48:313–324, 1972.

Kreidberg, J. A., H. Sariola, J. M. Loring, M. Maeda, J. Pelletier, D. Housman, and R. Jaenisch. WT-1 is required for early kidney development. *Cell* 74:679–691, 1993.

Little, M., G. Holmes, W. Bickmore, V. van Heyningen, N. Hastie, and B. Wainwright. DNA binding capacity of the WT1 protein is abolished by Denys-Drash syndrome WT1 point mutations. *Hum. Mol. Genet.* 4:351–358, 1995.

Little, M. H., J. Prosser, A. Condie, P.J. Smith, V. van Heyningen, and N. D. Hastie. Zinc finger point mutations within the WT1 gene in Wilms' tumor patients. *Proc. Natl. Acad. Sci. U.S.A.* 89:4791–4795, 1992.

Little, M. H., K. A. Williamson, M. Mannens, A. Kelsey, C. Gosden, N. D. Hastie, and V. van Heyningen. Evidence that WT1 mutations in Denys-Drash syndrome patients may act in a dominant-negative fashion. *Hum. Mol. Genet.* 2: 259–264, 1993.

Madden, S. L., D. L.M. Cook, J. F. Morris, A. Gashler, V. P. Sukhatme, F. J. Rauscher III. Trancriptional repression mediated by the WT1 Wilms tumor gene product. *Science* 253:1550–1554, 1991.

Morris, J. F., S. L. Madden, O. E. Tournay, D. M. Cook, V. P. Sukhatme, and F. Rauscher III. Characterization of the zinc finger protein encoded by the WT1 Wilms' tumor locus. *Oncogene* 6: 2339–2348, 1991.

Naruse, I., and Y. Kameyama. Prevention of manifestation of genetic expression of polydactyly in heterozygotes of Polydactyly Nagoya (Pdn) mice by cytosine arabinoside. *Environ. Med.* 28:89–92, 1984.

Naruse, I., and Y. Kameyama. Prevention of polydactyly manifestation in Polydactyly Nagoya (Pdn) mice by administration of cytosine arabinoside during pregnancy. *Teratology* 34:283–289, 1986.

Naruse, I., and Y. Kameyama. Prevention of genetic expression of polydactyly in mice by means of exo utero surgery. *Environ. Med.* 33:27–32, 1989.

Orenic, T. V., D. C. Slusarski, K. L. Kroll, and R. A. Holmgren. Cloning and characterization of the segment polarity gene cubitus interruptus Dominant of Drosophila. *Genes Dev.* 4:1053–1067, 1990.

Pelletier, J., W. Bruening, C. E. Kashtan, S. M. Mauer, J. C. Manivel, J. E. Striegel,

D. C. Houghton, C. Junien, R. Habib, L. Fouser, R. N. Fine, B. L. Silverman, D. A. Haber, and D. Housman. Germline mutations in the Wilms' tumor suppressor gene are associated with abnormal urogenital development in Denys-Drash syndrome. *Cell* 67:437–447, 1991a.

Pelletier, J., W. Bruening, F. P. Li, D. A. Haber, T. Glaser, and D. E. Housman. WT1 mutations contribute to abnormal genital system development and hereditary Wilms' tumor. *Nature* 353:431–434, 1991b.

Pelletier, J., M. Schalling, A. J. Buckler, A. Rogers, D. A. Haber, and D. Housman. Expression of the Wilms' tumor gene WT1 in the murine urogenital system. *Genes Dev.* 5:1345–1356, 1991c.

Pohl, T. M., M.-G. Mattei, and U. Ruther. Evidence for allelism of the recessive insertional mutation add and the dominant mouse mutation extra-toes (Xt). *Development* 110:1153–1157, 1990.

Pritchard-Jones, K., S. Fleming, D. Davidson, W. Bickmore, D. Porteous, C. Gosden, J. Bard, A. Buckler, J. Pelletier, D. Housman, V. van Heyningen, and N. Hastie. The candidate Wilms' tumor gene is involved in genitourinary development. *Nature* 346:194–197, 1990.

Rauscher, F., III, J. F. Morris, O. E. Tournay, D. M. Cook, and T. Curran. Binding of the Wilms' tumor WT1 zinc finger protein to the EGR-1 consensus sequence. *Science* 250:1259–1262, 1990.

Riccardi, V. M., E. Sujansky, A. C. Smith, and U. Francke. Chromosomal imbalance in the aniridia-Wilms tumor association: 11p interstitial deletion. *Pediatrics* 61:604–610, 1978.

Roberts, D. J., and C. Tabin. The genetics of human limb development. *Am. J. Hum. Genet.* 55:1–6, 1994.

Ruiz i Altaba, A. Catching a Gli-mpse of hedgehog. *Cell* 90:193–196, 1997.

Ruppert, J. M., K. W. Kinzler, A. J. Wong, S. H. Bigner, F. T. Kao, M. L. Law, H. N. Seuanez, S. J. O'Brien, and B. Vogelstein. The GLI-Kruppel family of human genes. *Mol. Cell. Biol.* 8:3104–3113, 1988.

Ruppert, J. M., B. Vogelstein, K. Arheden, and K. W. Kinzler. GLI3 encodes a 190-kilodalton protein with multiple regions of GLI similarity. *Mol. Cell. Biol.* 10:5408–5415, 1990.

Schimmang, T., M. Lemaistree, A. Vortkamp, and U. Ruther. Expression of the zinc finger gene Gli3 is affected in the morphogenetic mouse mutant extratoes (xt). *Development* 116:799–804, 1992.

Schimmang, T., F. van der Hoeven, and U. Ruther. Gli3 expression is affected in the morphogenetic mouse mutants add and Xt. *Prog. Clin. Biol. Res.* 383A: 153–161, 1993.

Schimmang, T., S. I. Oda, and U. Ruther. The mouse mutant Polydactyly Nagoya (Pdn) defines a novel allele of the zinc finger gene Gli3. *Mamm. Genome* 5: 384–386, 1994.

Schmickel, R. D. Contiguous gene syndromes: a component of recognizable syndromes. *J. Pediatr.* 109:231–241, 1986.

Scott, M. P. Hox genes, arms and the man. *Nat. Genet.* 15:117–118, 1997.

Stone, D. M., M. Hynes, M. Armanini, T. A. Swanson, Q. Gu, R. L. Johnson, M. P. Scott, D. Pennica, A. Goddard, H. Phillips, M. Noll, J. E. Hooper, F. De Sauvage, and A. Rosenthal. The tumour-suppressor gene patched encodes a candidate receptor for Sonic hedgehog. *Nature* 384:129–134, 1996.

Ton, C. C. T., V. Huff, K. Call, S. Cohn, L. C. Strong, D. E. Housman, and G. F. Saunders. Smallest region of overlap in Wilms' tumor deletions uniquely implicates an 11p13 zinc finger gene as the disease locus. *Genomics* 10:293–297, 1991.

van der Hoeven, F., T. Schimmang, A. Vortkamp, and U. Ruther. Molecular linkage of the morphogenetic mutant add and the zinc finger gene Gli3. *Mamm. Genome* 4:276–277, 1993.

van Heyningen, V., W. A. Bickmore, A. Seawright, J. M. Fletcher, J. Maule, G. Fekete, M. Gessler, G. A. Bruns, J. C. Huerre, C. Junien, B. R. G. Williams, and N. D. Hastie. Role of the Wilms tumor gene in genital development? *Proc. Natl. Acad. Sci. U.S.A.* 87:5383–5386, 1990.

Vortkamp, A., M. Gessler, and K.-H. Grzeschik. GLI3 zinc-finger gene interrupted by translocations in Greig syndrome families. *Nature* 352:539–540, 1991.

Vortkamp, A., T. Franz, M. Gessler, and K.-H. Grzeschik. Deletion of Gli3 supports the homology of the human Greig cephalopolysyndactyly syndrome (GCPS) and the mouse mutant extra toes (xt). *Mamm. Genome* 3:461–463, 1992.

Vortkamp, A., C. Heid, M. Gessler, and K.-H. Grzeschik. Isolation and characterization of a cosmid contig for the GCPS gene region. *Hum. Genet.* 95:82–88, 1995.

Wang, Z. Y., S. L. Madden, T. F. Deuel, and F. Rauscher III. The Wilms' tumor gene product, WT1, represses transcription of the platelet-derived growth factor A-chain gene. *J. Biol. Chem.* 207:21999–22002, 1992.

Zarkower, D., and J. Hodgkin. Molecular analysis of the C. elegans sex-determining gene tra-1; a gene encoding two zinc finger proteins. *Cell* 70:237–249, 1992.

PAX Proteins 7

As in the case of the HOX proteins (described in Chapter 9), the PAX proteins represent a family of transcription factors whose members appear to play key roles in the development of both invertebrates and vertebrates (reviewed by Chalepakis et al., 1993; Strachan and Read, 1994; Stuart and Gruss, 1995). Nine *PAX* genes have been identified to date in mice and humans (Fig. 7.1). Unlike the *HOX* genes, which are clustered at four loci in the human and mouse genomes, mapping of the *PAX* genes revealed no clustering even though several of the genes have similar genomic structure and coding sequences.

The proteins encoded by these genes have in common a unique 128-amino-acid DNA-binding domain, the paired domain. Although the paired domain contains three regions that are predicted to form α helices, there is no sequence similarity to the helix-turn-helix motif present in homeodomains. In addition to the paired domain, which is present in all nine PAX proteins, four of the proteins (PAX3, PAX4, PAX6, and PAX7) also contain a homeodomain that contributes to the affinity and specificity of DNA binding by these proteins. Curiously, three PAX proteins (PAX2, PAX5, and PAX8) contain truncated homeodomains of unknown function. PAX 1 and PAX9 lack homeodomain-related sequences altogether and must therefore rely entirely on the paired domain for DNA-binding activity.

In addition to the lack of clustered genes and the use of a paired domain rather than a homeodomain as the primary DNA-binding domain, PAX proteins also differ from HOX proteins in one other significant respect. Whereas heterozygosity for loss-of-function mutations in some *HOX* genes has little or no phenotypic effect (see Chapter 9), heterozygous loss-of-function mutations in *PAX* genes are associated with disease phenotypes in both humans and mice. Thus far, mutations af-

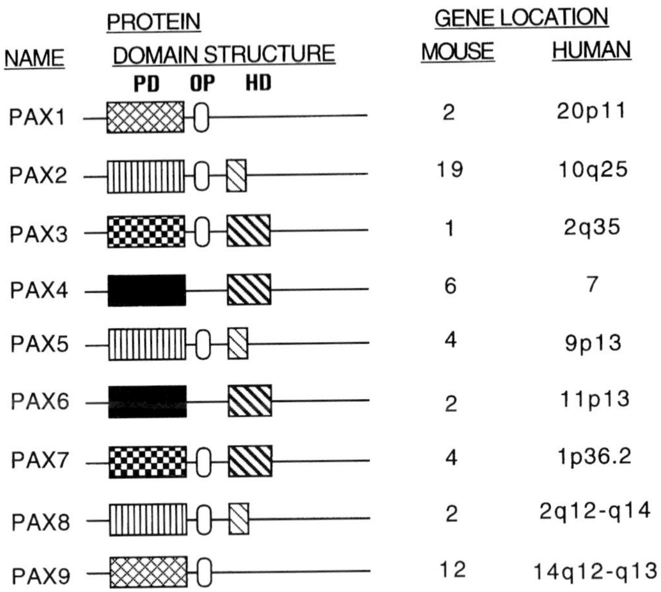

NAME	PROTEIN DOMAIN STRUCTURE	GENE LOCATION MOUSE	HUMAN
PAX1		2	20p11
PAX2		19	10q25
PAX3		1	2q35
PAX4		6	7
PAX5		4	9p13
PAX6		2	11p13
PAX7		4	1p36.2
PAX8		2	2q12-q14
PAX9		12	14q12-q13

FIGURE 7-1. *PAX* genes and their products. The chromosomal locations of the nine human *PAX* and mouse *Pax* genes are shown at right and the structure of their protein products is illustrated at left with the paired domain (PD), octapeptide (OP), and complete or truncated homeodomain (HD) motifs indicated schematically. Different patterns indicate proteins whose domain sequences show greatest similarity to one another. (Adapted from Stuart and Gruss, 1995.)

fecting PAX1, PAX2, PAX3, and PAX6 have been associated with malformation syndromes in humans and/or mice (Table 7.1).

PAX1

PAX1 is the only *PAX* gene that is not expressed in the nervous system (Chalepakis et al., 1993). In the mouse, *Pax1* expression is first detected at day E9 in the embryonic vertebral column and later in the intervertebral discs, sternum, and thymus (Deutsch et al., 1988).

Mutations in Murine Pax1: Undulated

The first malformation syndrome identified as due to a mutation in a *PAX* gene was *undulated (un)*, which is characterized by abnormal sternal and vertebral development. In *undulated* mice, the posterior segment of the vertebral bodies is hypoplastic and the intervertebral spaces are increased in size, resulting in a destabilization of the spinal column so that

TABLE 7.1. *PAX* gene-associated malformation syndromes

PAX Gene	Human Phenotype	Mouse Mutant
1	—	*undulated*
2	Renal-coloboma syndrome	*Pax2[1Neu]*
3	Waardenburg syndrome types I & III	*Splotch*
	Craniofacial-deafness-hand syndrome	
4	—	—
5	—	—
6	Aniridia; anophthalmia/CNS defects	*Small eye*
	Autosomal dominant keratitis	
	Isolated foveal hypoplasia	
	Peters' anomaly	
7	—	—
8	—	—
9	—	—

it assumes a wavy (undulated) appearance. *Pax1* was mapped to mouse chromosome 2 closely linked to *un*, and molecular analysis of *Pax1* revealed that the *un* allele represented a missense mutation (G15S) that resulted in the substitution of a conserved glycine residue within the paired domain that is present in all paired-domain proteins (Balling et al., 1988). The PAX1 protein binds to DNA via a paired domain only (Fig. 7.1), and the mutation greatly decreased the DNA-binding affinity as well as altering the DNA-binding specificity of PAX1 (Chalepakis et al., 1991).

un is a recessive allele, suggesting that the amino acid substitution does not fully eliminate DNA-binding activity. In contrast, the *Undulated short-tail (Un^s)* mutation is semi-dominant: *Un^s* heterozygotes have vertebral malformations similar to *un* homozygotes, whereas *Un^s* homozygotes completely lack vertebral bodies and intervertebral discs in the lumbar area, due to a complete deletion of the mouse *Pax1* gene (Balling et al., 1992), which of course would result in complete loss of function of the mutant allele. The comparison between *un* and *Un^s* thus provides a genotype-phenotype correlation that strongly supports the hypothesis that the pathophysiologic basis for these malformation syndromes is decreased PAX1 protein expression. Thus far, no human malformation syndromes have been associated with mutations in the *PAX1* gene (Balling et al., 1992).

PAX3

In contrast to PAX1, which contains only a paired domain, PAX3 binds to DNA through the combined activity of its paired and homeodomains

(Fig. 7.1). In mice, *Pax3* is expressed in the neural tube and developing brain, neural crest cells and their derivatives (e.g., within craniofacial mesectoderm and the heart), the dermomyotome of the developing somites, and the limb buds (Goulding et al., 1991).

Mutations in Murine Pax3: Splotch

Mutations at the *Splotch (Sp)* locus result in malformations involving neural crest–derived tissues (reviewed by Chalepakis et al., 1993; Gruss and Walther, 1992). *Sp/Sp* mice have exencephaly, spina bifida, limb defects, agenesis of melanoblasts, and dysgenesis of spinal ganglia and heart structures derived from neural crest. *Sp/+* mice have craniofacial malformations and pigmentary defects, the latter manifested as white splotches on the belly. Five different spontaneous or radiation-induced *Splotch* alleles have been shown to represent mutations affecting *Pax3*. The Sp^r and Sp^{4H} alleles represent very large (up to 14 cM) deletions that encompass the *Pax3* gene; the Sp^{2H} allele has a 32-bp frameshift deletion that results in protein truncation within the homeodomain; the *Sp* allele has a point mutation at a splice acceptor site that results in removal of exon 4 sequences from the mature mRNA, frameshift, and protein truncation within the paired domain; and the Sp^d allele has a missense mutation (G42R) in the paired domain (Epstein et al., 1991a, b, 1993; Goulding et al., 1993; Vogan et al., 1993).

As in the case of *Pax1* mutations, the phenotype is more severe in the homozygous than in the heterozygous state and the association of the phenotype with complete gene deletion provides strong evidence for loss of function as the molecular pathophysiologic basis for the observed malformations. However, because the deletions are likely to have resulted in loss of other genes in addition to *Pax3*, the severity of phenotype associated with complete gene deletion cannot be compared with the phenotype associated with a missense mutation that might result in residual biological activity of the mutant protein. Phenotype-genotype correlations have been more informative with respect to mutations affecting the human *PAX3* gene.

Mutations in Human PAX3: Waardenburg Syndrome and Related Disorders

Waardenburg syndrome (WS) is an autosomal dominant disorder with an incidence of 1 in 40,000, although more than 1% of congenitally deaf children are affected by WS (Waardenburg, 1951). In addition to sensorineural deafness, there are two characteristic features of WS: first, pigmentation defects of the hair, manifested by a white forelock or eyelashes, and of the iris, manifested by hypoisochromia (pale blue irises) or heterochromia irides (e.g., a brown iris on the left and a blue iris on the right) (Fig. 7.2); and second, hypoplastic alae nasi (small nasal openings). Heterochromia may represent a stochastic effect (the mutation increases the probability that an eye will be hypopigmented) or the presence of a second (somatic) mutation in melanoblasts responsible for pigmentation in one eye of affected individuals. Type 1 and type 2 WS (MIM 193500 and 193510, respectively) are distinguished by the presence of dystopia canthorum, which refers to lateral displacement of the inner canthus (inner corner of the eye), in individuals with type 1 WS and its absence in those with type 2 WS (Hageman and Delleman, 1977). Type 3 WS (Klein-Waardenburg syndrome; MIM 148820) is distinguished from type 1 WS by the presence of hypoplasia of the shoulder and arm musculature (reviewed by Klein, 1983).

WS type 1. Investigations of the human *PAX3* gene have revealed multiple mutations associated with type 1 WS (Baldwin et al., 1992, 1994; Butt et al., 1994; Farrer et al., 1994; Lalwani et al., 1995; Morell et al., 1992; Pierpont et al., 1994; Tassabehji et al., 1992, 1993, 1994, 1995; Zlotogora et al., 1995). These mutations include insertions and deletions that frameshift the translational reading frame, resulting in truncated proteins; splice site mutations; nonsense mutations; an 18-bp in-frame deletion that eliminates six amino acids from the paired domain; and mis-

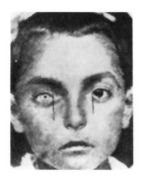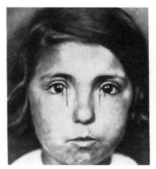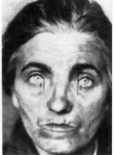

FIGURE 7-2. Heterozygosity for a mutation in the human *PAX3* gene: Waardenburg syndrome type 1. Left, a 4-year-old male with heterochromia irides. Right, a woman with hypoisochromia irides. Center, her 9-year-old niece manifests hypochromia only within the nasal upper quadrant of the right iris. The vertical lines indicate the presence of dystopia canthorum. (Reprinted with permission of the University of Chicago Press from Waardenburg, 1951. Copyright ©1951 by the American Society of Human Genetics. All rights reserved.)

sense mutations that involve conserved amino acid residues in the paired domain or homeodomain. These mutations, as in the case of the *Sp* alleles, all appear to result in loss of function. Moreover, the missense mutations indicate that both the paired domain (Fig. 7.3) and homeodomain are required for biological activity. However, a direct demonstration that missense mutations in the paired domain or homeodomain result in loss of DNA-binding activity has not been reported. Interestingly, mutations within the paired domain or homeodomain are found in patients with similar clinical presentations, suggesting that these mu-

```
                42 45 47 50     56    60 62                78  81 8485              99
PAX3    GQGRVNQLGGVFINGRPLPNHIRHKIVEMAHHGIRPCVISRQLRVSHGCVSKILCRYQFTGSIRPGAIGGSK

Spd     ---------R-----------------------------------------------------------

WS 1    -----------L---------------------------------------------------------

WS 3    -------------H-------------------------------------------------------

CDHS    -------------K-------------------------------------------------------

WS 1    -----------------L---------------------------------------------------

WS 1    ---------------------L-----------------------------------------------

WS 1    -----------------------------M---------------------------------------

WS 1    -------------------------------V-------------------------------------

WS 1    -----------------------------------------M---------------------------

WS 1    ---------------------------------------------------A-----------------

WS 1/3  ------------------------------------------------------F--------------

WS 1    ------------------------------------------------------E--------------

WS 1    -----------------------------------------------------------D-----
```

FIGURE 7-3. Missense mutations in the paired domain of *PAX3*. Amino acids 34 to 105 of the PAX3 protein are shown, representing the first 72 amino acids of the paired domain. Underscore indicates amino acids that are conserved in all known paired domains from mammalian PAX proteins to the PAIRED protein of *Drosophila melanogaster* (reviewed by Xu et al., 1995). Below the amino acid sequence are missense mutations in the paired domain associated with *Splotch* (*Sp*), Waardenburg syndrome types 1 and 3 (WS1 and WS3, respectively), and craniofacial-deafness-hand syndrome (CDHS). WS1/3 indicates that WS1 and WS3 phenotypes were associated with heterozygosity and homozygosity, respectively, for the mutant allele. A variety of other mutations (involving residues outside the paired domain) have also been identified in patients with WS1.

tations have the same effect, most likely loss of function due to loss of DNA-binding activity.

The history of the *Splotch* and Waardenburg discoveries is an instructive paradigm for the utilization of comparative genetics and gene mapping in the identification of human disease genes (Walter and Goodfellow, 1992). The mouse *Pax* genes were originally identified by crosshybridization with probes derived from the *paired* gene of *Drosophila melanogaster*. A human gene that was originally designated *HuP2* was found by nucleotide sequence analysis to be homologous to murine *Pax3*. The phenotypic similarities between Waardenburg syndrome and *Splotch* mice had been previously noted (Asher and Friedman, 1990; Foy et al., 1990). When *Splotch* mutations were mapped to *Pax3* and WS1 was mapped to chromosome 2q37 in the vicinity of *HuP2* (Farrer et al., 1992), this gene immediately became a candidate locus for WS1 and facilitated the rapid identification of disease-causing mutations in the (re-named) human *PAX3* gene.

WS type 2. Although initially a patient with WS type 2 was reported to have a mutation in *PAX3* (Tassahbehji et al., 1993), clinical reevaluation using revised diagnostic criteria resulted in this patient being reclassified as type 1 WS, and no other patient with type 2 WS has been shown to have a mutation in *PAX3* (Strachan and Read, 1994). Despite the remarkably similar phenotypes, type 2 WS was shown to map to chromosome 3p12-p14.1 (Hughes et al., 1994). Subsequent work demonstrated that WS type 2 was associated with mutations in the *MITF* gene, which encodes a basic helix-loop-helix leucine-zipper transcription factor (see Chapter 8).

WS type 3. Despite speculation that Klein-Waardenburg syndrome was etiologically distinct from type 1 and type 2 WS on clinical grounds (McKusick, 1986), type 3 WS was also mapped to the *PAX3* gene. Initially, the association of type 3 WS with a large deletion suggested that it might represent a contiguous gene syndrome (Pasteris et al., 1993; Tassabehji et al., 1993). However, subsequent analysis identified individuals with type 3 WS who carried missense mutations in the paired domain (e.g., N47H) similar to those seen in patients with type I WS (e.g., P50L) (Hoth et al., 1993) (Fig. 7.3). These mutations, although affecting amino acid residues located in close proximity to one another, might have different effects on PAX3 function, thus resulting in the phenotypic differences between type 1 and type 3 WS. Alternatively, alleles at other loci (modifier genes) may determine the phenotypic presentation. If such were the case, then it should be possible to identify families in which both type 1 and type 3 WS are segregating. If indeed complete gene deletions were associated with both type 1 and type 3 WS, this would provide strong evidence for effects of modifier genes on the WS presentation.

Craniofacial-deafness-hand syndrome. A rare autosomal dominant syndrome which, as in the case of WS type 3, is characterized by sensorineural deafness and craniofacial and limb anomalies is the Craniofacial-deafness-hand syndrome (CDHS; MIM 122880). Craniofacial malformations in CDHS include aplasia or hypoplasia of the nasal bones, small nose with thin nares, maxillary hypoplasia, short palpebral fissures, and hypertelorism; limb involvement includes limited mobility of the wrist joint and ulnar deviation of the digits (Sommer et al., 1983). In CDHS there is no limb hypoplasia such as is seen in WS type 3 and development of the nasal bones is not markedly affected in WS type 3. These two conditions were thus considered to be etiologically distinct (McKusick, 1986). Remarkably, however, analysis of the *PAX3* gene in DNA from three members of a family affected by CDHS revealed a missense mutation in the paired domain, N47K, (Asher et al., 1996b) that involves the same amino acid residue that was substituted in a case of WS3, N47H (Hoth et al., 1993) (Fig. 7.3). These data once again raise the question whether these three different phenotypes (WS1, WS3, and CDHS) are a reflection of the functional effects of different *PAX3* mutations or whether they represent the effects of modifier genes. Introduction of these mutations into the mouse germline, using new hit-and-run techniques of homologous recombination in embryonic stem cells, would be very informative in this regard because the phenotypic effect of mutations on different genetic backgrounds could be determined.

Heterozygosity and homozygosity for a PAX3 mutation. For most autosomal dominant conditions, homozygosity for the mutant allele results in a more severe phenotype than does heterozygosity. In experimental animals such as mice, in which one can examine both heterozygotes and homozygotes, even when the latter result in embryonic lethality, the term semi-dominant is often used to denote the difference in phenotype based on the difference in genotype. In humans, homozygosity is less often observed because of the low probability that two individuals carrying rare mutations at the same locus will mate and because of the difficulty of detecting fetal loss associated with homozygosity. However, as in the case of rare recessive disorders, the probability of detecting homozygosity for a rare dominant disorder is greatly increased by consanguinity or inbreeding. Under these circumstances, the probability that the prospective parents will carry a mutant allele that is identical-by-descent is a direct function of their degree of relatedness.

A family was identified in which the parents were first cousins and were both diagnosed as having mild WS1, manifested by dystopia canthorum without deafness, pigmentary defects, or limb anomalies, due to heterozygosity for a S84F missense mutation within the paired domain (Zlotogora et al., 1995) (Fig. 7.3). Their firstborn son was also heterozygous for the S84F mutation and WS type I was manifested by dystopia canthorum and heterochromia irides. Examination of their second-born son at 3 months of age revealed complete absence of pigment in his hair, eyebrows, and eyelashes; multiple craniofacial malformations; upper limb malformations including restricted mobility of the elbow, shoulder, and wrist joints, muscular hypoplasia, and axillary webbing; and liver dysfunction with cholestatic jaundice (Fig. 7.4). DNA analysis revealed that the child was homozygous for the S84F mutation (Zlotogora et al., 1995).

Thus, in this family, heterozygosity for a *PAX3* missense mutation resulted in a mild form of WS type 1 whereas homozygosity was associated with a severe form of WS type 3. One of Klein's original patients

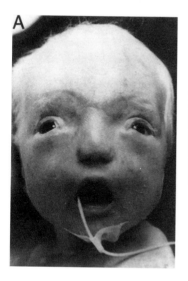
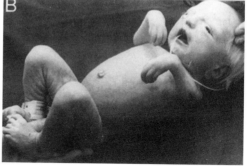

FIGURE 7-4. Homozygosity for a mutation in the human *PAX3* gene. The photographs are of a 3–month-old boy who was shown to be homozygous for an S84F missense mutation. Note the absence of pigmentation and severe craniofacial (A) and limb (B) malformations. (Reprinted with permission of The University of Chicago Press from Zlotogora et al., 1995. Copyright ©1995 by the American Society of Human Genetics. All rights reserved.)

displayed a similar phenotype of severe pigmentary and limb defects suggestive of homozygosity for *PAX3* mutations (Waardenburg, 1951) (Fig. 7.5). These results suggest that WS3 represents a more severe phenotypic manifestation of deficient PAX3 biological activity, which could result from decreased levels of active PAX3 protein and/or decreased activity of a modifier gene product, because the child with type 3 WS born to first cousins may have also been homozygous at a modifier locus. A comparison of the phenotypes associated with homozygosity for *PAX3* mutations in humans and mice is also instructive. First, whereas the child homozygous for S84F was alive at 3 months, homozygosity for any of

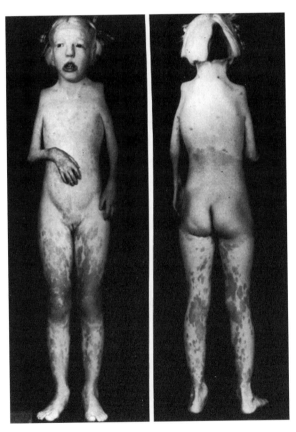

FIGURE 7-5. One of Klein's original patients (WS3; Klein-Waardenburg syndrome). Note the severe pigmentary and limb defects. (Reprinted with permission of The University of Chicago Press from Waardenburg, 1951. Copyright ©1951 by the American Society of Human Genetics. All rights reserved.)

the *Splotch* alleles results in prenatal or neonatal lethality (Chalepakis et al., 1993). However, the only missense allele, Sp^d (G42R), is associated with the longest survival, suggesting that the mutant PAX3 proteins (human S84F and mouse G42R) may have some residual biological activity that allows survival to term. Second, whereas homozygosity for any of the *Splotch* alleles results in neural tube defects (Chalepakis et al., 1993), this malformation was not observed in the human S84F homozygote. However, the Sp^d (G42R) allele again manifested a milder phenotype than other *Splotch* alleles, as exencephaly was associated with homozygosity for all *Splotch* alleles except Sp^d . It is not possible to determine from the available data whether differences in phenotype are due to differences in genotype at *PAX3* or modifier loci or whether they are due to stochastic effects. Resolving these types of questions represents a major challenge for mammalian and medical geneticists in the coming years.

Modifier loci. The identification of modifier loci that affect the presentation of rare genetic disorders cannot be accomplished in human populations with currently available methods of analysis. However, the availability of inbred mouse strains and wild mouse populations provide conditions of genetic uniformity and diversity that allow experimental investigation of this issue. The preliminary results of this type of analysis have recently been reported (Asher et al., 1996a). Heterozygosity for the Sp^d allele on the C57/BL6 (B6) genetic background was associated with a mild phenotype manifested by white belly spotting with 100% penetrance. However, when Sp^d/+ B6 females were mated to +/+ *Mus spretus* males and the F_1 Sp^d/+ females were mated to +/+ B6 males, the resulting progeny showed extremely variable phenotypes, ranging from absence of the white belly spot (32%) to prenatal lethality (24%). The penetrance and expressivity of the phenotype was influenced by sex and genetic background, with *Agouti* or a closely linked locus implicated as a specific modifier gene (Asher et al., 1996a). These results provide compelling evidence for the role of modifier genes in determining the phenotypic manifestations of a *Pax3* mutation and further studies of mice from these and other crosses should allow an extensive epistasis analysis to be performed.

Other neurocristopathies. Because many of the malformations observed in Waardenburg syndrome involve cells of neural crest origin and *Pax3* expression has been detected in neural crest cells and their derivatives, a variety of individuals with other auditory, pigmentary, or neural crest syndromes were studied. Of 36 individuals whose DNA was analyzed, none was found to have a mutation in *PAX3* (Tassabehji et al., 1995).

Analysis of Paired-Domain Mutations in Pax1 and Pax3/PAX3

As shown in Figure 7.3, all of the known missense mutations in the paired domain of human and mouse PAX3 that result in WS and *Splotch* phenotypes, respectively, have been localized to the amino-terminal half of the 128-residue domain. The same is also true for the *Pax1* mutation responsible for the *undulated* phenotype. The amino-terminal portion of the paired domain was shown to be sufficient for DNA binding (Chalepakis et al., 1991; Czerny et al., 1993; Treisman et al., 1991). Determination of the crystal structure of a complex between an oligonucleotide containing an optimized binding site and the paired domain of the *Drosophila* PAIRED protein indicated that the conserved residues, which are sites of mutation in PAX1 and PAX3, either directly contact DNA or stabilize the tertiary structure of the DNA-binding domain (Xu et al., 1995). For example, the G15S mutation in PAX1 affects a glycine residue in a β turn that directly contacts DNA in the minor groove. Substitution of this residue (which is equivalent to glycine-48 of PAX3; see Fig. 7.3) decreases DNA binding affinity because the residue lies too close to the DNA to accommodate any side chain other than the minimal hydrogen atom present in glycine. The N47H, N47K, and P50L mutations identified in WS type 3, CDHS, and WS type 1, respectively, are also located in or near this β turn (Xu et al., 1995). This analysis suggests that these mutations reduce or eliminate the ability of protein to bind to DNA, resulting in a loss of biological activity.

PAX6

As in the case of PAX3, PAX6 contains both a paired domain and a homeodomain (Fig. 7.1), and both *Pax3* and *Pax6* are expressed in the developing mouse central nervous system beginning at E8 (Chalepakis et al., 1993). However, these genes are expressed in different structures of the developing brain. In addition, *Pax6* is remarkable for its expression as early as E8.5 in the optic pit and subsequently in the differentiating eye vesicle, optic stalk, retina, lens, and cornea, representing all of the structures of the developing eye (Walther and Gruss, 1991). In addition, *Pax6* is expressed during all stages of development of the olfactory and nasal structures (Chalepakis et al., 1993). Remarkably, human and mouse PAX6 proteins consist of 422 amino acid residues of identical sequence (Glaser et al., 1992).

Mutations in Murine Pax6: Small eye

Mutations affecting PAX6 were first identified in mice as the cause of the *Small eye (Sey)* phenotype (Hill et al., 1991). In *Sey/+* mice, the eyes are smaller than normal and closure of the optic cup is incomplete, whereas in *Sey/Sey* mice, development of the eyes and nasal cavity does not occur. Molecular analysis (Hill et al., 1991) revealed that the *Sey* allele contained a nonsense mutation that is predicted to truncate synthesis of the PAX6 protein before the homeodomain, whereas the *Sey^Neu* allele has a splice junction mutation that would result in synthesis of a truncated protein lacking the carboxyl-terminal 115 amino acids, which are rich in proline, serine, and threonine (PST) residues, a characteristic of some transactivation domains (Fig. 7.6). In rats, the *rSey* allele is a splicing mutation that is predicted to cause translational termination at the beginning of the PST-rich region (Matsuo et al., 1993). These findings predict that the *Sey* mutant protein would be unable to bind to DNA, whereas the *Sey^Neu* and *rSey* proteins would be unable to activate transcription. Transcription studies have demonstrated that the PAX6 PST domain is a potent activator of transcription and that the *Sey^Neu* mutation results in a complete loss of transcriptional activity mediated

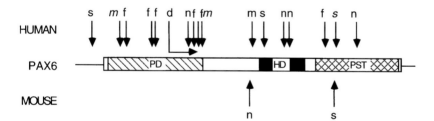

FIGURE 7-6. Mutations in *PAX6*. PAX6 mRNA is shown schematically with untranslated sequences depicted by a thin line and translated sequences by a box with paired domain (PD), homeodomain (HD), and proline-serine-threonine-rich domain (PST) indicated. Mutations in the human *PAX6* gene identified in patients with aniridia and other ocular disorders are indicated by the following abbreviations: d, in-frame deletion; f, frameshift mutation; m, missense mutation; *m*, missense mutation causing Peter's anomaly (R26G) or isolated foveal hypoplasia (R125C); n, nonsense mutation; s, mutation affecting RNA splicing; *s*, splicing mutation in autosomal dominant keratitis. Mutations in the mouse *Pax6* gene identified in *Small eye (Sey* and *Sey^Neu)* mice are also indicated. Note that splicing mutations in the same intron are responsible for *Sey^Neu* and autosomal dominant keratitis.

by this domain (Glaser et al., 1994). More severe phenotypes are associated with mouse Sey^H and Sey^{Dey} alleles, in which the entire $Pax6$ gene is deleted (Hill et al., 1991). In the case of Sey^H, other genes are deleted as well as $Pax6$ (including $Wt1$), which makes it difficult to determine which aspects of the phenotype are attributable to Pax6 deficiency only. However, comparison of the phenotypes of mice heterozygous as compared to homozygous for either Sey or Sey^{Neu} demonstrates a clear gene dosage effect.

In Sey homozygotes, how does loss of PAX6 function affect ocular and nasal development? The eye develops from neural ectoderm, which gives rise to the optic vesicle, and the overlying surface ectoderm, which gives rise to the cornea and lens. The optic vesicle invaginates to form a bilayered optic cup in which the inner layer gives rise to the neuroretina and the outer layer forms the retinal pigmented epithelium. Inductive interactions between the optic vesicle/cup and lens primordium are required for normal ocular development. Analysis of Sey homozygotes revealed that the optic vesicle formed (although its structure was not normal) but the lens placode did not, resulting in subsequent optic degeneration (Grindley et al., 1995). As in the case of the lens placode, the nasal cavities, which normally develop by invagination of surface ectoderm that expresses $Pax6$, also did not form in Sey homozygotes. These results suggest that $Pax6$ expression is required for differentiation of surface ectoderm into lens and nasal placodes (Grindley et al., 1995). Analysis of aggregation chimeras derived from wild-type and Sey/Sey 8-cell embryos demonstrated that $Pax6$ expression was required, in a cell-autonomous manner, for differentiation of the presumptive lens and nasal epithelia and that PAX6 was also essential for formation of the retinal pigmented epithelium (Quinn et al., 1996). These results provide direct evidence that PAX6 plays an important role in establishing the identity of cells derived both from surface ectoderm (lens and nasal placodes) and from neural ectoderm (retinal pigmented epithelium).

Whereas it is clear from these studies that loss of PAX6 activity results in ocular malformations, overexpression of PAX6 in transgenic mice results in ocular defects similar to those associated with PAX6 deficiency (Schedl et al., 1996). These results suggest that in order for normal ocular development to occur, PAX6 levels must be maintained within a narrow range. For example, PAX6 expression may be calibrated to different levels in different cell types in the developing eye so that either overexpression or underexpression would affect the identity of one or more cell types.

Mutations in Human PAX6: Aniridia

Despite its name, aniridia is a panocular disorder of variable severity and autosomal dominant inheritance with an incidence of approximately 1 in 80,000 (reviewed by Jordan et al., 1992). In addition to iris aplasia or hypoplasia, other ocular abnormalities including cataract, foveal dysplasia, glaucoma, lens dislocation, and optic nerve hypoplasia have been detected in affected individuals. A small minority of patients with aniridia also manifest the other findings of the WAGR syndrome (see Chapter 6). As predicted by the observation that *Pax6* and *Wt1* were closely linked in the mouse genome and the similarity of the *Small eye* and aniridia phenotypes, the human *PAX6* locus (originally named *AN*) was mapped to a position 700 kb telomeric to *WT1* on human chromosome 11p13 within the region that is deleted in patients with WAGR (Ton et al., 1991). In humans, as in the mouse, PAX6 mRNA was localized to structures of the developing human eye.

Analysis of genomic DNA from patients with isolated aniridia (MIM 106210), who did not have other findings of WAGR syndrome and did not have chromosome 11p13 deletions, resulted in the identification of mutations (Fig. 7.6) in the human *PAX6* gene (Davis and Cowell, 1993; Glaser et al., 1992, 1994; Hanson et al., 1993; Jordan et al., 1992; Martha et al., 1994a, b). All of the mutations identified in genomic DNA from patients with isolated aniridia predict the synthesis of a truncated, nonfunctional protein except for a single missense mutation (R208W) just amino-terminal to the homeodomain. In contrast to the analysis of *PAX3* in patients with Waardenburg syndrome and related disorders, no missense mutations have been identified in the paired domain of PAX6 in patients with aniridia. In the case of the nonsense mutation S353X that truncates the protein within the PST domain, transcriptional studies revealed that the mutated domain still retained residual transcriptional activity (Glaser et al., 1994). This is consistent with the observations that (1) the truncation is less extensive than in the Sey^{Neu} allele that results in complete loss of transcriptional activity and (2) heterozygosity for the S353X mutation was associated with a relatively mild clinical presentation (see below). These results therefore provide a correlation between the effect of the mutation on the ability of PAX6 to function as a transcriptional activator and the effect of the mutation on ocular development.

As in the case of *Small eye, Splotch,* and Waardenburg syndrome, homozygosity for mutant alleles at the human *PAX6* locus results in an extremely severe phenotype. In the single family that was investigated thoroughly at the molecular level (Glaser et al., 1994), the father was heterozygous for the S353X mutation and had relatively mild disease that manifested as neonatal cataracts, decreased visual acuity, nystagmus, and right exotropia (Fig. 7.7 c, d). The mother was heterozygous for a single nucleotide insertion at codon 103 at the end of the paired box that resulted in a frameshift termination codon. Her ophthalmologic examination revealed bilateral severe iris hypoplasia, cataracts, corneal and foveal hypoplasia, and reduced visual acuity (Fig. 7.7 a, b). Their offspring, who was a compound heterozygote due to inheritance of mutant alleles from both parents, died on the eighth day of life and manifested generalized growth retardation, bilateral anophthalmia, dysplastic nose with choanal atresia, micrognathia, and microcephaly with multiple central nervous system abnormalities including cerebral and cerebellar dys-

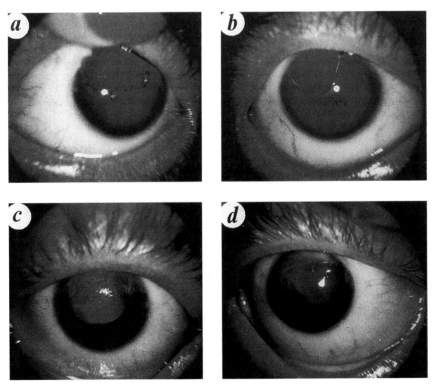

FIGURE 7-7. Aniridia in a husband and wife. Eyes of the female (*a*, *b*) demonstrate only a small rim of iris tissue whereas the eyes of the male (*c*, *d*) are notable for postsurgical defects in the iris following bilateral removal of the lens. (Reprinted with permission from Glaser et al., 1994.)

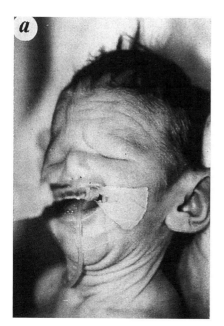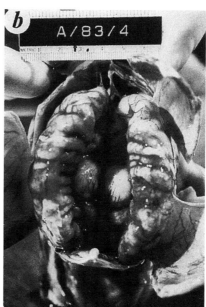

FIGURE 7-8. Homozygosity for mutation of the human *PAX6* gene. (*a*), Craniofacial malformations include microcephaly (small head), anophthalmia (absence of eyes) with fused eyelids, malformed nose with small nares, and mandibular hypoplasia (small jaw). (*b*), Postmortem examination of the brain demonstrated absence of the corpus callosum, reduction in size of the cerebral hemispheres, and presence of a large midline cavity with brainstem visible below. (Reprinted with permission from Glaser et al., 1994.)

plasia/hypoplasia, agenesis of the olfactory bulbs and corpus callosum, and a single open ventricular system (Fig. 7.8). The central nervous system and ocular defects were remarkably similar to those observed in homozygous Sey^{Neu} mice (Glaser et al., 1994).

Mutations in Human PAX6: Other Ocular Disorders

Peters' anomaly. In contrast to aniridia, the abnormalities that constitute Peters' anomaly are limited to structures of the anterior chamber (cornea, iris, and lens). Peters' anomaly can thus be considered a less severe developmental defect than aniridia. A missense mutation affecting the paired domain (R26G) was identified as a cause of this syndrome (Hanson et al., 1994). It will be interesting to determine whether this mutation affects development of only anterior structures because of dosage effects,

effects on binding to a subset of target genes, or effects on binding to a subset of coactivator proteins. It is difficult to attribute the difference in phenotype to the specific mutation because another patient was found to have complete deletion of *PAX6* and *WT1* (Hanson et al., 1994) (i.e., WAGR syndrome), but with Peters' anomaly rather than aniridia, suggesting that other genetic factors may play an important role in determining the phenotypic outcome when the activity of PAX6 is reduced in developing ocular structures. Examination of *Sey*/+ mice revealed variable presence of corneal adhesions that are a characteristic finding of Peters' anomaly (Hanson et al., 1994). These results suggest that in animals with *PAX6* mutations, the specific ocular malformations and their severity may, to a certain degree, be determined by stochastic mechanisms.

Isolated foveal hypoplasia. PAX6 mutations are also associated with an ocular malformation syndrome affecting the posterior chamber only. The fovea centralis is located at the posterior pole of the retina and is important for normal visual acuity. Isolated foveal hypoplasia is an autosomal dominant condition (MIM 136520) and a missense mutation in the paired domain of PAX6 (R125C) was shown to segregate with disease in multiple members of a single family (Azuma et al., 1996). The affected arginine (residue 23 of the paired domain) is at the same position as the arginine that is substituted in the mutant PAX3 (R56L) protein associated with WS type I (see Fig. 7.3). Arginine-23 of the paired domain has been shown to directly contact the sugar phosphate backbone of the DNA binding site (Xu et al., 1995), suggesting that the PAX3 (R56L) and PAX6 (R125C) missense mutations may adversely affect the ability of these proteins to bind to DNA.

Autosomal dominant keratitis. Another disorder of the anterior chamber is autosomal dominant keratitis (MIM 148190). Molecular genetic analysis of a family in which this disorder was segregating revealed a mutation at the *PAX6* intron 10 splice-acceptor site, AG → TG, which predicts the synthesis of a protein truncated within the PST domain (Mirzayans et al., 1995). The *Sey^Neu* mutation is a GT → TT substitution within the splice donor site of intron 10 of the mouse *Pax6* gene, which is also predicted to encode a protein truncated within the PST domain that is transcriptionally inactive (Glaser et al., 1994; Hill et al., 1991). The milder phenotype associated with the human compared to the mouse mutation may reflect utilization of cryptic splice sites that might introduce several novel amino acids into the protein without altering the translational reading frame (Mirzayans et al., 1995). The severity of ocular defects in affected family members varied significantly, suggesting that variation at other loci and/or environmental factors may modify the clinical presentation associated with a given *PAX6* genotype.

Mutations in Drosophila pax6: eyeless

The compound eye of insects such as *Drosophila melanogaster* differs greatly in structure from the mammalian eye with its single lens. It was therefore a surprise when the gene affected by the *Drosophila eyeless (ey)* mutation was identified as the fly homologue of the mammalian *PAX6* gene (Quiring et al., 1994). When compared to mammalian PAX6, the amino acid sequence of *Drosophila* PAX6 was 94% and 90% identical in the paired domain and homeodomain, respectively, a remarkable degree of conservation considering the approximately 500 million years of evolutionary divergence separating these species. However, the *Drosophila* protein, at 838 amino acids, is almost twice as large as its mammalian homologues. Two mutant alleles, ey^2 and ey^R, contained insertions of transposable elements into the same region of an intervening sequence, which prevented gene expression probably by disrupting an important *cis*-acting regulatory element (Quiring et al., 1994). The implications of these results with respect to evolutionary theories were significant. Prior to this report, it was assumed that ocular structures had evolved independently as many as several dozen times (reviewed by Zuker, 1994). These results provide compelling evidence that a gene encoding an ancestral PAX6 molecule was present at a very early stage in metazoan evolution.

As remarkable as these results were, further investigations led to equally amazing discoveries. When the *ey* gene was expressed ectopically in imaginal discs of developing flies, supernumerary eyes developed at the sites of *ey* expression, regardless of whether the location was the imaginal discs giving rise to antenna, leg, or wing (Halder et al., 1995) (Fig. 7.9). These eyes were functional, for illumination resulted in electrical activity in photoreceptor cells. Ectopic expression of the mouse *Pax6* gene in flies also resulted in ectopic eye formation, demonstrating conservation of function as well as sequence between the invertebrate and vertebrate proteins. Expression in *Drosophila* of *Pax6* gene isolated from the squid *Loligo opalescens* also resulted in the development of ectopic eyes (Tomarev et al., 1997). These results indicated that *PAX6* is a master regulatory gene capable of controlling all steps required for the formation of a functioning eye, regardless of the ocular structure, which varies greatly among fly, human, and squid (see Zuker, 1994). Thus,

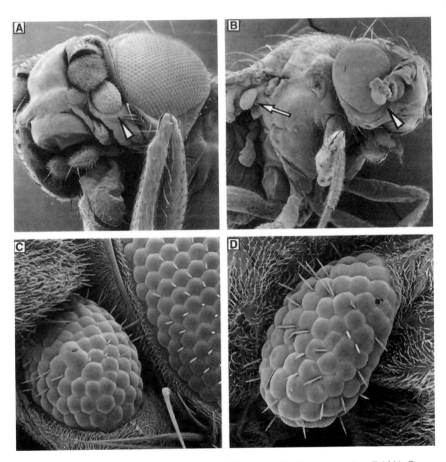

FIGURE 7-9. Formation of ectopic eyes in flies ectopically expressing PAX6. Scanning electron micrographs demonstrate ectopic eyes in the region formed by the antennal disc (A and C) and under the wing (B and D). Note that the structural organization of the normal and ectopic compound eyes is remarkably similar. (Reprinted with permission from Halder et al., 1995. Copyright ©1995 by the American Association for the Advancement of Science.)

whereas *HOX* genes appear to determine spatial identity within the developing embryo (see Chapter 9), *PAX6* appears to determine organ identity regardless of position.

PAX6 also participates in other developmental pathways in some species: in mammals the formation of brain and craniofacial structures requires PAX6 expression (Glaser et al., 1994; Hill et al., 1991). The PAX6 homologue in the roundworm *Caenorhabditis elegans* also plays a more general role in head morphogenesis and the formation of other sense organs (Chisholm and Horvitz, 1995; Zhang and Emmons, 1995). Because *C. elegans* has no photoreceptor cells, these results bring into question the model in which PAX6 expression is associated with photosensation. An alternate hypothesis is that PAX6 originally evolved to control development of head structures and later became involved in ocular development (Chisholm and Horvitz, 1995). Thus, the evolutionary debate has shifted from structural models of ocular development to genetic models of PAX6 function. These investigations of PAX6 illustrate how the use of powerful molecular biological techniques will result in rapid advances in our understanding of both development and evolution in the coming years.

Halder et al. (1995) estimated that more than 2500 genes are involved in ocular development and proposed that based on their results, all of these genes must be directly or indirectly controlled by PAX6. During the evolution of different species, it is likely that different target genes were brought under the control of PAX6 (by nucleotide sequence changes that resulted in the generation of a PAX6 binding site within *cis*-acting regulatory elements), thus allowing for a single master regulator to direct the formation of radically divergent structures that, however, were all designed to accomplish a similar function. Given the fact that PAX6 is also expressed in the nervous system, one wonders whether it is also involved in the development of visual processing centers within the brainstem and cortex in order to ensure that all aspects of light sensation are properly coordinated.

That the concept of a "master" regulatory gene may be too simple to represent the full story of ocular development is suggested by recent studies investigating the role of the *dachshund* gene in *Drosophila* ocular development (Shen and Mardon, 1997). Ectopic expression of the *dachshund* gene also resulted in ectopic eye formation, although not in 100% of transgenic flies as was described for the *eyeless* gene. However, in the absence of *dachshund* expression, flies developed with severely reduced or no eyes and *dachshund* expression was required for ectopic ocular development in response to ectopic *eyeless* expression. Ectopic expression of *dachshund* was induced by ectopic expression of *eyeless*. However, ectopic *dachshund* expression also induced ectopic *eyeless* expression. Taken together these results suggest that *dachshund* may be immediately downstream of *eyeless* and that an *eyeless-dachshund-eyeless* positive-regulatory loop may be important to ensure that the genetic program that controls ocular development is stably activated in the original *eyeless*-expressing cells and in all of their descendants. The identification of vertebrate homologues will provide additional evidence for the importance of *dachshund* in ocular development.

PAX2

Beginning at E10, the mouse *Pax2* gene is expressed in the developing central nervous system, eyes, ears, and urogenital system (Dressler et al., 1990; Nornes et al., 1990; Rowitch and McMahon, 1995). In contrast to PAX1, PAX3, and PAX6, PAX2 contains a paired domain and a truncated homeodomain (Fig. 7.1). PAX2 shares with PAX3, but not PAX6, the presence of a conserved octapeptide sequence located between the paired domain and homeodomain.

Mutation in Human PAX2

A syndrome of optic nerve coloboma, renal hypoplasia, and vesicoureteral reflux (renal-coloboma syndrome; MIM 120330) was identified in a father and three of his five children. A single nucleotide deletion was demonstrated in one copy of the *PAX2* gene in affected family members (Sanyanusin et al., 1995b). The frameshift mutation predicted the synthesis of a protein truncated within the octapeptide (see Fig. 7.1) and thus lacking the entire carboxyl-terminal half of the PAX2 polypeptide. In a second family with optic nerve coloboma and chronic renal failure, a single nucleotide-insertion frameshift mutation was identified in *PAX2* that would encode a truncated protein lacking most of the paired domain and downstream residues (Sanyanusin et al., 1995a).

Subsequently, a group of 40 patients who had multiple malformations that included ocular and renal defects but did not manifest the classic renal-coloboma syndrome were studied and four patients were found to be heterozygous for *PAX2* mutations (Schimmenti et al., 1997). Together with previous cases, a total of 10 patients could be compared with respect to phenotypic manifestations. Whereas all patients manifested renal hypoplasia/failure and retinal/optic nerve malformations of variable severity, three patients had central nervous system malformations including one case of microcephaly and mental retardation, three patients had sensorineural hearing loss, and seven patients had soft skin and/or joint laxity. This latter finding is unexplained, because PAX2 expression has not been detected in these tissues. Thus, PAX6 and PAX2 are expressed in the anterior-posterior and posterior chambers of the eye, respectively; both PAX3 and PAX2 are expressed in the inner ear; and PAX2, PAX3, and PAX6 are all expressed in the developing central nervous system. This study is instructive for clinical geneticists: at some frequency (in this case, 10%), mutations will be found in patients with nonclassical presentations of malformation syndromes. Thus, as techniques for gene screening become more efficient, so will our ability to obtain molecular diagnoses. Five of the ten patients had the same frame-shift mutation, insG619, yet manifested remarkably different phenotypes, including a mildly affected mother and severely affected son (Schimmenti et al., 1997). This result provides another didactic point: identification of a gene mutation will not tell us everything about the patient's disease.

Effects of Altered Levels of Pax2 Expression in Mice

A line of transgenic mice was identified in which transgene integration was associated with a malformation syndrome consisting of kidney and retinal defects (Keller et al., 1994). The insertional mutation *Krd* included a large deletion of approximately 7 cM on mouse chromosome 19 that included the *Pax2* locus. Renal abnormalities in *Krd/+* mice ranged from aplasia to hypoplasia to polycystic kidneys. Reduction in cell numbers were also seen in the retina. Although several other known genes and an indeterminate number of unknown genes were also deleted, the fact that abnormal ocular and renal development were also associated with loss of human PAX2 function suggested that these aspects of the phenotype were attributable to deletion of *Pax2*. If such were the case, then introduction of a *Pax2* transgene into the germline of *Krd* mice may result in normal ocular and renal development, but transgene correction of the phenotype has not been reported. Dysregulated expression of Pax2 from a cytomegalovirus promoter in transgenic mice is associated with renal cystic dysplasia (Dressler et al., 1993). Although these mice were reported to be born with their eyes open (abnormal for mice), no specific ocular malformations were reported. These results suggest that, as in the case of *Pax6* and ocular development (Schedl et al., 1996), both underexpression and overexpression of Pax2 can result in renal malformations.

Mice homozygous for a *Pax2* null allele manifested aplasia of the kidneys, ureters, and genital tract of both sexes (Torres et al., 1995). In addition, there was a high incidence of renal hypoplasia among heterozygotes. Homozygous *Pax2* mutant mice also had defective optic fissure closure, failure of optic nerve glial cell differentiation, and aplasia of the optic chiasm (Torres et al., 1996). These results demonstrate that PAX2 expression is required for normal genitourinary and ocular development.

A mouse mutant allele, *Pax2^{1Neu}*, was recently described containing a frameshift mutation that alters the amino acid sequence after codon 24 (Favor et al., 1996). Remarkably, this is the same mutation found in 5 of 10 patients with renal-coloboma syndrome and *PAX2* gene defects as described above. Both the human and mouse genes contain seven consecutive guanine residues at the site of the nucleotide insertion, suggesting that strand slippage during DNA replication may be responsible for this mutation in both species (Favor et al., 1996). *Pax2^{1Neu}* heterozygotes manifested optic disc dysplasia and kidney defects, whereas homozygotes manifested optic nerve hypoplasia, failure of metanephric kidney development, agenesis of the cerebellum and posterior mesencephalon, and inner ear defects including cochlear agenesis (Favor et al., 1996). The similarity between the phenotype of homozygous *Pax2^{1Neu}* and *Pax2* knockout mice suggests that the mouse (and therefore, human) frameshift mutation results in a loss of function.

The defects in development of the mid-hindbrain region in *Pax2^{1Neu}* homozygotes were similar to those observed in mice homozygous for null alleles of the *Wnt1* and *En1* genes, which encode a signaling molecule and transcription factor, respectively (McMahon and Bradley, 1990; Wurst et al., 1994). Several observations suggest that PAX2 may regulate expression of *Wnt1, En1,* and *En2*: (1) *Pax2* expression precedes expression of *En1, En2,* and *Wnt1* during mouse mid-hindbrain development (Kelly and Moon, 1995; Rowitch and McMahon, 1995); (2) injection of antibodies to block PAX2 function leads to reduced *En2* and *Wnt1* expression and mid-hindbrain malformations in zebrafish embryos (Krauss et al., 1992); and (3) potential PAX2 binding sites are required for *En2* expression in the embryonic brain (Song et al., 1996). Remarkably, in *Drosophila*, the *paired* gene product is required for expression of *wingless* and *engrailed*, the homologues of the mammalian *Wnt1* and *En1/En2* genes, respectively, suggesting that this genetic regulatory circuit has been conserved for over 500 million years (Favor et al., 1996).

Summary

Active research over the past decade has provided compelling evidence for the essential role of PAX proteins in mammalian development. Loss-of-function mutations in PAX1, PAX2, PAX3, and PAX6 have been associated with malformation syndromes (Table 7.1). The striking conservation of amino acid sequence and the strikingly similar phenotypic effects of mutations in the genes encoding these proteins in humans and mice provide further evidence of their importance for normal development. Whereas germline mutations in these genes result in malformation syndromes, somatic mutations in these same genes have been identified in human cancers, as will be described in Chapter 15.

References

Asher, J., and T. Friedman. Mouse and hamster mutants as models for Waardenburg syndromes in humans. *J. Med. Genet.* 27:618–626, 1990.

Asher, J. H., Jr., R. W. Harrison, R. Morell, M. L. Carey, and T. B. Friedman. Effects of Pax3 modifier genes on craniofacial morphology, pigmentation, and viability: a murine model of Waardenburg syndrome variation. *Genomics* 34:285–298, 1996a.

Asher, J. H., Jr., A. Sommer, R. Morell, and T. B. Friedman. Missense mutation in the paired domain of PAX3 causes craniofacial-deafness-hand syndrome. *Hum. Mutat.* 7:30–35, 1996b.

Azuma, N., S. Nishina, H. Yanagisawa, T. Okuyama, and M. Yamada. PAX6 missense mutation in isolated foveal hypoplasia. *Nat. Genet.* 13:141–142, 1996.

Baldwin, C. T., C. F. Hoth, J. A. Amos, E. O. da-Silva, and A. Milunsky. An exonic mutation in the HuP2 paired domain gene causes Waardenburg's syndrome. *Nature* 355:637–638, 1992.

Baldwin, C. T., N. R. Lipsky, C. F. Hoth, T. Cohen, W. Mamuya, and A. Milunsky. Mutations in PAX3 associated with Waardenburg syndrome type I. *Hum. Mutat.* 3:205–211, 1994.

Balling, R., U. Deutsch, and P. Gruss. Undulated, a mutation affecting development of the mouse skeleton, has a point mutation in the paired box of Pax-1. *Cell* 55:531–535, 1988.

Balling, R., C. F. Lau, S. Dietrich, J. Wallin, and P. Gruss. Development of the skeletal system. *Ciba Found. Symp.* 165:132–143, 1992.

Butt, J., J. Greenberg, I. Winship, S. Sellars, P. Beighton, and R. Ramesar. A splice junction mutation in PAX3 causes Waardenburg syndrome in a South African family. *Hum. Mol. Genet.* 3:197–198, 1994.

Chalepakis, G., R. Fritsch, H. Fickenscher, U. Deutsch, M. Goulding, and P. Gruss. The molecular basis of the undulated/Pax-1 mutation. *Cell* 65:873–884, 1991.

Chalepakis, G., A. Stoykova, J. Wijnholds, P. Tremblay, and P. Gruss. Pax: gene regulators in the developing nervous system. *J. Neurobiol.* 24:1367–1384, 1993.

Chisholm, A. D., and H. R. Horvitz. Patterning of the Caenorhabditis elegans head region by the Pax-6 family member vab-3. *Nature* 377:52–55, 1995.

Czerny, T., G. Schaffner, and M. Busslinger. DNA sequence recognition by Pax proteins: bipartite structure of the paired domain and its binding site. *Genes Dev.* 7:2048–2061, 1993.

Davis, A., and J. K. Cowell. Mutations in the PAX6 gene in patients with hereditary aniridia. *Hum. Mol. Genet.* 2:2093–2097, 1993.

Deutsch, U., G. R. Dressler, and P. Gruss. Pax1, a member of a paired box homologous murine gene family, is expressed in segmental structures during development. *Cell* 53:617–625, 1988.

Dressler, G. R., U. Deutsch, K. Chowdhury, H. O. Nornes, and P. Gruss. Pax 2, a new murine paired-box-containing gene and its expression in the developing excretory system. *Development* 109:787–795, 1990.

Dressler, G. R., J. E. Wilkinson, U. W. Rothenpieier, L. T. Patterson, L. Williams-Simons, and H. Westphal. Deregulation of Pax-2 expression in transgenic mice generates severe kidney abnormalities. *Nature* 362:65–67, 1993.

Epstein, D. J., D. Malo, M. Vekemans, and P. Gros. Molecular characterization of a deletion encompassing the Splotch mutation on mouse chromosome 1. *Genomics* 10:89–93, 1991a.

Epstein, D. J., M. Vekemans, and P. Gros. Splotch (Sp^{2h}), a mutation affecting development of the mouse neural-tube shows a deletion within the paired homeodomain of Pax-3. *Cell* 67:767–774, 1991b.

Epstein, D. J., K. J. Vogan, D. G. Trasler, and P. Gros. A mutation within intron-3 of the pax-3 gene produces aberrantly spliced messenger-RNA transcripts in the Splotch (Sp) mouse mutant. *Proc. Natl. Acad. Sci. U.S.A.* 90:532–536, 1993.

Farrer, L. A., K. S. Arnos, J. H. Asher, Jr., C. T. Baldwin, S. R. Diehl, T. B. Friedman, J. Greenburg, K. M. Grundfast, C. Hoth, A. K. Lalwani, B. Landa, K. Leverton, A. Milunsky, R. Morell, W. Nance, V. Newton, R. Ramesar, V. S. Rao, J. E. Reynolds, T. B. San Agustin, E. R. Wilcox, I. Winship, and A. P. Read. Locus heterogeneity for Waardenburg syndrome is predictive of clinical subtypes. *Am. J. Hum. Genet.* 55:728–737, 1994.

Farrer, L. A., K. M. Grundfast, J. Amos, K. S. Arnos, J. H. Asher, Jr., P. Beighton, S. R. Diehl, J. Fex, C. Foy, T. B. Friedman, J. Greenberg, C. Hoth, M. Marazita, A. Milunsky, R. Morell, W. Nance, V. Newton, R. Ramesar, T. B. San Agustin, J. Skare, C. A. Stevens, R. G. Wagner, Jr., E. R. Wilcox, I. Winship, and A. P. Read. Waardenburg syndrome (WS) type I is caused by defects at multiple loci, one of which is near ALPP on chromosome 2: first report of the WS consortium. *Am. J. Hum. Genet.* 50:902–913, 1992.

Favor, J., R. Sandaulache, A. Neuhauser-Klaus, W. Pretsch, B. Chatterjee, E. Senft, W. Wurst, V. Blanquet, P. Grimes, R. Sporle, and K. Schughart. The mouse Pax2[1Neu] mutation is identical to a human PAX2 mutation in a family with renal-coloboma syndrome and results in developmental defects of the brain, ear, eye, and kidney. *Proc. Natl. Acad. Sci. U.S.A.* 93:13870–13875, 1996.

Foy, C., V. Newton, D. Wellesley, R. Harris, and A. P. Read. Assignment of the locus for Waardenburg syndrome type I to human chromosome 2q37 and possible homology to the Splotch mouse. *Am J. Hum. Genet.* 46:1017–1023, 1990.

Glaser, T., L. Jepeal, J. G. Edwards, S. R. Young, J. Favor, and R. L. Maas. PAX6 gene dosage effect in a family with congenital cataracts, aniridia, anophthalmia and central nervous system defects. *Nat. Genet.* 7:463–471, 1994.

Glaser, T., D. S. Walton, and R. L. Maas. Genomic structure, evolutionary conservation, and aniridia mutations in the human PAX6 gene. *Nat. Genet.* 2: 232–239, 1992.

Goulding, M. D., G. Chalepakis, U. Deutsch, J. Erselius, and P. Gruss. Pax-3, a novel murine DNA binding protein expressed during early neurogenesis. *EMBO J.* 10:1135–1147, 1991.

Goulding, M., S. Sterrer, J. Fleming, R. Balling, J. Nadeau, K. J. Moore, S. D. M. Brown, K. P. Steel, and P. Gruss. Analysis of the pax-3 gene in the mouse mutant Splotch. *Genomics* 17:355–363, 1993.

Grindley, J. C., D. R. Davidson, and R. E. Hill. The role of Pax-6 in eye and nasal development. *Development* 121:1433–1442, 1995.

Gruss, P., and C. Walther. Pax in development. *Cell* 69:719–722, 1992.

Hageman, M. J., and J. W. Delleman. Heterogeneity in Waardenburg syndrome. *Am. J. Hum. Genet.* 29:468–485, 1977.

Halder, G., P. Callaerts, and W. J. Gehring. Induction of ectopic eyes by targeted expression of the eyeless gene in Drosophila. *Science* 267:1788–1792, 1995.

Hanson, I., J. M. Fletcher, T. Jordan, A. Brown, D. Taylor, R. J. Adams, H. H. Punnett, and V. van Heyningen. Mutations at the PAX6 locus are found in heterogeneous anterior segment malformations including Peters' anomaly. *Nat. Genet.* 6:168–173, 1994.

Hanson, I. M., A. Seawright, K. Hardman, S. Hodgson, D. Zaletayev, G. Fekete, and V. van Heyningen. PAX6 mutations in aniridia. *Hum. Mol. Genet.* 2:915–920, 1993.

Hill, R. E., J. Favor, B. L. M. Hogan, C. C. T. Ton, G. F Saunders, I. M. Hanson, J. Prosser, T. Jordan, N. D. Hastie, and V. van Heyningen. Mouse small eye results from mutations in a paired-like homeobox-containing gene. *Nature* 354:522–525, 1991.

Hoth, C. F., A. Milunsky, N. Lipsky, R. Sheffer, S. K. Clarren, and C. T. Baldwin. Mutations in the paired domain of the human PAX3 gene cause Klein-Waardenburg syndrome (WS-III) as well as Waardenburg syndrome type I (WS-I). *Am. J. Hum. Genet.* 52:455–462, 1993.

Hughes, A. E., V. E. Newton, X. Z. Liu, and A. P. Read. A gene for Waardenburg syndrome type 2 maps close to the human homologue of the microphthalmia gene at chromosome 3p12–p14.1. *Nat. Genet.* 7:509–512, 1994.

Jordan, T., I. Hanson, D. Zaletayev, S. Hodgson, J. Prosser, A. Seawright, N. Hastie, and V. van Heyningen. The human PAX6 gene is mutated in two patients with aniridia. *Nat. Genet.* 1:328–332, 1992.

Keller, S. A., J. M. Jones, A. Boyle, L. L. Barrow, P. D. Killen, D. G. Green, N. V. Kapousta, P. F. Hitchcock, R. T. Swank, and M. H. Meisler. Kidney and retinal defects (Krd), a transgene-induced mutation with a deletion of mouse chromosome 19 that includes the Pax2 locus. *Genomics* 23:309–320, 1994.

Kelly, G. M., and R. T. Moon. Involvement of wnt1 and pax2 in the formation of the midbrain-hindbrain boundary in the zebrafish gastrula. *Dev. Genet.* 17:129–140, 1995.

Klein, D. Historical background and evidence for dominant inheritance of the Klein-Waardenburg syndrome (type III). *Am. J. Med. Genet.* 14:231–239, 1983.

Krauss, S., M. Maden, N. Holder, and S. W. Wilson. Zebrafish pax[b] is involved in the formation of the midbrain-hindbrain boundary. *Nature* 360:87–89, 1992.

Lalwani, A. K., J. R. Brister, J. Fex, K. M. Grundfast, B. Ploplis, T. B. San Agustin, and E. R. Wilcox. Further elucidation of the genomic structure of PAX3 and identification of two different point mutations within the PAX3 homeobox that cause Waardenburg syndrome type I in two families. *Am. J. Hum. Genet.* 56:75–83, 1995.

Martha, A., R. E. Ferrell, H. Mintz-Hittner, L. A. Lyons, and G. F. Saunders. Paired box mutations in familial and sporadic aniridia predicts truncated aniridia proteins. *Am. J. Hum. Genet.* 54:801–811, 1994a.

Martha, A. D., R. E. Ferrell, and G. F. Saunders. Nonsense mutation in the homeobox region of the aniridia gene. *Hum. Mutat.* 3:297–200, 1994b.

Matsuo, T., N. Osumi-Yamashita, S. Noji, H. Ohuchi, E. Koyama, F. Myokai, N. Matsuo, S. Taniguchi, H. Doi, S. Iseki, Y. Ninomiya, M. Fujiwara, T. Watanabe, and K. Eto. A mutation in the pax-6 gene in rat small-eye is associated with impaired migration of midbrain crest cells. *Nat. Genet.* 3:299–304, 1993.

McKusick, V. A. *Mendelian Inheritance in Man: Catalogs of Autosomal Dominant, Autosomal Recessive, and X-linked Phenotypes.* Baltimore: The Johns Hopkins University Press, 1986.

McMahon, A. P., and A. Bradley. The Wnt-1 (int-1) proto-oncogene is required for development of a large region of the mouse brain. *Cell* 62:1073–1085, 1990.

Mirzayans, F., W. G. Pearce, I. M. MacDonald, and M. A. Walter. Mutation of the PAX6 gene in patients with autosomal dominant keratitis. *Am. J. Hum. Genet.* 57:539–548, 1995.

Morell, R., T. B. Friedman, S. Moeljopawiro, Hartono, Soervito, and J. H. Asher. A frameshift mutation in the HuP2 paired domain of the probable human homologue of murine Pax-3 is responsible for Waardenburg syndrome type I in an Indonesian family. *Hum. Mol. Genet.* 1:243–247, 1992.

Nornes, H. O., G. R. Dressler, E. W. Knapik, U. Deutsch, and P. Gruss. Spatially and temporally restricted expression of Pax 2 during murine neurogenesis. *Development* 109:797–809, 1990.

Pasteris, N. G., B. J. Trask, S. Sheldon, and J. L. Gorski. Discordant of two over-lapping deletions involving the PAX3 gene in chromosome 2q35. *Hum. Mol. Genet.* 2:953–959, 1993.

Pierpont, J. W., L. D. Doolan, G. R. Snead, and R. P. Erickson. A single base pair substitution within the paired box of PAX3 in an individual with Waarden-burg syndrome type I (WSI). *Hum. Mutat.* 4:227–228, 1994.

Quinn, J. C., J. D. West, and R. E. Hill. Multiple functions for Pax6 in mouse eye and nasal development. *Genes Dev.* 10:435–446, 1996.

Quiring, R., U. Walldorf, U. Kloter, and W. J. Gehring. Homology of the eyeless gene of Drosophila to the Small eye gene in mice and Aniridia in humans. *Science* 265:785–789, 1994.

Rowitch, D. H., and A. P. McMahon. Pax-2 expression in the murine neural plate precedes and encompasses the expression domains of Wnt-1 and En-1. *Mech. Dev.* 52:3–8, 1995.

Sanyanusin, P., L. A. McNoe, M. J. Sullivan, R. G. Weaver, and M. R. Eccles. Mutation of PAX2 in two siblings with renal-coloboma syndrome. *Hum. Mol. Genet.* 4:2183–2184, 1995a.

Sanyanusin, P., L. A. Schimmenti, L. A. McNoe, T. A. Ward, M. E. M. Pierpont, M. J. Sullivan, W. B. Dobyns, and M. R. Eccles. Mutation of the PAX2 gene in a family with optic nerve colobomas, renal anomalies and vesicoureteral reflux. *Nat. Genet.* 9:358–363, 1995b.

Schedl, A., A. Ross, M. Lee, D. Engelkamp, P. Rashbass, V. van Heyningen, and N. D. Hastie. Influence of PAX6 gene dosage on development: over-expression causes severe eye abnormalities. *Cell* 86:71–82, 1996.

Schimmenti, L. A., H. E. Cunliffe, L. A. McNoe, T. A. Ward, M. C. French, H. H. Shim, Y.-H. Zhang, W. Proesmans, A. Leys, K. A. Byerly, S. R. Braddock, M. Masuno, K. Imaizumi, K. Devriendt, and M. R. Eccles. Further delineation of renal-coloboma syndrome in patients with extreme variability of pheno-type and identical PAX2 mutations. *Am. J. Hum. Genet.* 60:869–878, 1997.

Shen, W., and G. Mardon. Ectopic eye development in Drosophila induced by directed dachshund expression. *Development* 124:45–52, 1997.

Sommer, A., T. Young-Wee, and T. Frye. Previously undescribed syndrome of craniofacial, hand anomalies, and sensorineural deafness. *Am. J. Med. Genet.* 15:71–77, 1983.

Song, D. L., G. Chalepakis, P. Gruss, and A. L. Joyner. Two Pax-binding sites are required for early embryonic brain expression of an Engrailed-2 transgene. *Development* 122:627–635, 1996.

Strachan, T., and A. P. Read. PAX genes. *Curr. Opin. Genet. Devel.* 4:427–438, 1994.

Stuart, E. T., and P. Gruss. PAX genes: what's new in developmental biology and cancer? *Hum. Mol. Genet.* 4:1717–1720, 1995.

Tassabehji, M., V. E. Newton, K. Leverton, K. Turnbull, E. Seemanova, J. Kunze, K. Sperling, T. Strachan, and A. P. Read. PAX3 gene structure and mutations: close analogies between Waardenburg syndrome and the Splotch mouse. *Hum. Mol. Genet.* 3:1069–1074, 1994.

Tassabehji, M., V. E. Newton, X. Z. Liu, A. Brady, D. Donnai, M. Krajewska-Walasek, V. Murday, A. Norman, E. Obersztyn, W. Reardon, J. C. Rice, R. Trembath, P. Wieacker, M. Whiteford, R. Winter, and A. P. Read. The mutational spectrum in Waardenburg syndrome. *Hum. Mol. Genet.* 4:2131–2137, 1995.

Tassabehji, M., A. P. Read, V. E. Newton, R. Harris, R. Balling, P. Gruss, and T. Strachan. Waardenburg's syndrome patients have mutations in the human homologue of the Pax-3 paired box gene. *Nature* 355:635–636, 1992.

Tassabehji, M., A. P. Read, V. E. Newton, M. Patton, P. Gruss, R. Harris, and T. Strachan. Mutations in the PAX3 gene causing Waardenburg syndrome type 1 and type 2. *Nat. Genet.* 3:27–30, 1993.

Tomarev, S. I., P. Callaerts, L. Kos, R. Zinovieva, G. Halder, W. Gehring, and J. Piatigorsky. Squid Pax-6 and eye development. *Proc. Natl. Acad. Sci. U.S.A.* 94:2421–2426, 1997.

Ton, C. C. T., H. Hirronen, H. Miwa, M. M. Weil, P. Monaghan, T. Jordan, V. van Heyningen, N. D. Hastie, H. Meijers-Heijboer, M. Drechsler, B. Royer-Pokora, F. Collins, A. Swaroop, L. C. Strong, and G .F. Saunders. Positional cloning and characterization of a paired box-and homeobox-containing gene farom the aniridia region. *Cell* 67:1059–1074, 1991.

Torres, M., E. Gomez-Pardo, G. R. Dressler, and P. Gruss. Pax-2 controls multiple steps of urogenital development. *Development* 121:4057–4065, 1995.

Torres, M., E. Gomez-Pardo, and P. Gruss. Pax-2 contributes to inner ear patterning and optic nerve trajectory. *Development* 122:3381–3391, 1996.

Treisman, J., E. Harris, and C. Desplan. The paired box encodes a second DNA-binding domain in the paired homeodomain protein. *Genes Dev.* 5:594–604, 1991.

Vogan, K. J., D. J. Epstein, D. G. Trasler, and P. Gros. The Splotch-delayed (Sp^d) mouse mutant carries a point mutation within the paired box of the pax-3 gene. *Genomics* 17:364–369, 1993.

Waardenburg, P. J. A new syndrome combining developmental anomalies of the eyelids, eyebrows, and nose root with pigmentary defects of the iris and head hair and with congenital deafness. *Am. J. Hum. Genet.* 3:195–253, 1951.

Walter, M. A., and P. N. Goodfellow. Disease and development. *Nature* 355:590–591, 1992.

Walther, C., and P. Gruss. Pax-6, a murine paired box gene, is expressed in the developing CNS. *Development* 113:1435–1449, 1991.

Wurst, W., A. B. Auerbach, and A. L. Joyner. Multiple developmental defects in Engrailed-1 mutant mice: an early mid-hindbrain deletion and patterning defects in forelimbs and sternum. *Development* 120:2065–2075, 1994.

Xu, W., M. A. Rould, S. Jun, C. Desplan, and C. O. Pabo. Crystal structure of a paired domain-DNA complex at 2.5 Å resolution reveals structural basis for pax developmental mutations. *Cell* 80:639–650, 1995.

Zhang, Y., and S. W. Emmons. Specification of sense-organ identity by a Caenorhabditis elegans Pax-6 homologue. *Nature* 377:55–59, 1995.

Zlotogora, J., I. Lerer, S. Bar-David, Z. Ergaz, and D. Abeliovich. Homozygosity for Waardenburg syndrome. *Am. J. Hum. Genet.* 56:1173–1178, 1995.

Zuker, C. S. On the evolution of eyes: would you like it simple or compound. *Science* 265:742–743, 1994.

bHLH Proteins 8

As described in Chapter 3, the basic helix-loop-helix (bHLH) proteins are a large superfamily of dimeric transcription factors in which the HLH motif mediates protein dimerization and the basic domain mediates DNA binding. In some bHLH families, such as the myogenic bHLH family consisting of MYOD, MYOGENIN, MYF5, and MRF4, the HLH domain is both necessary and sufficient to mediate dimerization. In other families, an additional domain that is present immediately carboxyl-terminal to the HLH domain is also required for dimerization. Thus, the bHLH-ZIP proteins contain a helix-loop-helix and an adjacent leucine zipper domain that are both required for proper protein dimerization. Because dimerization is a prerequisite for DNA binding, these domains are crucial for the biological activity of bHLH and bHLH-ZIP proteins.

MI/MITF

The Mouse Mi Gene and microphthalmia

Mouse *microphthalmia* mutations affect the development of the eyes, ears, skin, bones, and teeth in a semidominant manner. Mice heterozygous for the *mi* allele manifest white spotting of the belly, head, and tail and hypopigmentation of the iris. Homozygotes have microphthalmia; lack melanocytes in the iris, skin, and inner ear; are deficient in mast cells; and their osteoclasts do not function properly, leading to osteopetrosis and failure of incisor eruption (reviewed by Hodgkinson et al., 1993). The eyes are small and malformed as a result of failure of the optic fissure to close during development, secondary to abnormalities in the retinal pigmented epithelium. Multiple *mi* alleles have been described that all demonstrate melanocyte abnormalities but the severity of the phenotype varies greatly, with some alleles manifesting an abnormal phenotype only in the homozygous state. Furthermore, compound heterozygotes between different alleles may manifest phenotypes that are either more severe or less severe than either true homozygote.

The *mi* locus on mouse chromosome 6 was serendipitously identified as a consequence of transgene insertional mutagenesis, and the cloning of DNA flanking the transgene integration site led to the isolation of the intact *Mi* gene (Hodgkinson et al., 1993; Hughes et al., 1993; and references therein). *Mi* was found to encode a 419-amino-acid bHLH-ZIP protein that was almost identical within the bHLH-ZIP domain to the transcription factors TFE3, TFEB, and TFEC. MI can homodimerize or heterodimerize with TFE3, TFEB, or TFEC and bind to the DNA sequence 5'-CAYGTG-3' (Y = C or T) (Hemesath et al., 1994; Moore, 1995). In contrast to TFE3 and TFEB, which are ubiquitously expressed, MI mRNA was detected specifically in the pigment layer of the retina, in cells surrounding the otic vesicle, and in hair follicles of mouse embryos, which is consistent with the defects observed in *mi* mice (Hodgkinson et al., 1993).

The original *mi* mutation, delR215, results in the deletion of one of three consecutive arginine residues within the basic domain of the protein (Hodgkinson et al., 1993) (Fig. 8.1 and Table 8.1). The *Mi*[or] allele results in an arginine-to-lysine substitution (R216K) within the same arginine triad affected by the *mi* mutation (Fig. 8.1) and *Mi*[or] results in a phenotype that is similar to that associated with *mi* (Steingrimsson et al., 1994). The protein products of the *mi* and *Mi*[or] genes have been shown to lack DNA-binding activity in electrophoretic mobility-shift assays (Hemesath et al., 1994). *Mi*[wh] represents an I212N missense mutation in the basic domain (Fig. 8.1) and the mutant protein cannot bind to DNA as a homodimer (Hemesath et al., 1994; Steingrimsson et al., 1994). MI mRNA undergoes several alternative splicing events, one of which results in the presence (+) or absence (−) of six amino acids just amino-terminal to the basic region (Hodgkinson et al., 1993). The *Mi*[wh] (+) isoform can bind to DNA as a heterodimer with wild-type MI or TFE3, whereas the (−) isoform cannot (Hemesath et al., 1994). *mi*, *Mi*[or], and *Mi*[wh] behave as dominant-negative alleles, interfering with the DNA-binding activity of wild-type MI and TFE3 (Table 8.1), which may account for their semidominant inheritance (Hemesath et al., 1994), although these results do not rule out haploinsufficiency as the basis for the phenotypic manifestations.

In contrast, the *mi*[ce] mutation, R263X, introduces a stop codon at the beginning of the leucine zipper domain (Fig. 8.1), and the truncated poly-

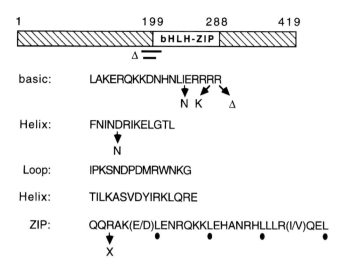

FIGURE 8-1. Structure of MI and MITF bHLH-ZIP proteins. The amino acid sequences of the basic (aa 199–217), helix (aa 218–230 and 245–260), loop (aa 231–244), and leucine zipper (aa 261–288) domains are shown. MITF and MI are identical in the bHLH domain and differ by only two substitutions (E266D and I285V) in the leucine zipper domain (Tachibana et al., 1994). The leucine residues of the heptad repeats are indicated by filled ovals. Mutations in the *Mi* gene associated with the *microphthalmia* phenotype are indicated: deletion (Δ) of amino acids 187–212 or 186–191; I212N, R216K, delR217, D222N, and R263X.

TABLE 8.1. *Microphthalmia* mutations

| Allele | Phenotype[a] | Mutation | Site | Effect on DNA Binding | | |
				homo	hetero[b]	dom-neg[c]
mi	SD	del R217	basic	−	−	+
mi^Or	SD	R216K	basic	−	−	+
mi^wh	SD	I212N	basic	−	+[d]	+[e]
mi^ce	R	R263X	ZIP-C term	−	−	−
mi^ew	R	del A187-I212	basic	−	−	+
mi^vit	R	D222N	helix 1	+	+	−
mi^sp	E	del T186-P191	alt. exon	+	+	−

[a] Phenotypes are semidominant (SD), recessive (R), or enhancing (E; affects phenotype only in the presence of a heterologous mutant allele).

[b] Ability to bind to DNA in the presence of wild-type MI or TFE3.

[c] Ability to inhibit DNA binding of wild-type MI.

[d] Binds to DNA only in the presence of the wild-type MI (+) isoform.

[e] Inhibits DNA binding of the wild-type MI (−) isoform only.

Data from Hemesath et al., 1994.

peptide cannot dimerize nor bind to DNA (Hemesath et al., 1994). These results demonstrate that the ZIP domain of MI, as in the case of TFE3 (Beckmann and Kadesch, 1991), is required for dimerization. The lack of dimerization eliminates the possibility of a dominant negative effect and it is therefore of interest that mi^{ce} is a recessive allele. The mi^{ws} allele contains an intragenic deletion such that the encoded polypeptide lacks 136 amino acids that are normally present amino terminal to the bHLH-ZIP domain. The mutant protein can thus dimerize and bind to DNA but may be deficient in transactivation. The semidominant inheritance of the mi^{ws} phenotype again suggests a dominant negative effect in which heterodimers containing the mutant protein may occupy MI binding sites but are unable to activate transcription. The allele that has the least severe effect on phenotype is mi^{sp}. mi^{sp}/mi^{sp} mice are normal and an effect on phenotype is observed only in compound heterozygotes carrying mi^{sp} and a different mi allele.

In mice carrying mutations in the Mi gene, there is a loss of melanocytes that results in white spotting of the fur. Melanocytes are also present within the stria vascularis of the cochlea (Steel and Barkway, 1989). Analysis of mouse embryos by in situ hybridization revealed the presence of MI mRNA within presumptive melanoblasts in the vicinity of the otic vesicle at E13.5, whereas MI-expressing cells could not be detected in embryos that were homozygous for the transgene insertion within the Mi gene (mi^{VGA-9}) and, in adult mi^{VGA-9} homozygotes, the stria vascularis was morphologically abnormal and lacked melanocytes (Hodgkinson et al., 1993; Moore, 1995). Microphthalmic mice with mutations in Mi have reduced pigmentation in the retinal pigmented epithelium (Moore, 1995).

Deficiency of MI also results in cell-autonomous defects in osteoclasts, mast cells, and natural killer cells (Stechschulte et al., 1987; Walker, 1975a, b). The presence of osteoclast dysfunction and osteopetrosis in mice with mutations in Mi is intriguing because of the fact that osteopetrosis has been detected in mice with a homozygous null mutation in the c-Fos gene, which encodes a bZIP component of the heterodimeric transcription factor AP-1 (Johnson et al., 1992; Wang et al., 1992). A bHLH-ZIP protein, FIP (Fos-interacting protein), was identified that could heterodimerize with C-FOS (Blanar and Rutter, 1992). It is possible that MI can heterodimerize with either C-FOS or FIP and that these interactions are disturbed in MI-deficient mice. In this regard, it is of interest that osteopetrosis is seen almost exclusively in mice with semidominant alleles (mi and Mi^{or}) with putative dominant-negative effects (Steingrimsson et al., 1994).

The Human MITF Gene and Waardenburg Syndrome Type 2

The human homologue of the mouse *Mi* gene was cloned, named *MITF* (microphthalmia-associated transcription factor), and localized to chromosome 3p12.3–p14.1 (Tachibana et al., 1994). The MI and MITF proteins are each 419 amino acids and their sequences are 94% identical, including complete identity in the bHLH domain. Linkage analysis of a large family with Waardenburg syndrome (WS) type 2 revealed a LOD score of 6.48 at 0% recombination with the marker *D3S1261*, which was mapped to chromosome 3p12-p14 (Hughes et al., 1994). Even prior to the isolation of *Mi* or *MITF*, microphthalmia had been proposed as a mouse model for WS (Asher and Friedman, 1990). Subsequent studies identified *MITF* mutations in patients with Waardenburg syndrome type 2 (Nokubuni et al., 1996; Tassabehji et al., 1994, 1995).

Analysis of DNA from one individual with WS type 2 revealed a mutation (delR217) that is exactly analogous to the mouse *mi* mutation (Tassabehji et al., 1995). However, in contrast to the mouse mutations in the *Mi* gene described above, most *MITF* mutations associated with the dominantly inherited WS type 2 phenotype appear to be loss-of-function mutations that lack dominant negative effects based on electrophoretic mobility-shift and transcriptional assays (Nokubuni et al., 1996). These data suggest that the molecular pathophysiology may differ in mouse and human and that in humans, melanocyte development is disrupted by smaller reductions in MITF compared to the reduction in MI expression required to significantly affect mouse melanocyte development. As in the case of *Pax3* mutations, it may be informative to explore the role of modifier loci in determining the phenotype of mice that are heterozygous for loss-of-function and dominant-negative *Mi* mutations.

In both WS type 1 (MIM 193500) and WS type 2 (MIM 193510), there is a deficiency of melanocytes, resulting in iris heterochromia and white spotting of the hair. In addition, there is a high incidence of hearing loss, which is caused by a loss of melanocytes from the stria vascularis of the cochlea (Steel and Barkway, 1989). Melanocytes are neural crest derivatives and in WS type 2 the deficiency of MITF appears to specifically affect melanocytes, compared to WS type 1, in which the additional presence of craniofacial malformations (dystopia canthorum) indicates that other neural crest cell derivatives are affected by the deficiency of PAX3. The etiology of WS type 2 appears to be genetically heterogeneous, as only approximately 20% of cases are associated with *MITF* mutations (Tassabehji et al., 1995), suggesting the existence of at least one other transcription factor besides MI/MITF and PAX3 that is specifically required for melanocyte development.

MI/MITF and Control of Melanocyte Development

Loss of cochlear, dermal, and ocular melanocytes results in deafness and hypopigmentation of hair and eyes in patients with WS type 2 and *microphthalmia* mice. Classical experiments utilizing melanoblast transplantation and aggregation chimeras demonstrated that the defect in *mi/mi* mice is a cell-autonomous loss of melanocyte development and/or survival (Silvers, 1979). To complement the loss-of-function studies associated with *Mi* mutations, NIH 3T3 embryonic fibroblasts were stably transfected with an expression vector encoding MITF (Tachibana et al., 1996). In contrast to the nontransfected cells, the transfectants exhibited morphological alterations, such as dendritic processes, that are characteristic of melanocytes and expressed melanocyte-specific mRNAs encoding tyrosinase and tyrosinase-related proteins 1 and 2, three enzymes involved in melanin biosynthesis that are expressed only after differentiation of melanocytes from the nonpigmented melanoblasts. Transfectants expressing the structurally related transcription factor TFE3 did not manifest morphological or genetic evidence of melanocytic differentiation (Tachibana et al., 1996). These results suggest that MI/MITF is not only necessary for melanocyte development but it is also sufficient for at least part of the melanocyte program of differentiation to be carried out in a heterologous cell type.

Expression of the gene encoding tyrosinase appears to be directly regulated by MI/MITF. A 39-bp *cis*-acting regulatory element located 1.8 kb 5' to the transcription initiation site directs melanocyte-specific transcription of a heterologous reporter gene and contains the 5'-CATGTG-3' MI/MITF binding-site sequence (Shibata et al., 1992). Two additional copies of the 5'-CATGTG-3' sequence were identified within the first 100 base pairs 5' to the transcription initiation site and transcription of reporter genes containing either the distal or proximal tyrosinase regulatory element was activated in nonmelanocytic HeLa cells by cotransfection of an MITF expression vector (Bentley et al., 1994; Yasumoto et al., 1994). In contrast, the tyrosinase promoter was not activated by expression of mutant forms of MITF (Nobukuni et al., 1996). An identical 11-bp "M-box" sequence 5'-AGT<u>CATGTG</u>CT-3' (MI/MITF core binding site is underlined) is present in the promoters of the genes encoding tyrosinase and tyrosinase-related protein 1 (Lowings et al., 1992; Shibahara et al., 1991; Yavuzer and Goding, 1994). Coexpression of MI activated transcription of a reporter plasmid containing four copies of the M-box cloned upstream of the otherwise minimally responsive SV40 promoter (Hemesath et al., 1994). Taken together, the available data indicate that MI/MITF is required for the survival, proliferation, and differentiation of melanocytes. In common with other master regulatory transcription factors, such as MYOD (see Chapter 3) and PAX6 (see Chapter 7), MI/ MITF appears to control both the process of cellular differentiation and the expression of cell-type-specific gene products within the final differentiated cell type.

TWIST and Saethre-Chotzen Syndrome

Saethre-Chotzen syndrome (acrocephalosyndactyly type III; MIM 101400) is an autosomal-dominant human malformation syndrome, which—as in the case of the Greig syndrome (see Chapter 6) and Boston-type craniosynostosis (see Chapter 9)—is characterized by craniofacial and limb anomalies. The craniofacial anomalies most typically include craniosynostosis (premature fusion of the coronal sutures). Other findings may include maxillary hypoplasia, cleft palate, conductive deafness, and enamel hypoplasia (Fig. 8.2). Limb anomalies include brachydactyly and cutaneous syndactyly. In some patients, cognitive development is also adversely affected. A locus for Saethre-Chotzen syndrome was mapped to chromosome 7p21-p22 by linkage analysis (van Herwerden et al., 1994; Lewanda et al., 1994a) and the identification of patients carrying chromosome translocations (Lewanda et al., 1994b and references therein).

The murine *Twist* gene, which encodes a bHLH transcription factor, was mapped to a region of chromosome 12 that demonstrates conservation of synteny with human chromosome 7p21-p22 (Mattei et al., 1993; DeBry and Seldin, 1996). Furthermore, mouse embryos homozygous for a null allele at the *Twist* locus died at E11.5 with defects in cranial neural tube closure, head mesenchyme, branchial arches, somites, and limbs (Chen and Behringer, 1995). The human *TWIST* gene was localized to the same genomic region as the Saethre-Chotzen locus and sequence analysis revealed *TWIST* gene mutations in multiple affected individuals (El Ghouzzi et al., 1997; Howard et al., 1997).

In one study, unique *TWIST* mutations were shown to segregate with the disease in five different families (Howard et al., 1997). In one of these families, an insertion of a single nucleotide resulted in a frameshift prior to the bHLH domain. The loss of the entire bHLH domain is predicted to result in a complete loss of protein function. In two families, in-frame duplications of 21 bp resulted in the addition of seven amino acids within the HLH domain, whereas in another family a deletion of

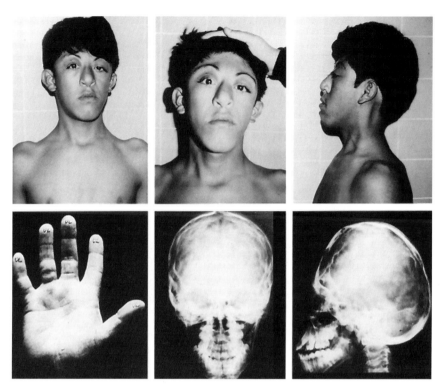

Figure 8-2. Saethre-Chotzen syndrome. Top row, clinical photographs (Q119P missense mutation heterozygote) demonstrating (left to right): facial asymmetry, left ptosis, and maxillary hypoplasia; low hairline; and malformed ear with prominent crus. Bottom row, hand photograph demonstrating brachydactyly (short fingers) (left); and radiographs demonstrating the combination of digital markings (center) and decreased anteroposterior diameter (right) of the skull that is indicative of coronal synostosis. (Reprinted with permission from Howard et al., 1997.)

23 bp resulted in a frameshift within the HLH domain. These mutations are also predicted to result in loss of function. Finally, a missense mutation (Q119P) within the basic domain was detected. The substitution of proline for a glutamine residue that is conserved in human, mouse, *Xenopus*, and *Drosophila* TWIST proteins (see Fig. 8.3 and Fig. 8.4) is predicted to destroy the α-helical structure of the basic domain and prevent DNA binding. This mutation may also interfere with conformation of the first α-helix of the HLH domain and thus prevent dimerization as well, representing another loss-of-function allele, rather than a dominant negative allele as would occur if the mutant protein was functional for di-

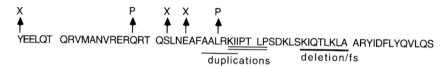

FIGURE 8-3. Mutations in the bHLH domain of TWIST associated with Saethre-Chotzen syndrome. The amino acid sequence of the human TWIST protein (residues 103–165) spanning the bHLH domain and preceding six residues, with sites of missense and nonsense mutations, 21–bp duplications; and 23–bp frameshift (fs) mutation.

merization but not for DNA binding, as in the case of several *Mi* alleles described earlier in this chapter. The observation that individuals carrying the frameshift mutation prior to the bHLH domain had the most severe phenotype is consistent with the hypothesis that all of the *TWIST* mutations reported result in disease by a loss-of-function mechanism.

In another study, nonsense and missense *TWIST* mutations were also reported (El Ghouzzi et al., 1997). Nonsense mutations were identified that would terminate translation prior to or within the bHLH domain. A missense mutation, L131P, in which a highly conserved leucine residue in helix I (see Fig. 8.3 and Fig. 8.4) was substituted by a helix-breaking proline residue, was also detected. In addition, two 21-bp duplications which differed by only one nucleotide were reported. One of these duplications was identical to the mutation described above, and both resulted in the duplication of the amino acid sequence KIIPTLP at the junction of the first helix and loop regions (El Ghouzzi et al., 1997). The presence of a 6-bp direct repeat immediately preceding and at the

Species	Basic	Helix	Loop	Helix
Human	QRVMANVRERQRT	QSLNEAFAALRKIIPT	LPSDKLSKIQTLKLA	ARYIDFLYQVLQS
Mouse	-------------	----------------	---------------	-------------
Xenopus	-------------	-------SS-------	---------------	S------C-----
Drosophila	-------------	----D--KS-QQ----	---------------	T------CRM-S-

FIGURE 8-4. The bHLH domains of vertebrate and invertebrate TWIST. The amino acid sequence of the human, mouse, *Xenopus*, and *Drosophila* TWIST proteins are shown. Hyphen: identity with human sequence. Underscore: site of missense mutation in Saethre-Chotzen syndrome.

end of the duplicated sequences may have predisposed to strand slippage during DNA replication. This group also reevaluated mice heterozygous for an inactivated *Twist* allele, which were previously considered to be normal, and found hindlimb digit I duplications and skull defects, including hypoplastic squamosal and hyperplastic interparietal bones (El Ghouzzi et al., 1997). Thus, heterozygosity for a loss-of-function allele encoding TWIST results in craniofacial and limb defects in both humans and mice.

TWIST was originally identified in *Drosophila melanogaster*, in which homozygosity for a *twist* mutation was associated with embryonic lethality due to defective gastrulation that resulted in the embryo having an abnormal, twisted appearance (Simpson, 1983). In *Drosophila*, *twist* encodes a protein of 490 amino acids, considerably larger than the mouse, human, and *Xenopus* TWIST proteins, which consist of 206, 202, and 166 amino acid residues, respectively (reviewed by Dixon, 1997). However, there is remarkable amino acid sequence conservation within the bHLH domain (which spans amino acids 109–165 of human TWIST) with complete sequence identity found in the basic and loop regions (Fig. 8.4). The two missense mutations identified in patients with Saethre-Chotzen syndrome affect invariant residues in the basic and loop regions as described above.

The phenotype of TWIST-deficient flies is similar to that observed in flies deficient for the fibroblast growth factor receptor DFR1, and *DFR1* expression is greatly reduced in TWIST-deficient embryos (Shishido et al., 1993). Remarkably, three other human craniosynostotic conditions, the Apert, Crouzon, and Jackson-Weiss syndromes, are caused by mutations in human genes encoding fibroblast growth factor receptors (reviewed in Howard et al., 1997). These results suggest that in both flies and humans, TWIST plays an important role in the developmentally regulated transcription of genes encoding fibroblast growth factor receptors. In some patients with Saethre-Chotzen syndrome, linkage to the *TWIST* locus on chromosome 7p21-p22 has been excluded, indicating genetic heterogeneity (Lewanda et al., 1994a; von Gernet et al., 1996). Identification of other genes that are mutated in Saethre-Chotzen syndrome will provide information about additional components of the genetic circuits required for proper craniofacial and limb development. Furthermore, the conservation of many of these genes in lower organisms should allow utilization of genetic techniques to establish epistatic relationships between the increasing number of genes (*FGFR1, FGFR2, FGFR3, GLI3, MSX2, TWIST*) that have already been implicated in these developmental systems.

References

Asher, J. H., and T. B. Friedman. Mouse and hamster mutants as models for Waardenburg syndrome in humans. *J. Med. Genet.* 27:618–626, 1990.

Beckmann, H. and T. Kadesch. The leucine zipper of TFE3 dictates helix-loop-helix dimerization specificity. *Genes Dev.* 5:1057–1066, 1991.

Bentley, N. J., T. Eisen, and C. R. Goding. Melanocyte-specific expression of the human tyrosinase promoter: activation by the microphthalmia gene product and role of the initiator. *Mol. Cell. Biol.* 14:7996–8006, 1994.

Blanar, M. A., and W. J. Rutter. Interaction cloning: identification of a helix-loop-helix zipper protein that interacts with c-Fos. *Science* 256:1014–1018, 1992.

Chen, Z-F., and R. R. Behringer. Twist is required in head mesenchyme for cranial neural tube morphogenesis. *Genes Dev.* 9:686–699, 1995.

DeBry, R. W., and M. F. Seldin. Human/mouse homology relationships. *Genomics* 33:337–351, 1996.

Dixon, M. J. Twist and shout. *Nat. Genet.* 15:3–4, 1997.

El Ghouzzi, V., M. Le Merrer, F. Perrin-Schmitt, E. Lajeunie, P. Benit, D. Renier, P. Bourgeois, A.-L. Bolcato-Bellemin, A. Munnich, and J. Bonaventure. Mutations of the TWIST gene in the Saethre-Chotzen syndrome. *Nat. Genet.* 15: 42–46, 1997.

Hemesath, T. J., E. Steingrimsson, G. McGill, M. J. Hansen, J. Vaught, C. A. Hodgkinson, H. Arnheiter, N. G. Copeland, N. A. Jenkins, and D. E. Fisher. microphthalmia, a critical factor in melanocyte development, defines a discrete transcription factor family. *Genes Dev.* 8:2770–2780, 1994.

Hodgkinson, C. A., K. J. Moore, A. Nakayama, E. Steingrimsson, N. G. Copeland, N. A. Jenkins, and H. Arnheiter. Mutations at the mouse microphthalmia locus are associated with defects in a gene encoding a novel basic-helix-loop-helix-zipper protein. *Cell* 74:395–404, 1993.

Howard, T. D., W. A. Paznekas, E. D. Green, L. C. Chiang, N. Ma, R. I. Ortiz de Luna, C. G. Delgado, M. Gonzalez-Ramos, A. D. Kline, and E. W. Jabs. Mutations in TWIST, a basic helix-loop-helix transcription factor, in Saethre-Chotzen syndrome. *Nat. Genet.* 15:36–41, 1997.

Hughes, A. E., V. E. Newton, X .Z. Liu, and A. P. Read. A gene for Waardenburg syndrome type 2 maps close to the human homologue of the microphthalmia gene at chromosome 3p12-p14.1. *Nat. Genet.* 7:509–512, 1994.

Hughes, M. J., J. B. Lingrel, J. M. Krakowsky, and K. P. Anderson. A helix-loop-helix transcription factor-like gene is located at the mi locus. *J. Biol. Chem.* 268:20687–20690, 1993.

Johnson, R. S., B. M. Spiegelman, and V. Papaionnou. Pleiotropic effects of a null mutation in the c-fos proto-oncogene. *Cell* 71:577–586, 1992.

Lewanda, A. F., M. M. Cohen, Jr., C. E. Jackson, E. W. Taylor, X. Li, M. Beloff, D. Day, S. K. Clarren, R. Ortiz, C. Garcia, and E. W. Jabs. Genetic heterogeneity among craniosynostosis syndromes: mapping the Saethre-Chotzen syndrome locus between D7S513 and D7S516 and exclusion of Jackson-Weiss and Crouzon syndrome loci from 7p. *Genomics* 19:115–119, 1994a.

Lewanda, A. F., E. D. Green, J. Weissenbach, H. Jerald, E. Taylor, M. L. Summar, J. A. Phillips III, M. Cohen, M. Feingold, W. Mouradian, S. K. Clarren, and E. W. Jabs. Evidence that the Saethre-Chotzen syndrome locus lies between

D7S664 and D7S507, by genetic analysis and detection of a microdeletion in a patient. *Am. J. Hum. Genet.* 55:1195–1201, 1994b.

Lowings, P., U. Yavuzer, and C. R. Goding. Positive and negative elements regulate a melanocyte-specific promoter. *Mol. Cell. Biol.* 12:3653–3662, 1992.

Mattei, M. G., C. Stoetzel, and F. Perrin-Schmitt. The B-HLH protein encoding the M-twist gene is located by in situ hybridization on murine chromosome 12. *Mamm. Genome* 4:127–128, 1993.

Moore, K. J. Insight into the microphthalmia gene. *Trends Genet.* 11:442–448, 1995.

Nokubuni, Y., A. Watanabe, K. Takeda, H. Skarka, and M. Tachibana. Analyses of loss-of-function mutations of the MITF gene suggest that haploinsufficiency is a cause of Waardenburg syndrome type 2A. *Am. J. Hum. Genet.* 59: 78–83, 1996.

Shibahara, S., H. Taguchi, R. M. Muller, K. Shibata, T. Cohen, Y. Tomita, and H. Tagami. Structural organization of the pigment cell-specific gene located at the brown locus in mouse: its promoter activity and alternatively spliced transcript. *J. Biol. Chem.* 266:15895–15901, 1991.

Shibata, K., Y. Muraosa, Y. Tomita, H. Tagami, and S. Shibahara. Identification of a cis-acting element that enhances the pigment cell-specific expression of the human tyrosinase gene. *J. Biol. Chem.* 267:20584–20588, 1992.

Shishido, E., S. Higashijima, Y. Emori, and K. Saigo. Two FGF-receptor homologues of Drosophila: one is expressed in mesodermal primordium in early embryos. *Development* 117:751–761, 1993.

Silvers, W. K. *The Coat Colors of Mice: A Model for Mammalian Gene Action and Interaction.* New York: Springer-Verlag, 1979.

Simpson, P. Maternal-zygotic gene interactions during formation of the dorsoventral pattern in Drosophila embryos. *Genetics* 105:615–632, 1983.

Steel, K. P., and C. Barkway. Another role for melanocytes: their importance for normal stria vascularis development in the mammalian inner ear. *Development* 107:453–463, 1989.

Stechschulte, D. J., R. Sharma, K. N. Dileepan, K. M. Simpson, N. Aggarwal, J. Clancy Jr., and R. L. Jilka. Effect of the mi allele on mast cells, basophils, natural killer cells, and osteoclasts in C57Bl/6J mice. *J. Cell Physiol.* 132:565–570, 1987.

Steingrimsson, E., K. J. Moore, M. L. Lamoreux, A. R. Ferre-D'Amare, S. K. Burley, D. C. Zimring, L. C. Skow, C. A. Hodgkinson, H. Arnheiter, N. G. Copeland, and N. A. Jenkins. Molecular basis of mouse microphthalmia (mi) mutations helps explain their developmental and phenotypic consequences. *Nat. Genet.* 8:256–263, 1994.

Tachibana, M., L. A. Perez-Jurado, A. Nakayama, C. A. Hodgkinson, X. Li, M. Schneider, T. Miki, J. Fex, U. Francke, and H. Arnheiter. Cloning of MITF, the human homolog of the mouse microphthalmia gene and assignment to chromosome 3p14.1-p12.3. *Hum. Mol. Genet.* 3:553–557, 1994.

Tachibana, M., K. Takeda, Y. Nobukuni, K. Urabe, J. E. Long, K. A. Meyers, S. A. Aaronson, and T. Miki. Ectopic expression of MITF, a gene for Waardenburg syndrome type 2, converts fibroblasts to cells with melanocyte characteristics. *Nat. Genet.* 14:50–54, 1996.

Tassabehji, M., V. E. Newton, X.-Z. Liu, A. Brady, D. Donnai, M. Krajewska-Walasek, V. Murday, A. Norman, E. Obersztyn, W. Reardon, J. C. Rice, R. Trembath, P. Wieacker, M. Whiteford, R. Winter, and A. P. Read. The mutational spectrum in Waardenburg syndrome. *Hum. Mol. Genet.* 4:2131–2137, 1995.

Tassabehji, M., V. E. Newton, and A. P. Read. Waardenburg syndrome type 2 caused by mutations in the human microphthalmia (MITF) gene. *Nat. Genet.* 8:252–255, 1994.

van Herwerden, L., C. S. P. Rose, W. Reardon, W. A. Brueton, J. Weissenbach, S. Malcolm, and R. M. Winter. Evidence for locus heterogeneity in acrocephalosyndactyly: a refined localization for the Saethre-Chotzen syndrome locus on distal chromosome 7p—and exclusion of Jackson-Weiss syndrome from craniosynostosis loci on 7p and 5q. *Am. J. Hum. Genet.* 54:669–674, 1994.

von Gernet, S., S. Schuffenhauer, A. Golla, P. Lichtner, S. Balg, W. Muhlbauer, J. Murken, J. Fairley, and T. Meitinger. Craniosynostosis suggestive of Saethre-Chotzen syndrome: clinical description of a large kindred and exclusion of candidate regions on 7p. *Am. J. Med. Genet.* 63:177–184, 1996.

Walker, D. G. Bone resorption restored in osteopetrotic mice by transplants of normal bone marrow and spleen cells. *Science* 190:784–785, 1975a.

Walker, D. G. Spleen cells transmit osteopetrosis in mice. *Science* 190:785–787, 1975b.

Wang, Z. Q., C. Ovitt, A. E. Grigoriadis, U. Mohle-Steinlein, U. Ruther, and E. F. Wagner. Bone and hematopoietic defects mice lacking c-fos. *Nature* 360: 741–745, 1992.

Yasumoto, K.-I., K. Yokoyama, K. Shibata, Y. Tomita, and S. Shibahara. Microphthalmia-associated transcription factor as a regulator for melanocyte-specific transcription of the human tyrosinase gene. *Mol. Cell. Biol.* 14:8058–8070, 1994.

Yavuzer, U., and C. R. Goding. Melanocyte-specific gene expression: role of repression and identification of a melanocyte-specific factor, MSF. *Mol Cell Biol.* 14:3494–3503, 1994.

9 Homeodomain Proteins

As described in Chapter 3, homeodomain proteins are transcription factors that are characterized by the presence of a 60-amino-acid DNA-binding domain. The structure of the homeodomain consists of a flexible amino-terminal arm followed by three α helices (Fig. 9.1) with the second and third helices forming a helix-turn-helix motif that is structurally similar to the DNA binding domain of several prokaryotic transcriptonal repressors (Harrison and Aggarwal, 1990). The carboxyl-terminal third helix of the homeodomain makes direct base contacts with the major groove of the double helix (and is thus known as the recognition helix), the amino-terminal arm makes contact in the minor groove, and there are extensive contacts with the sugar-phosphate backbone (Kissinger et al., 1990; Otting et al., 1990; Wohlberger et al., 1991).

Homeodomain proteins are divided into HOX and non-HOX factors. The HOX proteins each contain a homeodomain with sequence similarity to the proteins encoded by the *HOM-C* gene clusters of *Drosophila melanogaster* (reviewed by Ruddle et al., 1994). The 39 HOX proteins are encoded by genes that are organized into four clusters located on different chromosomes (reviewed by Scott, 1997; Zeltser et al., 1996) (Fig. 9.2). *Hox* genes are expressed in the developing nervous system, somites, and limbs but are not expressed in the head rostral to the hindbrain. The expression of genes within a *Hox* cluster is restricted to domains within the developing embryo that are colinear with the order of genes within the cluster, so that genes at the 5' end of the cluster are expressed in posterior regions relative to genes at the 3' end of the cluster (Gaunt et al., 1988; reviewed by Izpisua-Belmonte and Duboule, 1992). Thus, 3' genes in groups 1–4 of each cluster (Fig. 9.2) are expressed in the branchial arches and rhombencephalon; genes in the middle groups 5–8 are expressed in the thoracic region; and 5' genes of

```
              HELIX 1                    HELIX 2              HELIX 3
              ‾‾‾‾‾‾‾                    ‾‾‾‾‾‾‾              ‾‾‾‾‾‾‾
Antp   RKRGRQTYTRYQTLELEKEFHFNRYLTRRRRIEIAHALCLTERQIKIWFQNRRMKWKKEN
HOXA6  GR-------------------------------------N----------------------
AbdB   VRKK-KP-SKP---------L--A-VSKQK-W-L-RN-Q-----V----------L--MS
HOXB9  SRKK-CP--K---------L--M----D--H-V-RL-N-S---V----------M--M-
Dfd    P--Q-TA---H-I--------Y--------------T-V-S---V------------D-
HOXA4  P--S-TA---Q-V-----------------------T---S---V------------DH
Lab    NNS--TNF-NK-L--------------A------NT-Q-N-T-V----------Q--RV
HOXA1  PNAV-TNF-TK-LT---------K----A--V---AS-Q-N-T-V----------Q--RE
Msh    NRKP-TPF-TQ-L-S---K-REQK--SIAE-A-FSSS-R---T-V--------PRQASPG
MSX1   NRKP-TPF-TA-L-A--RK-RQKQ--SIAE-A-FSSS-S---T-V--------A-A-RLQ
```

FIGURE 9-1. Amino acid sequence of homeodomains. The location of the three α helices of the Antp protein, as determined by x-ray crystallography, are shown. Note the striking homology between the homeodomain sequences from human HOX and *Drosophila* HOM-C proteins. Note also the divergence of the *Drosophila* MSH and human MSX1 homeodomain sequences from those of the HOX/HOM-C proteins. (Adapted from Shashikant et al., 1991.)

groups 9–13 are expressed in the lumbosacral and anogenital regions. The correlation between gene location and spatial expression is also a feature of the *Drosophila* HOM-C gene clusters (Lewis, 1978). However, whereas the temporal expression pattern of *HOM-C* genes is not colinear with their order in the cluster, *Hox* genes do show temporal colinearity (Izpisua-Belmonte et al., 1991; reviewed by Duboule, 1992). *Hox* expression is essential for the establishment of positional identity along the anteroposterior axis of the body and limbs (reviewed by Krumlauf, 1994).

In contrast, the many non-HOX homeodomain proteins are expressed in the brain and a variety of other organs during development and are encoded by genes that are not organized into clusters. Examples of non-HOX homeodomain proteins that are discussed elsewhere in the text are PAX3 and PAX6 (Chapter 7) and members of the POU transcription factor family (Chapter 11). The PAX and POU proteins contain a second domain that is required for DNA binding (the paired and POU$_S$ domain, respectively), whereas for the proteins described in this chapter the homeodomain is necessary and sufficient for DNA binding.

Whereas the *Hox* genes are expressed throughout the trunk and limbs during development, the rostral border of expression is the third rhombomere (r3) of the embryonic hindbrain (Hunt et al., 1991; Hunt and Krumlauf, 1991). The craniofacial skeleton forms primarily from

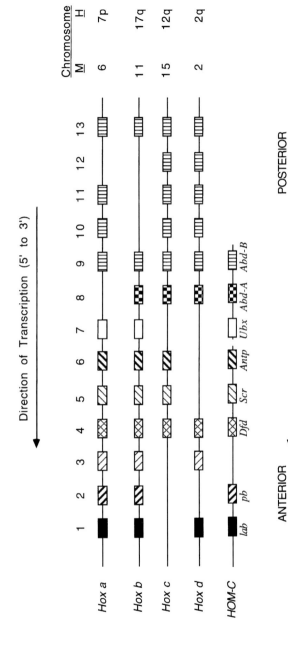

FIGURE 9-2. Organization of *Hox* genes in the mammalian genome. The four clusters of *Hox* genes present in the human (H) and mouse (M) genomes are shown with their chromosomal localization indicated at right. The bottom line shows the two *HOM-C* clusters present in the genome of *Drosophila melanogaster*. Shading indicates paralagous genes that share similar amino acid coding sequences, location within the cluster, and temporospatial expression pattern along the anteroposterior axis of the developing embryo. Note that the direction of transcription is the same for all genes (with the exception of *Dfd*). Intergenic and intragenic distances are not drawn to scale. See Scott (1992) for a discussion of past and present HOX gene nomenclature. (Data from Ruddle et al., 1994; Zeltser et al., 1996.)

neural crest cells that migrate from the hindbrain rhombomeres into the branchial arches. Cranial neural crest cells from r1 and r2 migrate into the first arch, whereas cells from r4 and r6 migrate into the second and third branchial arches, respectively (Lumsden et al., 1991). *Hox* genes, including *Hoxa1* (Lufkin et al., 1991), *Hoxa2* (Gendron-Maguire et al., 1993; Rijli et al., 1993), and *Hoxa3* (Chisaka and Capecchi, 1991) play a role in the development of craniofacial structures that are derived from the second and third branchial arches, but they are not involved in the patterning of first arch derivatives. Several other genes encoding non-HOX homeodomain proteins are expressed in cranial neural crest cells that migrate into the first branchial arch, including *Gsc* (Gaunt et al., 1993), *MHox* (Cserjesie et al., 1992), and members of the *Dlx* (*Dlx-1, Dlx-2, Dlx3, Dlx-5,* and *Dlx-6*) (Porteus et al., 1991; Price et al., 1991; Robinson and Mahon, 1994; Simeone et al., 1994a) and *Msx* (*Msx-1* and *Msx-2*) (Hill et al., 1989; MacKenzie et al., 1991a, b, 1992; Mina et al., 1995; Robert et al., 1989) gene families. Homozygous loss-of-function mutations in several of these genes are associated with craniofacial malformations in mice (Martin et al., 1995; Qiu et al., 1995; Rivera-Perez et al., 1995; Satokata and Maas, 1994).

MSX1 and MSX2

Msx1 and *Msx2* (previously designated *Hox7.1* and *Hox8.1*, respectively) are particularly remarkable for their patterns of expression within many of the developing craniofacial structures in which epithelial-mesenchymal interactions occur, including the developing eyes, ears, tooth buds, nasal, maxillary, and mandibular processes, and skull bones (Hill et al., 1989; Jabs et al., 1993; Jowett et al., 1993; MacKenzie et al., 1991b, 1992; Monaghan et al., 1991; Robert et al., 1989). The mesenchymal cells involved are cranial neural crest derivatives that interact with the epithelium lining the branchial arches to initiate the complex processes of craniofacial morphogenesis (Takahashi et al., 1991). Neural crest cells migrating into the developing craniofacial processes form mesenchymal condensations that differentiate into cartilage and bone of endochondral and membranous skull, respectively, in response to epithelial signals (Hall and Miyake, 1992).

Important determinative events occur even prior to the migration of cranial neural crest cells out of the hindbrain (Noden, 1983). Whereas cranial neural crest cells from rhombomeres r1, r2, r4, and r6 migrate to the branchial arches, neural crest cells from r3 and r5 undergo programmed cell death or apoptosis (Graham et al., 1993). In response to a signal generated by cells in the surrounding even-numbered rhombomeres, expression of bone morphogenetic protein 4 (BMP4) is induced, resulting in *Msx2* expression and apoptosis of neural crest cells in r3 and r5 (Graham et al., 1994). MSX2 may therefore play a key role in determining the number and nature of cranial neural crest cells that populate that branchial arches and that play essential roles in craniofacial morphogenesis.

The MSX1 and MSX2 proteins are 97% identical (58/60 residues) in the homeodomain (Jabs et al., 1993), suggesting that they recognize similar or identical binding site sequences in DNA. This prediction was confirmed at least in the context of in vitro electrophoretic mobility shift assays (Semenza et al., 1995). However, MSX1 and MSX2 amino acid sequences diverge outside the residues immediately flanking the homeodomain, suggesting that these proteins may have distinct biological functions. However, in the context of in vitro transcription assays, MSX1 and MSX2 both function as repressors (Catron et al., 1996; Semenza et al., 1995). In addition, *Msx1* and *Msx2* expression patterns during craniofacial development, although not identical, appear to overlap considerably.

MSX1 and Tooth Agenesis

Agenesis of one or more teeth is one of the most common developmental anomalies in humans, with an incidence exceeding 1% (Vastardis et al., 1996). *Msx1* and *Msx2* gene expression is temporospatially correlated with the epithelial-mesenchymal inductive interactions that are required for odontogenesis (Jowett et al., 1993; MacKenzie et al., 1991b, 1992). Furthermore, mice deficient for MSX1 because of gene targeting have a complete failure of mandibular and maxillary alveolar bone and tooth development (Satokata and Maas, 1994). Analysis of a large four-generation pedigree with autosomal-dominant agenesis of permanent teeth (premolars and molars only; Fig. 9.3) demonstrated linkage to *MSX1* at 0% recombination with a LOD score of 6.29, and an arginine-to-proline missense mutation (R196P) was identified affecting amino acid 196, which is residue 31 of the MSX1 homeodomain (Vastardis et al., 1996). Arginine is present at this position in all chicken, human, mouse, quail, sea urchin, and Xenopus MSX1 and MSX2 proteins studied, as well as in closely-related *Drosophila* and zebrafish proteins (Bell et al., 1993; Vastardis et al., 1996). The conservation of this residue in proteins from species separated by greater than 500 million years of evolution suggests that it plays a critical functional role. Arginine-31 is located within the second helix of the homeodomain, where it has been proposed to interact

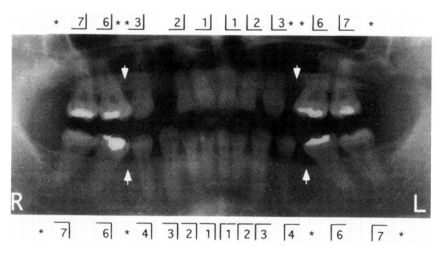

FIGURE 9-3. Familial tooth agenesis. Dental radiograph from proband of pedigree segregating autosomal dominant tooth agenesis due to an *MSX1* missense mutation. Arrowheads indicate the positions of missing teeth with numbering of maxillary and mandibular teeth shown above and below the radiograph, respectively. (Reproduced with permission from Vastardis et al., 1996.)

directly with DNA, suggesting that the mutation may affect DNA-binding affinity or specificity.

It is unclear whether the pathogenesis involves a loss-of-function, gain-of-function, or dominant-negative mechanism. Loss-of-function (haploinsufficiency) is an unlikely explanation for the phenotype because $Msx1^{+/-}$ mice have normal dentition (Satokata and Maas, 1994). However, it is clear that in *MSX1 R196P* heterozygotes, the biological activity of MSX1 is selectively affected. Mice homozygous for a null allele have complete absence of teeth and a variety of other craniofacial malformations, including cleft secondary palate and abnormalities of the nasal, frontal, and parietal bones (Satokata and Maas, 1994). In contrast, in family members heterozygous for the *MSX1* missense mutation, premolars and molars were affected but there were no abnormalities involving incisors or canines and no other craniofacial malformations (Vastardis et al., 1996).

MSX2 and Craniosynostosis

Craniosynostosis, the premature closure of one or more sutures that results in an abnormally shaped skull, is another relatively common craniofacial malformation, occurring with an incidence of 1 in 3000 infants. As in the case of tooth agenesis, the etiology of craniosynostosis is extremely heterogeneous (Gorlin et al., 1990). In a single large three-generation pedigree, an autosomal-dominant craniosynostosis phenotype was shown to segregate with a missense mutation that resulted in a proline-to-histidine substitution at residue 148 (P148H) of the human MSX2 protein (Jabs et al., 1993). The amino acid substitution involved residue 7 of the homeodomain, which is proline in all vertebrate MSX proteins as well as in the related MSH protein of *Drosophila melanogaster*. The P148H mutation segregated with the autosomal-dominant "Boston-type" craniosynostosis phenotype in a large kindred (Jabs et al., 1993). Affected individuals suffered varying degrees of craniofacial malformation ranging from mild fronto-orbital recession to severe cloverleaf skull malformation (Fig. 9.4); cleft soft palate was also identified in one family member (Warman et al., 1993). Both wild-type and mutant MSX2 were shown to specifically recognize a high-affinity MSX1 binding site and both proteins repressed reporter gene expression in transcription assays, suggesting that the P148H mutation may exert its pathophysiologic effects on craniofacial development by a gain-of-function, rather than a loss-of-function or dominant-negative, mechanism (Semenza et al., 1995). Recently, the MSX2 (P148H) protein was demonstrated to have increased DNA binding stability (decreased off-rate) compared to wild-type MSX2,

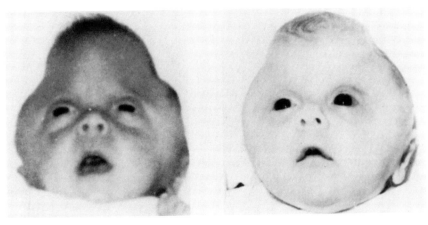

FIGURE 9-4. Boston-type craniosynostosis. Two affected half-brothers with severe cloverleaf skull malformations. (Reproduced with permission from Warman et al., 1993. Copyright ©1993 by Wiley-Liss, Inc., a subsidiary of John Wiley & Sons, Inc.)

without any detectable change in DNA binding specificity (Ma et al., 1996), suggesting that *MSX2 P148H* represents a hypermorphic allele.

Expression of MSX2 in Transgenic Mice

Expression of mouse *Msx2* coding sequences (either wild-type or containing the same missense mutation identified in human *MSX2*) from a ubiquitously expressed cytomegalovirus promoter in transgenic mice was associated with abnormal sutural morphology (Liu et al., 1995). Because the endogenous mouse *Msx2* genes were intact in these animals, and overexpression of wild-type or mutant MSX1 resulted in a similar phenotype, these results are most consistent with a gain-of-function mechanism.

The conclusions that can be drawn from these transgenic experiments must be tempered by the fact that a heterologous promoter was utilized and the transgene may therefore have been expressed in cell types in which the endogenous *Msx2* gene is not expressed. In order to maximize the probability that an *MSX2* transgene would be expressed with the temporospatial specificity exhibited by the endogenous gene, a 34-kb genomic fragment encompassing the human *MSX2* gene as well as 11 kb of 5'-flanking DNA and 14 kb of 3'-flanking DNA was isolated and the P148H missense mutation was introduced by site-directed mutagenesis. Inheritance of either a wild-type *MSX2* or *MSX2(P148H)* transgene was associated with perinatal lethality and multiple craniofacial malformations of varying severity including mandibular hypoplasia, cleft secondary palate, exencephaly, midline maxillonasofacial clefts, and ocular malformations (Winograd et al., 1997). More severe defects were observed in mice transgenic for *MSX2 (P148H)* and aplasia of the interparietal bone of the skull was also observed exclusively in these mice.

If the missense mutation resulted in increased biological activity of the MSX2 protein as suggested by the biochemical assays described above (Ma et al., 1996), then overexpression of the wild-type protein (as a consequence of increased gene dosage in transgenic mice) might have similar phenotypic effects. The presence of craniofacial malformations in both *MSX2* and *MSX2 (P148H)* transgenic mice was consistent with this hypothesis. However, the observed mouse malformations were more severe than those observed in humans with Boston-type craniosynostosis (Jabs et al., 1993; Warman et al., 1993). Two likely explanations that are not mutually exclusive involve *MSX2* gene dosage and genetic background. All transgenic lines contained multiple copies of the human *MSX2* gene in addition to the endogenous mouse *Msx2* genes and it is likely that expression of MSX2 protein (human + murine) was greatly increased in the transgenic mice and that the effect of this overexpression on craniofacial development was considerably greater than the effect of heterozygosity for the *MSX2 (P148H)* allele.

A second likely contributory factor is the effect of genetic background. In the case of the Boston kindred, marked variability was observed in the severity of the phenotype among affected family members (Warman et al., 1993). Similarly, in the transgenic mice two mutually exclusive phenotypic presentations, cleft secondary palate and exencephaly, were identified. The founder transgenic mice arose from microinjected embryos that were generated by the mating of (C57BL/6 x SJL)F_1 mice. It seems likely that genetic differences between the C57BL/6 and SJL strains segregating in the F_1 transgenic mice influenced the phenotypic presentation (Winograd et al., 1997).

As described above, the similarity of MSX1 and MSX2 homeodomain structure and expression patterns suggested that they might be functionally redundant. It was therefore surprising that the phenotype of mandibular hypoplasia, cleft secondary palate, respiratory insufficiency, and perinatal lethality was shared by *MSX2* transgenic mice and $Msx1^{-/-}$ knockout mice. The similar phenotypic effects of MSX1 deficiency and MSX2 overexpression raise the possibility that, in at least some tissues, these two factors may have antagonistic effects. Mice deficient for both MSX1 and MSX2 manifest exencephaly and cleft secondary palate, whereas these phenotypes are not observed in mice deficient for MSX2 alone (R. Maas, personal communication). The similar effects of MSX2 overexpression and MSX1 or MSX1/MSX2 deficiency suggest a complex functional interaction between these two factors during craniofacial development.

In addition to sharing phenotypic similarities with several knockout mice, the phenotype associated with inheritance of an *MSX2* transgene is also remarkably similar to the effects of teratogens. Exposure of mouse embryos to ethanol on E8 or E9 resulted in the development of cleft palate, exencephaly, mandibular hypoplasia, and midline facial clefts (Kotch et al., 1995; Kotch and Sulik, 1992a; Sulik et al., 1988). Analysis of these mice revealed that at sites of developmentally programmed cell death there was an increased number of dying cells. In the rhombencephalon, r3 and r5 in particular were sites of increased cell death (Kotch and Sulik, 1992b). Exposure of mouse embryos to retinoic acid at E8 or E9 also resulted in increased death of rhombencephalic neural crest cells, leading to cleft secondary palate and mandibular and maxillary deficiencies (Sulik et al., 1988). As described above, expression of *Msx2* in the rhombencephalon has been temporally and spatially correlated with the selective apoptosis of neural crest cells in r3 and r5 (Graham et al., 1993, 1994). Taken together, these results suggest that in *MSX2* transgenic mice, the combined levels of murine and human MSX2 may induce the death of an increased number of neural crest cells, resulting in a deficiency of cells that would normally populate the branchial arches and participate in craniofacial morphogenesis. MSX2 may thus regulate a balance between survival and apoptosis of multiple populations of rhombencephalic neural crest–derived cells that is required for proper craniofacial development. One intriguing hypothesis that follows from these conclusions is that the increased death of neural crest–derived cells that is associated with the development of craniofacial malformations may involve an induction of *MSX2* expression within apoptotic cells. Recently, exposure of mouse embryos to ethanol on E8 was shown to result in loss of *Msx2* expression throughout the embryo by E11, suggesting that ethanol suppresses, rather than induces, *Msx2* expression (Rifas et al., 1997). However, because *Msx2* expression was analyzed 3 days after ethanol exposure, it remains possible that the lack of *Msx2* expression on E11 was due to the death of *Msx2*-expressing cells between E8 and E11.

EMX2 and Schizencephaly

Schizencephaly is a rare developmental defect characterized by a full-thickness cleft within one or both cerebral hemispheres with communication between the ventricular and subarachnoid spaces (Fig. 9.5) representing a deficiency of brain tissue possibly due to abnormal neuronal proliferation and/or migration (Boncinelli, 1997; Yakovlev and Wadsworth, 1946). The clinical presentation varies widely and in severe cases includes seizures and major neurological deficits. Although most cases are isolated, several instances of familial recurrence have been reported (Hillburger et al., 1993; Hosley et al., 1992; Robinson, 1991). In one family, two sisters were affected (Hillburger et al., 1993), suggesting autosomal recessive inheritance (see MIM 269160). Four homeobox genes, *EMX1, EMX2, OTX1,* and *OTX2,* were considered candidate genes for this disorder, based on their expression in the cerebral cortex of mouse embryos (Simeone et al., 1992). Genomic DNA from eight severely affected patients was analyzed for mutations within exons of all four genes. Whereas no mutations were detected in *EMX1, OTX1,* and *OTX2,* three patients were heterozygous for mutations in *EMX2.* One mutation caused a frameshift within the homeodomain coding sequences, and the other two prevented normal splicing of intron 1 (Brunelli et al., 1996). Four other patients showed heterozygous nucleotide substitutions of un-

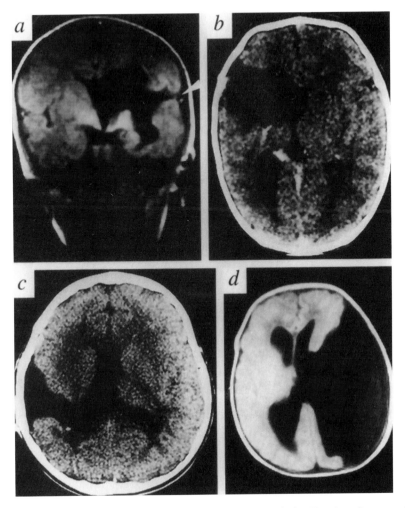

Figure 9-5. Radiographic appearance of schizencephaly. Varying degrees of schizencephaly are demonstrated by computed tomography (*a*, *d*) or magnetic resonance imaging (*b*, *c*), ranging from localized fronto-temporal (*a*, *b*; same patient) and temporo-parietal (*c*) defects to involvement of virtually an entire hemisphere (*d*). (Reprinted with permission from Brunelli et al., 1996.)

certain functional significance, including three patients with a synonymous nucleotide substitution that clearly represented a neutral polymorphism for it did not change the amino acid codon and was present in the patients' unaffected mothers.

    These results suggest that either schizencephaly is genetically heterogeneous or the ascertainment of mutations was incomplete because only exon sequences were screened. Based on the potentially incomplete ascertainment and the fact that all eight individuals represented isolated cases with no family history of the disorder, it is not possible to determine the inheritance pattern. However, the frameshift shift mutation occurred *de novo* in the affected individual, as it was not present in the genomic DNA of either parent (Brunelli et al., 1996). The identification of a new mutation strongly suggests a dominant inheritance pattern and the types of mutations identified suggest a loss-of-function (haploinsufficiency) mechanism for the pathophysiologic effects, as previously described for the *PAX* genes (see Chapter 7). The instance of apparent recessive inheritance described in the preceding paragraph may indicate germinal mosaicism, nonpenetrance, or genetic heterogeneity in schizencephaly.

However, generation of a null allele at the mouse *Emx2* locus by homologous recombination revealed the effect of a *bona fide* loss-of-function allele. Heterozygous mutant embryos developed normally whereas homozygous mutant embryos died after birth with urogenital abnormalities, reduced size of the cerebral hemispheres, hippocampus, and medial limbic cortex, and absence of the dentate gyrus (Pellegrini et al., 1996). In wild-type mice, *Emx2* expression was detected in proliferating neuronal progenitor cells and expression was downregulated at the transition from proliferation to differentiation (Gulisano et al., 1996). Thus the cerebral hypoplasia observed in the mutant mice is likely due to decreased proliferation of neuronal progenitor cells.

The human and mouse genotype-phenotype comparisons suggest that either the human mutations have a dominant negative effect or haploinsufficiency for EMX2 has a greater effect on human than on mouse central nervous system development. In this respect it should be noted that analysis of mice with a null mutation in the related *Otx2* gene revealed that presence of brain malformations in heterozygous mutant mice was dependent on the particular genetic background (Ang et al., 1996). Targeted introduction of human mutations into the mouse *Emx2* gene will increase our understanding of the pathophysiology of the human disorder. The identification of mutations in *EMX2* as a cause of a specific brain malformation represents an important advance toward defining the many genetic causes of mental retardation.

HOX Genes and Limb Development

HOXD13 and Synpolydactyly

Synpolydactyly (MIM 186000) is an autosomal dominant disorder involving both supernumerary digits (polydactyly) and bony or soft-tissue fusion of digits (syndactyly) of the upper and/or lower extremities.

Genes at the 5' end of the *HOXD* cluster (Fig. 9.2) are expressed in the developing distal limbs (Fig. 9.6) in a nested pattern that may determine the identity of specific digits (reviewed by Roberts and Tabin, 1994). In four pedigrees, synpolydactyly was shown to segregate with an unusual mutation in the *HOXD13* gene (Akarsu et al., 1996; Muragaki et al., 1996). In unaffected individuals, the degenerate trinucleotide sequence 5'-GCN-3' (where N = any nucleotide) is repeated 15 times in tandem, encoding a polyalanine stretch in the HOXD13 protein. In affected family members, the polyalanine stretch was increased by 7 to 10 residues. Another case represented a new mutation in which the affected individual was heterozygous for an expansion that increased the polyalanine stretch by 8 residues, whereas neither of his unaffected parents carried the mutant allele. The finding of a polyalanine expansion is unusual because the trinucleotide repeat expansions that have been associated with neurodegenerative disorders usually involve perfect rather than degenerate trinucleotide repeats and, when present within amino acid–coding sequences, usually encode glutamine. Further, the degree of the polyalanine tract expansion is modest and stable over many generations. Polyalanine tracts have been identified in several *Drosophila* proteins that function as transcriptional repressors (Han and Manley, 1993).

A striking example of gene dosage was documented in one of the families (Muragaki et al., 1996). An affected son who was heterozygous for the Ala_{22} allele (expansion by an additional seven alanine residues) had synpolydactyly that was manifested by a duplication of the third digit (III) of the hand with separate phalanges and a single, fused Y-shaped metacarpal (Fig. 9.7B). Cutaneous syndactyly between digits IIIa, IIIb, and IV was present at birth, and was partially corrected surgically by the release of IIIa from IIIb-IV, which shared a partially duplicated

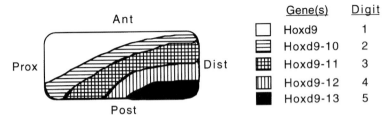

FIGURE 9-6. Expression of *Hoxd* genes in the developing limb. Nested patterns of gene expression along the anteroposterior axis of the developing limb bud (indicated by shading) are correlated with the positions of the presumptive digits. Ant, anterior; Dist, distal; Post, posterior; Prox, proximal. (Adapted from Roberts and Tabin, 1994.)

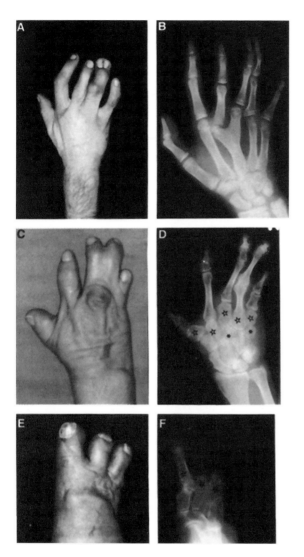

FIGURE 9-7. Heterozygosity and homozygosity for a mutant *HOXD13* gene. (A) Photograph and (B) radiograph of the hand of the heterozygous son. (C) Photograph and (D) radiograph of the hand of his homozygous mother. Star, hypoplastic metacarpal; asterisk, supernumerary carpal bone. (E) Photograph and (F) radiograph of the mother's foot. Star, hypoplastic metatarsal. (Reproduced with permission from Muragaki et al., 1996. Copyright ©1996 by the American Association for the Advancement of Science.)

(fused) fingernail (Fig. 9.6A). In contrast, his mother demonstrated syndactyly of digits III, IV, and V, marked hypoplasia of phalanges and metacarpals, and two additional carpal bones (Figs. 9.7 C and D). Her foot contained only three digits, with the replacement of metatarsals III, IV, and V by a single rudimentary bone that resembled a tarsal rather than a metatarsal (Figs. 9.7 E and F). DNA analysis revealed that she was homozygous for the mutant Ala_{22} allele as a result of consanguinity (her parents were first cousins). The Ala_{22} allele thus has the remarkable property of resulting in an excess of digits in the heterozygous state and a deficiency of digits in the homozygous state. Pedigree analysis in these families also revealed nonpenetrant individuals who were heterozygous for the repeat expansion but did not manifest synpolydactyly.

Analysis of 16 additional pedigrees revealed that the total length of the polyalanine tract varied among families from 22 to 29 residues in affected individuals (with no intrafamilial variation), whereas in unaffected individuals, only Ala_{15} tracts were identified (Goodman et al., 1997). Comparison of phenotype as a function of genotype revealed that there was a statistically significant increase in the penetrance and expressivity of alleles as the size of the repeat expansion increased. In the pedigree segregating the largest expansion (Ala_{29}), there were no nonpenetrant individuals. Affected individuals had the most severe phenotype, as the malformations extended anteriorly to include the first digit, and proximally to include the carpal bones. In contrast, individuals heterozygous for shorter expansions demonstrated malformations of the posterior digits (III, IV, and V) only. Two males in this family also manifested hypospadias, which is of interest given the involvement of *HOXA13* in the hand-foot-genital syndrome (see below).

Knowledge of the *HOXD13* genotype was not, however, sufficient to explain all aspects of the phenotype, for malformations varied among family members. Intrafamilial variation was greatest in families with the smallest repeat expansions, suggesting a greater influence of genetic background and/or environment in these cases (Goodman et al., 1997). However, variation was present even within the same individual, because unilateral involvement or involvement of the hands but not the feet was common, suggesting that the developmental process was also affected by stochastic processes.

From these data it is very difficult to decide whether the observed malformations reflect loss-of-function, dominant-negative, or gain-of-function effects of the mutant protein. In addition to HOXD13, polyalanine tracts have been identified in several mammalian homeodomain proteins, including MSX1, MSX2, and HOXA13 (Catron et al., 1996; Mortlock et al., 1996). In *Drosophila*, several transcriptional repressors, including

KRUPPEL, contain alanine-rich domains that are required for activity (Licht et al., 1990, 1994). It is possible that the increased size of the polyalanine tract may result in progressive increase in transcriptional repression mediated by HOXD13, which could be viewed as a gain-of-function (transcriptional repression) or dominant-negative (loss of activation of target genes) mechanism. This hypothesis is supported by mouse genetic studies described below.

Inactivation of Hoxd Gene Function by Homologous Recombination

In knockout mice homozygous for a disrupted *Hoxd13* gene, abnormalities of all four limbs were detected (Dolle et al., 1993). The size of all forelimb digits was reduced primarily because of involvement of the second phalanx, which was either hypoplastic (digits III and IV) or aplastic (digits II and V). In the hindlimbs, the metatarsals were short and thick and the second phalanges of digits II and V were absent (Fig. 9.8). In addition, a rudimentary sixth digit was present on a forelimb or hindlimb of some of the *Hoxd13*$^{-/-}$ mice and a supernumerary carpal bone was also occasionally present. The finding of reduced size and shape of affected bones suggests that *Hoxd13* regulates cellular proliferation, differentiation, and/or survival. Furthermore, the supernumerary digit and carpal indicate effects on pattern formation along the anteroposterior axis, whereas the reduction of second phalanges can also be interpreted as an effect on pattern formation along the proximodistal axis, suggesting that patterning along both of these axes may be determined by *Hox* gene expression (Dolle et al., 1993). However, it should be noted that the selective effects of HOXD13 deficiency on the growth of digits II and V are difficult to reconcile with the hypothesis that the pattern of *Hox* gene expression transmits positional information that determines digit identity. An alternative hypothesis is that *Hox* genes instead control limb patterning by regulating the timing and rate of cellular growth (Dolle et al., 1993).

The limb abnormalities detected in mice homozygous for a disrupted *Hoxd13* gene were less severe than those observed in the patient who was homozygous for the *HOXD13(Ala$_{22}$)* allele. One possible explanation for these results is that the mutant HOXD13(Ala$_{22}$) protein interfered with the activity of other HOXD proteins. To further explore the role of *Hoxd* genes in limb development, two lines of mice were developed. The first, targeted (*Targ*), line contained a *Hoxd11/lacZ* transgene located 5' to *Hoxd13* whereas in the second, deleted (*Del*), line the endogenous *Hoxd13*, *Hoxd12*, and *Hoxd11* genes were deleted so that the *Hoxd11/lacZ* transgene was located 5' to *Hoxd10* (see Fig. 9.2). In the *Targ/*

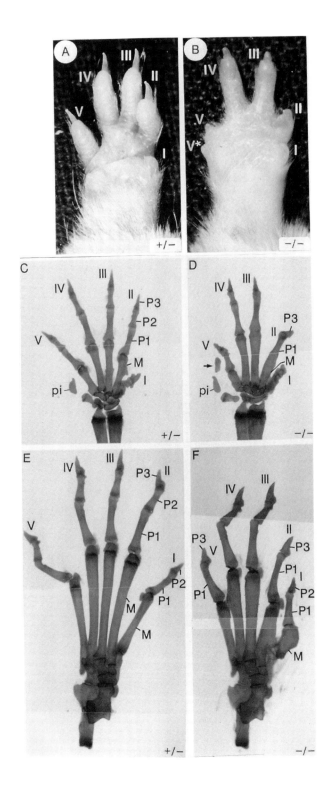

228

+ and *Del/+* mice, *lacZ* expression paralleled expression of *Hoxd13* and *Hoxd11*, respectively, indicating that the expression of the reporter gene depended on its position within the *Hoxd* gene cluster (Zakany and Duboule, 1996). In *Del/Del* mice, reduction of the presumptive digits could be identified as early as E11, polydactyly could be detected after digit condensation on E14, and at birth both brachydactyly and polydactyly were present (Fig. 9.9). Whereas *Del/+* mice manifested reduced size of digits II and V, *Del/Del* mice manifested reduction in size and number of digits and carpal bones. Synpolydactyly also arose as the result of fusion of hypoplastic proximal digits.

The phenotype of mice deficient for HOXD13, HOXD12, and HOXD11 is thus similar to the phenotype associated with homozygosity for *HOXD13 (Ala$_{22}$)* and is much more severe than that associated with deficiency of HOXD13 alone. Deficiency of either HOXD12 or HOXD11 alone resulted in mild hypoplasia of phalanges, metacarpals, and carpals (Davis and Capecchi, 1994, 1996; Favier et al., 1995). Taken together, these results suggest that the human HOXD13(Ala$_{22}$) protein interfered with the function of wild-type HOXD13, HOXD12, and HOXD11 and thus exerted its pathophysiologic effect by a dominant-negative mechanism. One possibility is that the HOXD13(Ala$_{22}$) protein may compete with HOXD13, HOXD12, and HOXD11 for common binding sites within regulatory regions of target genes but once bound may function differently—for example, as a repressor rather than an activator of transcription. In addition, these studies indicate that HOXD13, HOXD12, and HOXD11 determine the formation, proliferation, and ossification of digit condensations within the developing limb.

Hoxa13 and Hypodactyly

Hypodactyly (*Hd*) is a semidominant mutation that, in heterozygotes, results in shortening of the first digit of all four limbs (Fig. 9.10) and, in homozygotes, results in embryonic lethality with severe limb reduction

---

FIGURE 9-8. Limb malformations associated with deficiency of HOXD13. Top and middle rows, forelimbs from *Hoxd13$^{+/-}$* (A, C) and *Hoxd13$^{-/-}$* (B, D) mice. Metacarpal (M), pisiform bone (pi), and proximal (P1), middle (P2), and distal (P3) phalanges are indicated. Arrow in (D) demonstrates supernumerary bone associated with digit V*. Bottom row, hindlimbs from *Hoxd13$^{+/-}$* (E) and *Hoxd13$^{-/-}$* (F) mice. Note both hypoplasia and malformation of multiple bones. (Reproduced with permission from Dolle et al., 1993. Copyright ©1993 by Cell Press.)

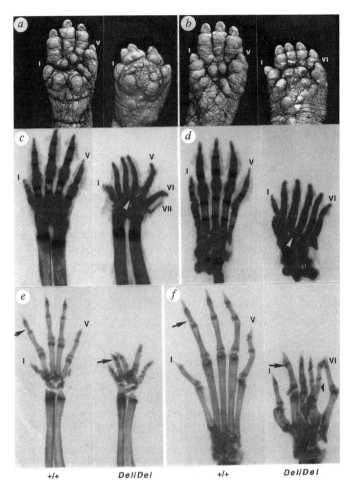

+/+   DelIDel   +/+   DelIDel

FIGURE 9-9. Limb malformations associated with deficiency of HOXD13, HOXD12, and HOXD11. Each panel is a comparison of +/+ (left) and *Del/Del* (right) mice. Top row, scanning electron micrographs of fore- (*a*) and hind- (*b*) limbs of newborn mice. Middle row, (*c*) and (*d*) are cleared skeletal preparations of specimens shown in (*a*) and (*b*), respectively. Arrowheads indicate two digits articulating with a single carpal (*c*) or tarsal (*d*) bone. Bottom row, adult fore- (*e*) and hind- (*f*) limbs. *Del/Del* mice manifest phalangeal hypoplasia (arrows) and synpolydactyly (arrowhead). (Reproduced with permission from Zakany and Duboule, 1996. Copyright ©1996 by Macmillan Magazines Limited.)

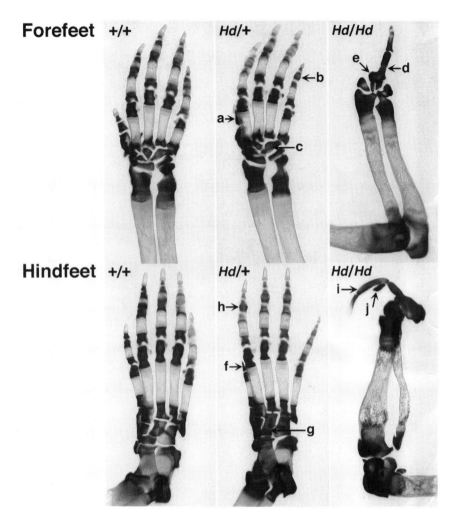

FIGURE 9-10. Limb malformations in *hypodactyly* mice. Skeletal preparations from the forelimb (upper panels) and hindlimbs (lower panels) of wild-type (+/+), heterozygous (Hd/+), and homozygous-mutant (Hd/Hd) mice are shown. (Reproduced with permission from Mortlock et al., 1996.)

defects so that the autopod (that part of the limb distal to the long bones) consists of only a few hypoplastic carpal/tarsal bones and a single digit (Hummel, 1970). As described above, the 5' members of the *Hoxa* and *Hoxd* gene clusters are expressed in a nested pattern in the developing mouse limb bud, so that the expression of the 5'-most genes occurs later and in more distal/posterior domains. *Hoxa13*, the 5'-most gene of the *Hoxa* cluster, is expressed across the entire distal tip of the limb bud

(Haack and Gruss, 1993). In *hypodactyly* mice, a 50–bp deletion was identified in exon 1 of *Hoxa13*, resulting in a frameshift at codon 25, prior to the homeobox, so that a functional HOXA13 protein could not be produced from the mutant allele (Mortlock et al.., 1996). The deletion was bounded by a 10-bp direct repeat, 5'-CGGCGGCGGC-3', suggesting that the deletion occurred via unequal crossing-over or strand slippage during DNA replication.

The most likely effect of the deletion is loss of function with a gene dosage effect manifesting as a mild and severe phenotype in the heterozygote and homozygote, respectively. However, dominant-negative and gain-of-function pathogenetic mechanisms are not ruled out by the present data. Generation of mice in which the entire *Hoxa13* coding region is deleted by homologous recombination to create a true null allele will be necessary to confirm that the phenotypes are strictly caused by loss of HOXA13 function.

Thus, mutations affecting the 5'-most members of the *Hoxa* (*Hoxa13*) and *Hoxd* (*Hoxd13*) gene clusters result in malformations of the autopod on all four limbs along both the anterior-posterior and proximal-distal axes. However, the malformations in *Hoxd13*$^{-/-}$ mice are less severe than in *Hd/Hd* mice. *Hoxd13*$^{-/-}$ mice are viable and demonstrate loss of a single phalanx in digits II and V as well as general shortening of all digits and dysplasia of carpal/tarsal bones, as described above. This is consistent with the observation that the expression pattern of *Hoxa13* is more extensive than that of *Hoxd13* (Mortlock et al., 1996). *Hoxd13* is expressed only in the digits, whereas *Hoxa13* is expressed throughout the autopod (Dolle et al., 1991, 1993; Yokouchi et al., 1991). It is also possible that HOXA13 regulates *Hoxd13* expression, so that the *Hd* mutation may result in decreased levels of functional HOXA13 and HOXD13 protein, but the analysis of *Hoxd13* expression in *Hd/Hd* compared to wild-type mice has not been reported.

HOXA13 and Hand-Foot-Genital Syndrome

Originally described (Stern et al., 1970) as the hand-foot-uterus syndrome (MIM 140000), this condition is characterized by the following malformations: (1) hand: hypoplasia of the first metacarpal, distal phalanx of the thumb, and middle phalanx of the fifth finger, as well as carpal bone abnormalities (Fig. 9.11); (2) foot: markedly reduced great toes due to hypoplasia of the first metatarsal and distal phalanx; (3) genital: in females, defects of müllerian duct fusion leading to development of a bicornuate uterus, longitudinal vaginal septum, and urinary tract malformations; and in males, hypospadias (ventrally displaced urethral orifice).

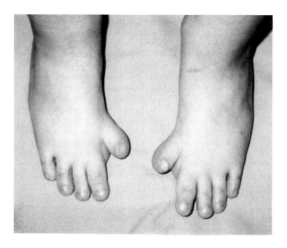

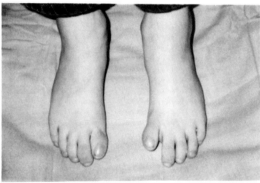

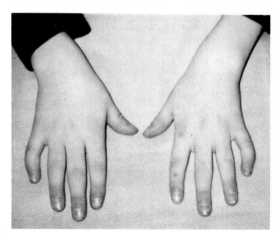

FIGURE 9-11. Limb malformations in hand-foot-genital syndrome. The great toes are reduced and medially deviated (upper and middle panels). The thumbs are reduced and there is clinodactyly (deviation) of the fifth fingers (bottom panel). (Reproduced with permission from Mortlock and Innis, 1997.)

The limb malformations are strikingly similar to those described in *Hd/* + mice. Furthermore, female *Hd/Hd* mice exhibited hypoplasia of the vagina and clitoris and occcasional urologic defects (Mortlock et al., 1996).

These observations suggested that the hand-foot-genital syndrome might be caused by mutations in the human *HOXA13* gene, and molecular analysis of the original hand-foot-uterus pedigree reported by Stern et al. (1970) revealed that affected individuals were heterozygous for a nonsense mutation that would truncate the last 20 amino acids of the gene product (Mortlock and Innis, 1997). The nonsense mutation involved the codon for a tryptophan residue within the third (recognition) helix of the homeodomain, which is the only amino acid that is invariant in all known homeodomain proteins. It is likely that this mutation results in a loss of HOXA13 biological activity, but dominant-negative and gain-of-function mechanisms have not been formally excluded. However, the similar effects of two very different types of mutations in humans and mice strongly suggest that limb malformations result from haploinsufficiency for HOXA13. Furthermore, whereas HOXA13 clearly plays an important role in the development of the autopod, these results also suggest that HOXA13 can now be added to a growing list of transcription factors, including AR, DAX1, and SF1 (Chapter 5), WT1 (Chapter 6), PAX2 (Chapter 7), and SOX9 and SRY (Chapter 10), whose function is important for normal genitourinary development. Indeed, the extreme conservation of *HOXA13* (and other *HOX* genes) during evolution may reflect essential roles in genital development (reviewed by Dickman, 1997). *Hoxa10* mutant mice also have reduced fertility due to uterine malformations (Benson et al., 1996). The fact that mutations in these genes can adversely affect reproductive function may explain why the presence of five digits on vertebrate limbs has remained virtually invariant for over 300 million years.

Rieger Syndrome

Autosomal dominant inheritance of dental hypoplasia and malformations of the ocular anterior chamber was first reported by Rieger (1935). Ocular malformations in Rieger syndrome (MIM 180500, 601499) include microcornea with opacity, iris hypoplasia, and anterior synechiae leading to glaucoma (Fig. 9.12). Craniofacial malformations include telecanthus, maxillary hypoplasia, and dysplastic ears. The spectrum of dental malformations includes cone-shaped teeth, hypodontia, and microdontia. An additional striking feature is incomplete involution of the periumbilical

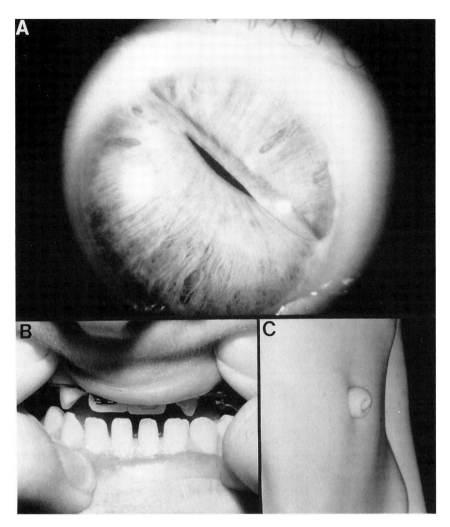

FIGURE 9-12. Clinical presentation of Rieger syndrome. (*a*) Ocular abnormalities. Note the pupillary distortion associated with iris malformation. (*b*) Dental abnormalities. The maxillary (upper) lateral incisors are absent and the mandibular (lower) central incisors are hypoplastic. (*c*) Umbilical abnormalities. Note the protruding umbilicus resulting from failed involution of periumbilical skin. (Reproduced with permission from Semina et al., 1996.)

skin and an increased incidence of umbilical herniae (Jorgenson et al., 1978).

Several patients with Rieger syndrome and cytogenetic deletions involving chromosome 4q25-q27 were identified (Fryns and van den Berghe, 1992; Shiang et al., 1987; Vaux et al., 1992). Consistent with these results, linkage of Rieger syndrome to genetic markers on chromosome 4q25 was reported (Murray et al., 1992). However, Rieger syndrome is clearly a genetically heterogeneous disorder. In addition to the locus at chromosome 4q25 (MIM 180500), a second locus has been mapped to chromosome 13q14 (MIM 601499) based on the identification of patients with cytogenetic deletions as well as linkage analysis of a single four-generation pedigree (Phillips et al., 1996). In the family studied by linkage analysis, affected individuals had the additional finding of hydrocephalus but lacked umbilical abnormalities. Additional loci may be implicated in Rieger syndrome, based on the identification of other cytogenetic abnormalities (reviewed by Phillips et al., 1996).

Analysis of genomic DNA from two patients with translocation breakpoints at chromosome 4q25 that were within 50 kb of one another facilitated a directed search for DNA sequences in this region that were expressed during craniofacial development, leading to the isolation of the *RIEG* gene (Semina et al., 1996). *RIEG* encoded a 271-amino-acid protein containing a homeodomain of the BICOID class, based on the presence of a Lys residue at homeodomain residue 50 within the third (recognition) helix that determines DNA binding specificity. Database searches revealed that RIEG and PTX1 (POTX1) were 97% identical in the 60-amino-acid homeodomain and 100% identical in a 14-amino-acid sequence of unknown function located C-terminal to the homeodomain (Semina et al., 1996). Both *RIEG* and *PTX1 (POTX1)* are expressed during craniofacial development. *Rieg* expression was demonstrated in E11 mouse embryos in developing ocular, maxillary, and mandibular structures, dental lamina, and umbilical cord, which was consistent with the involvement of *RIEG* in the pathogenesis of Rieger syndrome (Semina et al., 1996). This involvement was confirmed by the identification of heterozygous mutations in *RIEG* in affected individuals from six of ten families in which Rieger syndrome was segregating, including missense mutations in homeodomain helices 1, 2, and 3; two splicing mutations within the intron interrupting the homeobox; and a nonsense mutation just C-terminal to the homeodomain (Semina et al., 1996). Taken together with the cytogenetic abnormalities that presumably delete all or part of *RIEG*, these results suggest that Rieger syndrome results from haploinsufficiency for RIEG in these families. The translocation breakpoints were mapped 5–15 and 55–65 kb 5' to *RIEG*, respectively (Semina et al., 1996).

Thus, *RIEG* can be added to the list of genes encoding transcription factors in which deletions or translocations distal to the gene are presumed to result in transcriptional inactivation, including *GLI3* (Chapter 6), *PAX6* (Chapter 7), and *SOX9* (Chapter 10).

Multiple homeobox genes are expressed during craniofacial development, including *CART1, CHX10, HOXA1, HOXA2, HOXA3, MSX1, MSX2, OTP, PAX2, PAX3, PAX6, PRX1 PRX2, PTX1 (POTX)*, and *RIEG* (Chalepakis et al., 1993; Chisaka and Capecchi, 1991; Gendron-Maguire et al., 1993; Hill et al., 1989, 1991; Leussink et al., 1995; Liu et al., 1994; Lufkin et al., 1991; MacKenzie et al., 1991a, b, 1992; Mina et al., 1995; Rijli et al., 1993; Robert et al., 1989; Semina et al., 1996; Simeone et al., 1994b; Zhao et al., 1994). The complexity of mammalian craniofacial development will undoubtedly be controlled by a correspondingly large number of transcription factors. The identification of genes that, when mutated, result in similar malformations provides the potential to assemble genetic pathways underlying craniofacial morphogenesis. For example, heterozygous loss-of-function mutations at the *MSX1* or *RIEG* loci can result in oligodontia (missing teeth) and other dental abnormalities, whereas heterozygous loss-of-function mutations at the *PAX2, PAX6* or *RIEG* loci can result in ocular malformations. Given the sequence similarity between RIEG and PTX1, it will be interesting to learn whether mutations of *PTX1* also result in Rieger syndrome.

Short Stature Associated with Pseudoautosomal Deletions of *SHOX*

Terminal deletions of the short arm of the X or Y chromosome are associated with short stature and analysis of DNA from individuals with sex chromosome rearrangements who were of either normal or reduced height implicated a 170-kb region in the pseudoautosomal region (Rao et al., 1997). This DNA segment was deleted in all 36 individuals with short stature and a chromosomal rearrangement involving Xp22 or Yp11.3, whereas the segment was not deleted in 30 individuals with an Xp22 or Yp11.3 rearrangement and normal stature. A single gene was identified in this region using cDNA selection and exon amplification techniques as well as nucleotide sequence analysis of 140 kb. No cDNAs were identified by selection techniques or by screening (using three amplified exons as probes) 14 million clones from 14 libraries involving 12 different tissue types. Reverse-transcription PCR assays were successfully employed to amplify from placenta, skeletal muscle, and bone marrow fibroblasts cDNA sequences that encoded a homeodomain protein that was designated SHOX (short-stature homeobox) (Rao et al., 1997).

As expected, analysis of cell lines containing only an active X, inactive X, or Y chromosome revealed that *SHOX* was not subject to X inactivation. Because of the possibility that another undetected gene in the 170-kb interval was responsible for short stature, it was important to identify an intragenic mutation in *SHOX* associated with short stature. A nonsense mutation was identified in one of 91 individuals studied. Analysis of this individual's family revealed the presence of the mutation in all five short-statured and none of the normal-statured family members.

These results provide evidence that suggests, but not does not definitively establish, a role for SHOX in control of linear growth. Among the shortcomings (no pun intended) of this work are the absence of *de novo* mutations associated with short stature or a sufficient number of familial mutations to allow linkage analysis. In addition, expression of the gene has not been demonstrated in an appropriate cell type, such as developing bone or cartilage. Of interest is the fact that hemizygosity for this gene may account for the short stature observed in Turner syndrome, which is due to the presence of a 45, X0 chromosome constitution. A putative mouse homologue of *SHOX, Og-12a*, was also identified and mapped to an autosome, similar to two other genes present in the human pseudoautosomal region and consistent with the involvement of *SHOX* in Turner syndrome because in mice the X0 karyotype is not associated with short stature (Rao et al., 1997). Further studies will be required to identify additional *SHOX* mutations in humans with short stature, to analyze expression of *SHOX/Og-12a* during development, and to determine the effect of loss of *Og-12a* expression on linear growth in mice.

Pancreatic Agenesis Associated with Homozygosity for an *IPF1* Mutation

A homeodomain protein designated IPF1, IDX1, STF1, and PDX1 by various laboratories was identified as a transcriptional activator of the genes encoding insulin and somatostatin in pancreatic islet cells (Leonard et al., 1993; Miller et al., 1994; Ohlsson et al., 1993). IPF1 (insulin-promoter factor 1) was shown to be expressed in both endocrine and exocrine cells of the developing pancreas and epithelial cells of the duodenum and pancreatic duct (Guz et al., 1995). Mice homozygous for a null allele at the *Ipf1* locus manifested pancreatic agenesis (Jonnson et al., 1994). These results indicate that IPF1 is a transcription factor that controls both organ formation and the expression of specific products of terminally differentiated cells within the organ. This is similar to the role of PIT1 (Chapter 11), which also contains a homeodomain and is required for both anterior pituitary development and the expression of growth hormone and prolactin.

Pancreatic agenesis is a very rare and usually fatal disorder in humans, but a child was diagnosed soon after birth and provided with replacement insulin therapy and pancreatic enzymes, allowing survival (Wright et al., 1993). DNA analysis revealed homozygosity for a single nucleotide deletion in the *IPF1* gene resulting in a frameshift allele encoding a truncated protein lacking the homeodomain (Stoffers et al., 1997). This truncated protein is likely to be nonfunctional because it lacks amino acid sequences required for nuclear localization and DNA binding. Both parents were heterozygous for the mutation and, despite the absence of known consanguinity, extended haplotype analysis indicated that the parental alleles were probably inherited from a common ancestor, as is often observed with extremely rare genetic disorders.

Perhaps the most interesting aspect of this analysis was the finding that both the maternal and paternal families (including the parents themselves) had a very strong history of non-insulin dependent diabetes mellitus (Stoffers et al., 1997). This observation suggests that heterozygosity for the *IPF1* mutation predisposes to the development of NIDDM, an hypothesis that can be tested by genotype analysis of additional unaffected and affected family members, as well as unrelated individuals with NIDDM, and by the analysis of heterozygous mutant mice for evidence of NIDDM. Mutations in genes encoding the transcription factors HNF1α and HNF4α have already been demonstrated in a variant form of NIDDM, maturity-onset diabetes of the young (see Chapter 12). These results further emphasize that master control genes such as HNF1α, HNF4α, IPF1, and PIT1 play absolutely essential roles in both organ development and physiology from embryonic through adult life.

References

Akarsu, A. N., I. Stoilov, E. Yilmaz, B. S. Sayli, and M. Sarfarazi. Genomic structure of HOXD13 gene: a nine polyalanine duplication causes synpolydactyly in two unrelated families. *Hum. Mol. Genet.* 5:945–952, 1996.

Ang, S. L., O. Jin, M. Rhinn, N. Daigle, L. Stevenson, and J. Rossant. A targeted mouse Otx2 mutation leads to severe defects in gastrulation and formation of axial mesoderm and to deletion of rostral brain. *Development* 122:243–252, 1996.

Bell, J. R., A. Noveen, Y. H. Liu, L. Ma, S. Dobias, R. Kundu, W. Luo, Y. Xia, A. Lusis, M. L. Snead, and R. Maxson. Genomic structure, chromosomal location, and evolution of the mouse *Hox 8* gene. *Genomics* 16:123–131, 1993.

Benson, G. V., H. Lim, B. C. Paria, I. Satokata, S. K. Dey, and R. L. Maas. Mechanisms of reduced fertility in Hoxa-10 mutant mice: uterine homeosis and loss of maternal Hoxa-10 expression. *Development* 122:2687–2696, 1996.

Boncinelli, E. Homeobox genes and disease. *Curr. Opin. Genet. Dev.* 7:331–337, 1997.

Brunelli, S., A. Faiella, V. Capra, V. Nigro, A. Simeone, A. Cama, and E. Boncinelli. Germline mutations in the homeobox gene EMX2 in patients with severe schizencephaly. *Nat. Genet.* 12:94–96, 1996.

Catron, K. M., H. Wang, G. Hu, M. M. Shen, and C. Abate-Shen. Comparison of MSX-1 and MSX-2 suggests a molecular basis for functional redundancy. *Mech. Dev.* 55:185–199, 1996.

Chalepakis, G., A. Stoykova, J. Wijnholds, P. Tremblay, and P. Gruss. Pax: gene regulators in the developing nervous system. *J. Neurobiol.* 24:1367–1384, 1993.

Chisaka, O., and M. R. Capecchi. Regionally restricted developmental defects resulting from targeted disruption of the mouse homeobox gene *hox-1.5.* *Nature* 350:473–479, 1991.

Cserjesi, P., B. Lilly, L. Bryson, Y. Wang, D. Sassoon, and E. N. Olson. MHox: a mesodermally restricted homeodomain protein that binds an essential site in the muscle creatine kinase enhancer. *Development* 115:1087–1101, 1992.

Davis, A. P., and M. R. Capecchi. Axial homeosis and appendicular skeleton defects in mice with a targeted disruption of hoxd-11. *Development* 120:2187–2198, 1994.

Davis, A. P., and M. R. Capecchi. A mutational analysis of the 5' HoxD genes: dissection of genetic interactions during limb development in the mouse. *Development* 122:1175–1185, 1996.

Dickman, S. HOX gene links limb, genital defects. *Science* 275:1568, 1997.

Dolle, P., A. Dierich, M. LeMeur, T. Schimmang, B. Schuhbaur, P. Chambon, and D. Duboule. Disruption of the Hoxd-13 gene induces localized heterochrony leading to mice with neotenic limbs. *Cell* 75:431–441, 1993.

Dolle, P., J.-C. Izpisua-Belmonte, E. Boncinelli, and D. Duboule. The Hox-4.8 gene is localised at the 5' extremity of the HOX-4 complex and is expressed in the most posterior parts of the body during development. *Mech. Dev.* 36:3–14, 1991.

Duboule, D. The vertebrate limb: a model system to study the HOX/HOM gene network during development and evolution. *Bioessays* 14:375–384, 1992.

Favier, B., M. LeMeur, P. Chambon, and P. Dolle. Axial skeleton homeosis and forelimb malformations in Hoxd-11 mutant mice. *Proc. Natl. Acad. Sci. U.S.A.* 92:310–314, 1995.

Fryns, J. P., and H. van den Berghe. Rieger syndrome and interstitial 4q26 deletion. *Genetic Counseling* 3:153–154, 1992.

Gaunt, S. J., M. Blum, and E. M. De Robertis. Expression of the mouse *goosecoid* gene during mid-embryogenesis may mark mesenchymal cell lineages in the developing head, limbs, and body wall. *Development* 117:769–778, 1993.

Gaunt, S. J., P. T. Sharpe, and D. Duboule. Spatially restricted domains of homeogene transcripts in mouse embryos: relation to a segmented body plan. *Development* (Suppl.) 104:71–82, 1988.

Gendron-Maguire, M., M. Mallo, M. Zhang, and T. Gridley. *Hoxa-2* mutant mice exhibit homeotic transformation of skeletal elements derived from cranial neural crest. *Cell* 75:1317–1331, 1993.

Goodman, F. R., S. Mundlos, Y. Muragaki, D. Donnai, M. L. Giovannucci-Uzielli, E. Lapi, F. Majewski, J. McGaughran, C. McKeown, W. Reardon, J. Upton,

R. M. Winter, B. R. Olsen, and P. J. Scambler. Synpolydactyly phenotypes correlate with size of expansions in HOXD13 polyalanine tract. *Proc. Natl. Acad. Sci. U.S.A.* 94:7458–7463, 1997.

Gorlin, R. J., M. M. Cohen, Jr., and L. S. Levin. *Syndromes of the Head and Neck.* New York: Oxford University Press, 1990.

Graham, A., P. Francis-West, P. Brickell, and A. Lumsden. The signaling molecule BMP4 mediates apoptosis in the rhombencephalic neural crest. *Nature* 372: 684–686, 1994.

Graham, A., I. Heyman, and A. Lumsden. Even-numbered rhombomeres control the apoptotic elimination of neural crest cells from odd-numbered rhombomeres in the chick hindbrain. *Development* 119:233–245, 1993.

Gulisano, M., V. Broccoli, C. Pardini, and E. Boncinelli. Emx1 and Emx2 show different patterns of expression during proliferation and differentiation of the developing cerebral cortex. *Eur. J. Neurosci.* 8:1037–1050, 1996.

Guz, Y., M. R. Montminy, R. Stein, J. Leonard, L. W. Gamer, C. V. Wright, and G. Teitelman. Expression of murine STF-1, a putative insulin gene transcription factor, in beta cells of pancreas, duodenal epithelium and pancreatic exocrine and endocrine progenitors during ontogeny. *Development* 121:11–18, 1995.

Haack, H., and P. Gruss. The establishment of murine Hox-1 expression domains during patterning of the limb. *Dev. Biol.* 157:410–422, 1993.

Hall, B. K., and T. Miyake. The membranous skeleton: the role of cell condensations in vertebrate skeletogenesis. *Anat. Embryol.* 186:107–124, 1992.

Han, K., and J. L. Manley. Transcriptional repression by the Drosophila even-skipped protein: definition of a minimal repression domain. *Genes Dev.* 7: 491–503, 1993.

Harrison, S. C., and A. K. Aggarwal. DNA recognition by proteins with the helix-turn-helix motif. *Annu. Rev. Biochem.* 59:933–969, 1990.

Hill, R. E., J. Favor, B. L. M. Hogan, C. C. T. Ton, G. F. Saunders, I. M. Hanson, J. Prosser, T. Jordan, N. D. Hastie, and V. van Heyningen. Mouse small eye results from mutations in a paired-like homeobox-containing gene. *Nature* 354:522–535, 1991.

Hill, R. E., P. F. Jones, A. R. Rees, C. M. Sime, M. J. Justice, N. G. Copeland, N. A. Jenkins, E. Graham, and D. R. Davidson. A new family of mouse homeo box-containing genes: molecular structure, chromosomal location, and developmental expression of *Hox-7.1. Genes Dev.* 3:26–37, 1989.

Hillburger, A. C., J. K. Willis, E. Bouldin, and A. Henderson-Tilton. Familial schizencephaly. *Brain Dev.* 15: 234–236, 1993.

Hosley, M. A., I. F. Abroms, and R. L. Ragland. Schizencephaly: case report of familial incidence. *Pediat. Neurol.* 8: 148–150, 1992.

Hummel, K. Hypodactyly, a semidominant lethal mutation in mice. *J. Hered.* 61: 219–220, 1970.

Hunt, P., M. Gulisano, M. Cook, M.-H Sham, A. Faiella, D. Wilkinson, E. Boncinelli, and R. Krumlauf. A distinct *Hox* code for the branchial region of the vertebrate head. *Nature* 353: 861–864, 1991.

Hunt, P., and Krumlauf, R. Deciphering the Hox code: clues to patterning branchial regions of the head. *Cell* 66:1075–1078, 1991.

Izpisua-Belmonte, J.-C., and D. Duboule. Homeobox genes and pattern formation in the vertebrate limb. *Dev. Biol.* 152:26–36, 1992.

Izpisua-Belmonte, J.-C., H. Falkenstein, P. Dolle, A. Renucci, and D. Duboule. Murine genes related to the Drosophila AbdB homeotic gene are sequentially expressed during development of the posterior part of the body. *EMBO J.* 10:2279–2289, 1991.

Jabs, E. W., U. Muller, X. Li, L. Ma, W. Luo, I. Haworth, I. Klisak, R. Sparkes, M. L. Warman, J. B. Mulliken, M. Snead, and R. Maxson. A mutation in the homeodomain of the human MSX2 gene in a family affected with autosomal dominant craniosynostosis. *Cell* 75:443–450, 1993.

Jonnson, J., L. Carlsson, T. Edlund, and H. Edlund. Insulin-promoter factor 1 is required for pancreas development in mice. *Nature* 371:606–609, 1994.

Jorgenson, R. J., L. S. Levin, H. E. Cross, F. Yoder, and T. E. Kelly. The Rieger syndrome. *Am. J. Med. Genet.* 2:307–318, 1978.

Jowett, A. K., S. Vainio, M. W. J. Ferguson, P. T. Sharpe, and I. Thesleff. Epithelial-mesenchymal interactions are required for *msx 1* and *msx 2* gene expression in the developing murine molar teeth. *Development* 117:461–470, 1993.

Kissinger, C. R., B. Liu, E. Martin-Blanco, T. B. Kornberg, and C. O. Pabo. Crystal structure of an engrailed homeodomain-DNA complex at 2.8 Å resolution: a framework for understanding homeodomain-DNA interactions. *Cell* 63: 579–590, 1990.

Kotch, L. E., S.-Y. Chen, and K. K. Sulik. Ethanol-induced teratogenesis: free radical damage as a possible mechanism. *Teratology* 52:128–136, 1995.

Kotch, L. E., and K. K. Sulik. Experimental fetal alcohol syndrome: proposed pathogenic basis for a variety of associated facial and brain anomalies. *Am. J. Med. Genet.* 44: 168–176:1992a.

Kotch, L. E., and K. K. Sulik. Patterns of ethanol-induced cell death in the developing nervous system of mice: neural fold states through the time of anterior neural tube closure. *Int. J. Dev. Neurosci.* 10:273–279, 1992b.

Krumlauf, R. Hox genes in vertebrate development. *Cell* 78:191–201, 1994.

Leonard, J., B. Peers, T. Johnson, K. Ferreri, S. Lee, and M. R. Montminy. Characterization of somatostatin transactivating factor-1, a novel homeobox factor that stimulates somatostatin expression in pancreatic islet cells. *Mol. Endocrinol.* 7:1275–1283, 1993.

Leussink, B., A. Brouwer, M. el Khattabi, R. E. Poelmann, A. C. Gittenberger-de Groot, and F. Meijlink. Expression patterns of the paired-related homeobox genes MHox/Prx1 and S8/Prx2 suggest roles in development of the heart and the forebrain. *Mech Dev.* 52:51–64, 1995.

Lewis, E. B. A gene complex controlling segmentation in Drosophila. *Nature* 276: 565–570, 1978.

Licht, J. D., M. J. Grossel, J. Figge, and U. M. Hansen. Drosophila Kruppel protein is a transcriptional repressor. *Nature* 346:76–79, 1990.

Licht, J. D., W. Hanna-Rose, J. C. Reddy, M. A. English, M. Ro, M. Grossel, R. Shaknovich, and U. Hansen. Mapping and mutagenesis of the amino-terminal transcription repression domain of the Drosophila Kruppel protein. *Mol. Cell. Biol.* 14:4057–4066, 1994.

Liu, I. S., J. D. Chen, L. Ploder, D. Vidgen, D. van der Kooy, V. I. Kalnins, and R. R. McInnes. Developmental expression of a novel murine homeobox gene (Chx10): evidence for roles in determination of the neuroretina and inner nuclear layer. *Neuron* 13:377–393, 1994.

Liu, Y. H., R. Kundu, L. Wu, W. Luo, M. A. Ignelzi, Jr., M. L. Snead, and R. E. Maxson, Jr. Premature suture closure and ectopic cranial bone in mice expressing *Msx2* transgenes in the developing skull. *Proc. Natl. Acad. Sci. U.S.A.* 92:6137–6141, 1995.

Lufkin, T., A. Dierich, M. LeMeur, M. Mark, and P. Chambon. Disruption of the *Hox-1.6* homeobox gene results in defects in a region corresponding to its rostral domain of expression. *Cell* 66:1105–1119, 1991.

Lumsden, A., N. Sprawson, and A. Graham. Segmental origin and migration of neural crest cells in the hindbrain region of the chick embryo. *Development* 113:1281–1291, 1991.

Ma, L., S. Golden, L. Wu, and R. Maxson. The molecular basis of Boston-type craniosynostosis: the Pro148→His mutation in the N-terminal arm of the MSX2 homeodomain stabilizes DNA binding without altering nucleotide sequence preferences. *Hum. Mol. Genet.* 5:1915–1920, 1996.

MacKenzie, A., M. W. J. Ferguson, and P. T. Sharpe. *Hox-7* expression during murine craniofacial development. *Development* 113:601–611, 1991a.

MacKenzie, A., M. W. J. Ferguson, and P. T. Sharpe. Expression patterns of the homeobox gene, *Hox-8*, in the mouse embryo suggest a role in specifying tooth initiation and shape. *Development* 115:403–420, 1992.

MacKenzie, A., G. L. Leeming, A. K. Jowett, M. W. J. Ferguson, and P. T. Sharpe. The homeobox gene Hox 7.1 has specific regional temporal expression patterns during early murine craniofacial embryogenesis, especially tooth development in vivo and in vitro. *Development* 111:269–285, 1991b.

Martin, J. F., A. Bradley, and E. N. Olson,. The *paired*-like homeo box gene *MHox* is required for early events of skeletogenesis in multiple lineages. *Genes Dev.* 9:1237–1249, 1995.

Miller, C. P., R. McGehee, and J. F. Habener. IDX-1: a new homeodomain transcription factor expressed in rat pancreatic islets and duodenum that transactivates the somatostatin gene. *EMBO J.* 13:1145–1156, 1994.

Mina, M., J. Gluhak, W. B. Upholt, E. J. Kollar, and B. Rogers. Experimental analysis of *Msx-1* and *Msx-2* gene expression during chick mandibular morphogenesis. *Dev. Dyn.* 202:195–214, 1995.

Monaghan, A. P., D. R. Davidson, C. Sime, E. Graham, R. Baldock, S. S. Bhattacharya, and R. E. Hill. The *Msh*-like homeobox genes define domains in the developing vertebrate eye. *Development* 112:1053–1061, 1991.

Mortlock, D. P., and J. W. Innis. Mutation of HOXA13 in hand-foot-genital syndrome. *Nat. Genet.* 15:179–180, 1997.

Mortlock, D. P., L. C. Post, and J. W. Innis. The molecular basis of hypodactyly (Hd): a deletion in Hoxa13 leads to arrest of digital arch formation. *Nat. Genet.* 13:284–289, 1996.

Muragaki, Y., S. Mundlos, J. Upton, and B. R. Olsen. Altered growth and branching patterns in synpolydactyly caused by mutations in HOXD13. *Science* 272:548–551, 1996.

Murray, J. C., S. R. Bennett, A. E. Kwitek, K. W. Small, A. Schinzel, W. L. M. Alward, J. L. Weber, G. I. Bell, and K. H. Buetow. Linkage of Rieger syndrome to the region of the epidermal growth factor gene on chromosome 4. *Nat. Genet.* 2:46–49, 1992.

Noden, D. M. The role of the neural crest in patterning of avian cranial skeletal, connective, and muscle tissues. *Dev. Biol.* 96:144–165, 1983.

Ohlsson, H., K. Karlsson, and T. Edlund. IPF1, a homeodomain-containing transactivator of the insulin gene. *EMBO J.* 12:4251–4259, 1993.

Otting, G., Y. Q. Qian, B. Milleter, M. Mueller, M. Affolter, W. J. Gehring, and K. Wuthrich. Protein-DNA contacts in the structure of a homeodomain-DNA complex determined by nuclear magnetic resonance spectroscopy in solution. *EMBO J.* 9:3085–3092, 1990.

Pellegrini, M. A. Mansouri, A. Simeone, E. Boncinelli, and P. Gruss. Dentate gyrus formation requires Emx2. *Development* 122:3893-3898, 1996.

Phillips, J. C., E. A. Del Bono, J. L. Haines, A. M. Pralea, J. S. Cohen, L. J. Greff, and J. L. Wiggs. A second locus for Rieger syndrome maps to chromosome 13q14. *Am. J. Hum. Genet.* 59:613–619, 1996.

Porteus, M. H., A. Bulfone, R. D. Ciaranello, and J. L. R. Rubenstein. Isolation and characterization of a novel cDNA clone encoding a homeo domain that is developmentally regulated in the ventral forebrain. *Neuron* 7:221–229, 1991.

Price, M., M. Lemaistre, M. Pischetola, R. D. Lauro, and D. Duboule. A mouse gene related to *Distal-less* shows a restricted expression in the developing forebrain. *Nature* 351:748–751, 1991.

Qiu, M., A. Bulfone, S. Martinez, J. J. Meneses, K. Shimamura, R. A. Pedersen, and J. L. R. Rubenstein. Null mutation of *Dlx-2* results in abnormal morphogenesis of proximal first and second branchial arch derivatives and abnormal differentiation of the forebrain. *Genes Dev.* 9:2523–2538, 1995.

Rao, E., B. Weiss, M. Fukamik, A. Rump, B. Niesler, A. Mertz, K. Muroya, G. Binder, S. Kirsch, M. Winkelmann, G. Nordsiek, U. Heinrich, M. H. Breuning, M. B. Ranke, A. Rosenthal, T. Ogata, and G. A. Rappold. Pseudoautosomal deletions encompassing a novel homeobox gene cause growth failure in idiopathic short stature and Turner syndrome. *Nat. Genet.* 16:54–63, 1997.

Rieger, H. Beitraege zur kenntnis seltener missbildungen der iris: ueber hypoplasie des irisvorderblattes mit verlagerung und entrundung der pupille. *Albrecht von Graefes Arch. Klin. Exp. Ophthal.* 133:602–635, 1935.

Rifas, L., D. A. Towler, and L. V. Avioli. Gestational exposure to ethanol suppresses msx2 expression in developing mouse embryos. *Proc. Natl. Acad. Sci. U.S.A.* 94:7549–7554, 1997.

Rijli, F. M., M. Mark, S. Lakkaraju, A. Dierich, P. Dolle, and P. Chambon. A homeotic transformation is generated in the rostral branchial region of the head by disruption of *Hox-a2*, which acts as a selector gene. *Cell* 75:1333–1349, 1993.

Rivera-Perez, J. A., M. Mallo, M. Gendron-Maguire, T. Gridley, and R. R. Behringer. *goosecoid* is not an essential component of the mouse gastrula organizer but is required for craniofacial and rib development. *Development* 121:3005–3012, 1995.

Robert, R., D. Sassoon, B. Jacq, W. Gehring, and M. Buckingham. *Hox-7*, a mouse homeobox gene with a novel pattern of expression during embryogenesis. *EMBO J.* 8:91–100, 1989.

Roberts, D. J., and C. Tabin. The genetics of human limb development. *Am. J. Hum. Genet.* 55:1–6, 1994.

Robinson, G. W., and K. A. Mahon. Differential and overlapping expression domains of *Dlx-2* and *Dlx-3* suggest distinct roles for *Distal-less* homeo box genes in craniofacial development. *Mech. Dev.* 48:199–215, 1994.

Robinson, R. O. Familial schizencephaly. *Dev. Med. Child Neurol.* 33: 1010–1014, 1991.

Ruddle, F. H., J. L. Bartels, K. L. Bentley, C. Kappen, M. T. Murtha, and J. W. Pendleton. Evolution of HOX genes. *Annu. Rev. Genet.* 28:423–442, 1994.

Satokata, I., and R. Maas. *Msx1* deficient mice exhibit cleft palate and abnormalities of craniofacial and tooth development. *Nat. Genet.* 6:348–355, 1994.

Scott, M. P. Vertebrate homeobox gene nomenclature. *Cell* 71:551–553, 1992.

Scott, M. P. Hox genes, arms and the man. *Nat. Genet.* 15:117–118, 1997.

Semenza, G. L., G. L. Wang, and R. Kundu. DNA binding and transcriptional properties of wild-type and mutant forms of the homeodomain protein MSX2. *Biochem. Biophys. Res. Commun.* 209:257–262, 1995.

Semina, E. V., R. Reiter, N. J. Leysens, W. L. M. Alward, K. W. Small, N. A. Datson, J. Siegel-Bartelt, D. Bierke-Nelson, P. Bitoun, B. U. Zabel, J. C. Carey, and J. C. Murray. Cloning and characterization of a novel bicoid-related homeobox transcription factor gene, RIEG, involved in Rieger syndrome. *Nat. Genet.* 14:392–399, 1996.

Shashikant, C. S., M. F. Utset, S. M. Violette, T. L. Wise, P. Einat, J. W. Pendleton, K. Schughart, and F. H. Ruddle. Homeobox genes in mouse development. *Crit. Rev. Eukaryot. Gene Expr.* 1:207–245, 1991.

Shiang, R., G. Bell, J. E. Divelbiss, A. Haskins-Olney, J. Overhauser, J. Wasmuth, and Murray, J. C. Mapping of ADH3, EGF, and IL2 in a patient with Riegers-like phenotype and 4q23-q27 deletion. *Am. J. Hum. Genet.* 41: A185, 1987.

Simeone, A., D. Acampora, M. Gulisano, A. Stornaiuolo, and E. Boncinelli. Nested expression domains of four homeobox genes in the developing rostral brain. *Nature* 358:687–690, 1992.

Simeone, A., D. Acampora, M. Pannese, M. D'Esposito, A. Stornaiuolo, M. Gulisano, A. Mallamaci, K Kastury, T. Druck, K Huebner, and E. Boncinelli. Cloning and characterization of two members of the vertebrate *Dlx* gene family. *Proc. Natl. Acad. Sci. U.S.A.* 91:2250–2254, 1994a.

Simeone, A., M. R. D'Apice, V. Nigro, J. Casanova, F. Graziani, D. Acampora, and V. Avantaggiato. Orthopedia, a novel homeobox-containing gene expressed in the developing CNS of both mouse and Drosophila. *Neuron* 13: 83–101, 1994b.

Stern, A. M., J. C. Gall, Jr., B. L. Perry, C. W. Stimson, L. R. Weitkamp, and A. K. Poznanski. The hand-foot-uterus syndrome: a new hereditary disorder characterized by hand and foot dysplasia, dermatoglyphic abnormalities, and partial duplication of the female genital tract. *J. Pediat.* 77: 109–116, 1970.

Stoffers, D. A., N. T. Zinkin, V. Stanojevic, W. L. Clarke, and J. F. Habener. Pancreatic agenesis attributable to a single nucleotide deletion in the human IPF1 gene coding sequence. *Nat. Genet.* 15:106–110, 1997.

Sulik, K. K., C. S. Cook, and W. S. Webster. Teratogens and craniofacial malformations: relationships to cell death. *Development* 103 (suppl.):213–232, 1988.

Takahashi, Y., M. Bontoux, and N. M. Le Douarin. Epithelio-mesenchymal interactions are critical for *Quox 7* expression and membrane bone differentiation in the neural crest derived mandibular mesenchyme. *EMBO J.* 10:2387–2393, 1991.

Vastardis, H., N. Karimbux, S. W. Guthua, J. G. Seidman, and C. E. Seidman. A human *MSX1* homeodomain missense mutation causes selective tooth agenesis. *Nat. Genet.* 13:417–421, 1996.

Vaux, C., L. Sheffield, C. G. Keith, and L. Voullaire. Evidence that Rieger syndrome maps to 4q25 or 4q27. *J. Med. Genet.* 29:256–258, 1992.

Warman, M. L., J. B. Mulliken, P. G. Hayward, and U. M. Muller,. Newly recognized autosomal dominant craniosynostotic syndrome. *Am. J. Med. Genet.* 46:444–449, 1993.

Winograd, J., M. P. Reilly, R. Roe, J. Lutz, E. Laughner, L. Hu, T. Asakura, C. vander Kolk, J. D. Strandberg, and G. L. Semenza. Perinatal lethality and multiple craniofacial malformations in MSX2 transgenic mice. *Hum. Mol. Genet.* 6:369–379, 1997.

Wolberger, C., A. K. Vershon, B. Liu, A. D. Johnson, and C. O. Pabo. Crystal structure of a MATα2 homeodomain-operator complex suggests a general model for homeodomain-DNA interactions. *Cell* 67:517–528, 1991.

Wright, N. M., D. L. Metzger, S. M. Borowitz, and W. L. Clarke. Permanent neonatal diabetes mellitus and pancreatic exocrine insufficiency resulting from congenital pancreatic agenesis. *Am. J. Dis. Child.* 147:607–609, 1993.

Yakovlev, P. I., and R. C. Wadsworth. Schizencephalies: a study of the congenital clefts in the cerebral mantle. I. Clefts with fused lips. *J. Neuropathol. Exp. Neurol.* 5: 116–130, 1946.

Yokouchi, Y., H. Sasaki, and A. Kuroiwa. Homeobox gene expression correlated with the bifurcation process of limb cartilage development. *Nature* 353:443–445, 1991.

Zakany, J., and D. Duboule. Synpolydactyly in mice with a targeted deficiency in the HoxD complex. *Nature* 384:69–71, 1996.

Zeltser, L., C. Desplan, and N. Heintz. Hoxb-13: a new Hox gene in a distant region of the HOXB cluster maintains colinearity. *Development* 122:2475–2484, 1996.

Zhao, G. Q., H. Eberspaecher, M. F. Seldin, and B. de Crombrugghe. The gene for the homeodomain-containing protein Cart-1 is expressed in cells that have a chondrogenic potential during embryonic development. *Mech. Dev.* 48:245–254, 1994.

HMG Domain Proteins   **10**

As described in Chapter 3, transcriptional regulators containing an HMG-type DNA-binding domain appear to function as architectural factors whose primary function is to bend DNA. The HMG domain is an 80-amino-acid motif that was first identified in the High Mobility Group nuclear proteins HMG1 and HMG2 and the RNA Pol I transcription factor UBF (Jantzen et al., 1990), which bind to DNA in a non-sequence-specific manner. The HMG domain has subsequently been shown to define a large superfamily of DNA-binding proteins containing over 100 members from eukaryotic species that include yeast, plants, and animals spanning one billion years of evolutionary time (Grosschedl et al., 1994; Laudet et al., 1993). Phylogenetic analysis identified two large subfamilies consisting of sequence-specific DNA binding proteins containing a single HMG domain and non-sequence-specific DNA-binding proteins containing multiple HMG domains (Laudet et al., 1993). All of the sequence-specific HMG-domain proteins that have been analyzed bind to DNA in the minor groove and recognize the consensus sequence 5'-(A/T)(A/T)CAA(A/T)G-3' (reviewed by Pevny and Lovell-Badge, 1997). In this chapter, SRY and SOX9, two HMG domain–containing proteins that bind to DNA in a sequence-specific manner and are essential for normal testicular determination and differentiation, will be described.

SRY

In mammals, the presence or absence of a Y chromosome determines the nature of sexual development. In the absence or presence of a Y chromosome, the undifferentiated fetal genital ridge (indifferent gonad) develops into an ovary or testis, respectively. Testicular differentiation is characterized by the secretion of müllerian inhibiting substance (MIS)/

anti-müllerian hormone (AMH) by Sertoli cells and the secretion of testosterone by Leydig cells. Secretion of MIS/AMH results in the regression of the müllerian duct, which in females gives rise to the uterus,
fallopian tubes, and upper vagina, whereas testosterone secretion results
in the development of the wolffian duct into vas deferens, seminal ves-
icles, and epididymis, and the masculinization of the external genitalia.
The differentiation of Sertoli cells appears to be a critical step, as these
cells may produce factors that trigger other cells in the indifferent gonad
to undergo testicular differentiation (Lovell-Badge and Hacker, 1995).

A locus on the short arm of the Y chromosome (Yp) was hypothesized to encode a testis-determining factor, based on genetic analysis of
individuals with sex reversal: Yp deletions were identified in XY females
and a Y:22 translocation was identified in an XX male (Page et al., 1987).
The gene encoding the testis determining factor was shown to be *SRY*
(sex-determining region of the Y chromosome), which was identified
within a region of less than 35 kb that was inherited by four XX males
and which encodes an HMG domain protein (Sinclair et al., 1990). The
mouse homologue, *Sry*, was shown to be deleted in a strain of sex-
reversed XY female mice and to be expressed in wild-type male mouse
embryos within somatic cells of the indifferent urogenital ridge between
E10.5 and E12, just prior to morphologic testicular differentiation (Gubbay et al., 1990; Hacker et al., 1995; Jeske et al., 1995; Koopman et al.,
1990). Finally, the introduction into XX mouse embryos of a 14-kb genomic DNA fragment from the Y chromosome that encompassed *Sry*
was sufficient to induce testis differentiation and male development in
the resulting transgenic mice (Koopman et al., 1991). In contrast, a 25-kb
fragment of human DNA encompassing the *SRY* gene did not cause sex
reversal in XX transgenic mice. The human and mouse SRY proteins
differ considerably with respect to amino acid sequence, as there are 23
substitutions in the HMG domain and little sequence conservation elsewhere in the proteins (Whitfield et al., 1993). The proteins also differ
with respect to their functional properties as mouse, but not human, SRY
contains a transactivation domain (Dubin and Ostrer, 1994). Thus, human SRY may be unable to interact with important DNA or protein
targets in mouse genital ridge cells.

Further analysis of patients with sex reversal revealed that 15% to
20% of XY females carried mutations at the *SRY* locus (Berta et al., 1990;
Harley et al., 1992; Hawkins et al., 1992; Jager et al., 1990; McElreavey
et al., 1992; Poulat et al., 1994; Schmitt-Ney et al., 1995). All of the *SRY*
gene defects reported to date are missense, nonsense, or frameshift mutations within the HMG box. Wild-type SRY protein was shown to bind

to the DNA sequences 5'-AACAAAG-3', 5'-AACAAG-3', and 5'-AACAAT-3' in electrophoretic mobility-shift assays and DNA binding of mutant SRY protein was absent or reduced in all five cases tested (Dubin and Ostrer, 1994; Haqq et al., 1994; Harley et al., 1992). Based on the binding properties of the HMG-domain protein LEF-1 (Giese et al., 1992), SRY is believed to contact DNA in the minor groove of the double helix and induce a sharp bend at the site of binding (Ferrari et al., 1992). In the case of the proteins HMG1 and HMG-D, DNA bending is mediated by the presence of three α helices in the HMG domain that assume an L-shaped configuration at an angle of 80° (Jones et al., 1994; Weir et al., 1993). There is no evidence that the human SRY protein contains a transactivation domain, suggesting that it may regulate transcription by altering the architecture of promoter or enhancer elements in such a way as to stabilize the binding of other DNA-binding proteins that contain transactivation domains. Alternatively, SRY may complex with another protein containing a transactivation domain. The HMG domain proteins XTCF-3 and TCF-4 were recently shown to associate with β-catenin to form transcriptional activators in *Xenopus* and human cells, respectively, with TCFs contributing the DNA-binding domain and β-catenin providing the transactivation domain (Korinek et al., 1997; Molenaar et al., 1996).

An isoleucine side chain at HMG domain position 68 of SRY contacts the DNA minor groove and intercalates between specific A:T base pairs, which interrupts base stacking but not base pairing (King and Weiss, 1993; Haqq et al., 1994). Each backbone phosphate on both strands of the binding site DNA was shown to interact with SRY, requiring partial unwinding of the double helix as well as bending and widening of the minor groove (Haqq et al., 1994). An I68T substitution, which was identified in an XY patient with gonadal dysgenesis, was shown to reduce the DNA-binding affinity of SRY by greater than 50-fold and increase the kinetic instability of the DNA-protein complex by more than 40-fold (Haqq et al., 1994).

MIS/AMH is expressed immediately following SRY expression in the indifferent gonad of male embryos and a putative SRY binding site was identified in the *MIS* gene promoter (Haqq et al., 1993). Transcription from the *MIS* promoter was activated by expression of wild-type SRY but not SRY (I68T), but mutation of the putative SRY binding site in the promoter did not eliminate the transcriptional activity mediated by coexpressed SRY (Haqq et al., 1994). These results suggest that SRY regulates *MIS* gene transcription indirectly, perhaps by activating transcription of an intermediate transcription factor. Thus, whereas the importance of SRY in initiating the genetic program of testicular determination and differentiation is well established, the precise molecular mechanisms by which this effect is achieved remain obscure.

SOX9

The indirect effect of SRY on expression of MIS, the observation that less than 20% of XY females contain mutations in the *SRY* gene, the identification of XX males that do not express SRY (Berkovitz et al., 1992; Turner et al., 1995), and the identification of pedigrees in which XY sex reversal demonstrates X-linked or autosomal recessive inheritance (Simpson et al., 1981) all indicate that factors in addition to SRY must play important roles in testicular differentiation. One factor identified thus far appears to share both structural and functional properties with SRY. This protein, SOX9, is encoded by a member of a large family of SRY-type HMG-box (*SOX*) genes (Gubbay et al., 1990; Stevanovic et al., 1993; Wright et al., 1993), which now contains at least 20 members (Meyer et al., 1996). A *SOX* gene is defined as encoding a protein that contains an HMG domain with at least 50% identity to the SRY HMG domain (Goodfellow and Lovell-Badge, 1993; Pevny and Lovell-Badge, 1997).

As in the case of *SRY*, the identification of patients with chromosomal rearrangements provided the initial mapping of an autosomal locus for XY sex reversal to chromosome 17q24.3-q25.1 (Tommerup et al., 1993; Young et al., 1992). The patients were all affected by a rare skeletal malformation syndrome, campomelic dysplasia, which has an incidence of approximately 1 per 100,000 newborns and in which three quarters of 46,XY individuals have abnormalities of genital development ranging from ambiguous genitalia to normal female genitalia (Kwok et al., 1995; Mansour et al., 1995). The term campomelia (or camptomelia) refers to the congenital bowing of long bones, especially the femur and tibia, that is characteristic of this disorder (Maroteaux et al., 1971; Hall and Spranger, 1980) (Fig. 10.1). In addition, the pelvis, ribs, vertebrae, scapulae, palate, and mandible are dysplastic or hypoplastic and there are generalized defects in cartilage formation (Mansour et al., 1995). Nonskeletal malformations in addition to XY sex reversal include aplasia of the olfactory bulbs/tracts, cerebral ventricular dilatation, and an increased incidence of cardiac and renal defects. The disease often results in neonatal lethality due to respiratory insufficiency.

The assignment of the *Sox9* gene to a region of mouse chromosome 11 with conserved synteny to the distal region of human chromosome 17q (Wright et al., 1993) and the demonstration that *Sox9* was expressed

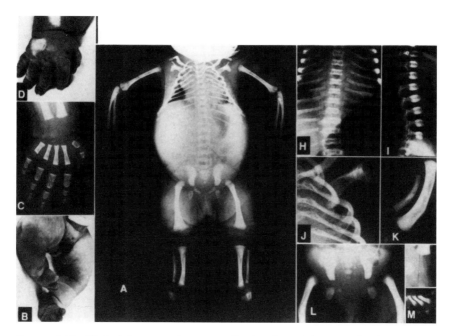

FIGURE 10-1. Clinical features of campomelic dysplasia. Photographs demonstrate bowing of the legs with equinovarus deformity (B) and shortening of the fingers (D). Radiographs demonstrate: bowing of the long bones (A) including tibiae (K) and femurs (L); shortened phalanges with widened distal tips (C); non-mineralized thoracic pedicles (H) but normal lower thoracic and lumbar spine (I); and hypoplastic scapula (J). (Reprinted with permission from Hall and Spranger, 1980. Copyright ©1980 by the American Medical Association.)

during chondrogenesis in mouse embryos (Wright et al., 1995) implicated human *SOX9* as a candidate gene for campomelic dysplasia and XY sex reversal. Isolation of human SOX9 sequences from a testis cDNA library revealed an open reading frame encoding a polypeptide of 509 amino acids, including an HMG domain with 71% similarity to SRY (Foster et al., 1994). Mutations in one *SOX9* allele were identified in patients with campomelic dysplasia without translocation (Foster et al., 1994; Kwok et al., 1995; Meyer et al., 1997; Wagner et al., 1994). These mutations included missense substitutions within the HMG box as well as frameshift, nonsense, and splice site mutations throughout the gene that were predicted to inactivate the protein product of the mutant allele (Fig. 10.2). Whereas the *SRY* mutations identified in XY females all result in loss of HMG-domain DNA-binding activity, nonsense mutations (e.g., Y440X)

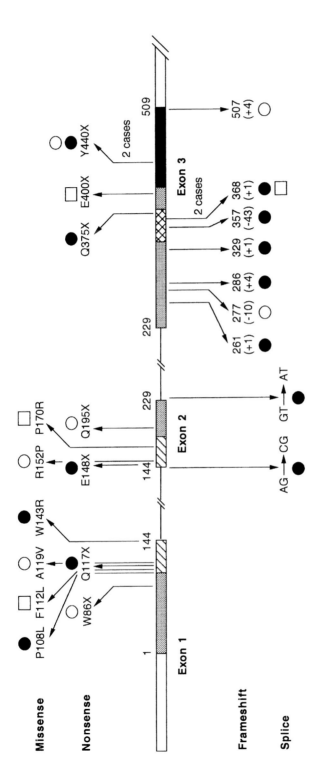

FIGURE 10-2. Mutations in *SOX9* responsible for campomelic dysplasia and XY sex reversal. Exons of the *SOX9* gene are indicated by boxes with untranslated and translated sequences shown as open and stippled boxes, respectively, except for the HMG domain (striped), proline-glutamine-alanine domain (cross-hatched), and transactivation domain (solid). Missense, nonsense, frameshift, and splice site mutations are shown from top to bottom, respectively, as indicated at left. Open and closed circles represent mutations detected in XX and XY females, respectively, whereas open squares represent mutations identified in XY males. (Reprinted with permission of Oxford University Press from Meyer et al., 1997.)

that only truncate the carboxyl-terminal transactivation domain of SOX9 (described below) have been identified (Meyer et al., 1997; Sudbeck et al., 1996).

No mutations within the *SOX9* gene were found in patients with translocations, suggesting that the rearrangement resulted in a transcriptional silencing of the *SOX9* gene in *cis*, as proposed for translocations near the *GLI3* and *PAX6* genes associated with Greig syndrome (see Chapter 6) and aniridia (see Chapter 7), respectively. As in these other malformation syndromes, the translocations associated with campomelic dysplasia occur quite far (50 kb or more) from the gene (Wagner et al., 1994). Several patients with campomelic dysplasia due to translocation have survived early childhood (Foster et al., 1994), suggesting that there may be residual expression from the affected allele, resulting in a milder phenotype. Taken together, these data suggest that campomelic dysplasia and sex reversal are due to haploinsufficiency for SOX9. Two 46,XY campomelic patients were identified with the same frameshift mutation, only one of whom was sex-reversed (Kwok et al., 1995), indicating that the lack of complete penetrance for sex reversal is probably not a function of the nature of the mutation but may be due to differences at other genetic loci or a reflection of stochastic processes.

The expression pattern of *Sox9* during mouse development provided further evidence for its key role in chondrogenesis and gonadogenesis. *Sox9* expression, first detected between E9 and E10, precedes the deposition of cartilage throughout the axial and appendicular skeleton and expression is no longer detected after deposition of cartilage is completed, suggesting that SOX9 may be responsible for the determination and differentiation of chondroblasts (Wright et al., 1995). In male embryos, *Sry* is expressed only from E10.5 to E12 within somatic cells of the genital ridge (Jeske et al., 1995; Hacker et al., 1995; Koopman et al., 1991) and is presumed to be responsible for the determination of Sertoli cell identity. However, because *Sry* is expressed only briefly, the maintenance of Sertoli cell differentiation must be due to the expression of downstream genes. *Sox9* is expressed in the genital ridge of both XY and XX mouse embryos prior to *Sry*, its expression becomes restricted to the genital ridges of XY embryos only at the time of *Sry* expression, and *Sox9* continues to be expressed in developing testes long after *Sry* expression is extinguished (Morais da Silva et al., 1996). These changes in *Sry* and *Sox9* expression represent the earliest differences in gene expression between male and female embryos. *Sox9* expression precedes the onset of *Mis/Amh* gene expression; thus, it is possible that SOX9, rather than SRY, may directly activate transcription of this gene (Morais da Silva et al., 1996).

TABLE 10.1. Comparison of amino acid
sequences in human and mouse

Protein	Percent Identity
SRY	27
SRY (HMG domain only)	71
DAX1	66
SOX9	96

In contrast to SRY, the amino acid sequence of SOX9 is highly conserved (Table 10.1) and contains a proline- and glutamine-rich transactivation domain, the loss of which is associated with XY sex reversal
(Foster et al., 1994; Meyer et al., 1997; Sudbeck et al., 1996; Wagner et
al., 1994; Wright et al., 1995). Notably, the transactivation domain is as
highly conserved (>90% identity) as the HMG domain. SOX9 may functionally interact with SRY in pre–Sertoli cells of the genital ridge, or
alternately, SOX9 may be expressed in cells that interact with SRY-
expressing pre-Sertoli cells to form a testis (Foster et al., 1994). The latter
hypothesis is appealing because mesenchymal cells migrating from the
mesonephros to the genital ridge are required for testis formation and
mesenchymal cells also give rise to chondroblasts and osteoblasts. Thus,
decreased SOX9 expression in mesenchymal cells might provide a uni-
fying etiology for campomelic dysplasia and sex reversal. SOX9 is coexpressed with type II collagen during chondrogenesis and activates transcription via an enhancer element from the gene encoding pro-αI(II)
collagen (Lefebre et al., 1997; Ng et al., 1997), providing evidence that
SOX9 controls both cell-type determination and the expression of gene
products specific to the differentiated state, a characteristic feature of
other master regulatory factors such as IPF1 (Chapter 9) and PIT1 (Chapter 11).

In addition to haploinsufficiency for SOX9 and loss of SRY function,
XY sex reversal has also been associated with duplication of a chromo-

TABLE 10.2. Mechanisms of sex reversal

Gene	Alteration	Effect on Sex Determination
SRY	Inactivating mutation	XY female
SRY	Translocation	XX male
SOX9	Inactivating mutation	XY female
DAX1	Duplication	XY female

some Xp21 locus termed *DSS* (dosage-sensitive sex reversal), which may be identical to *DAX1* (Bardoni et al., 1994; Swain et al., 1996; Zanaria et al., 1994), as described in Chapter 5 (Table 10.2). The downregulation of *Sox9* in the genital ridge of XX embryos may be due to transcriptional repression by DAX1, which is overcome in XY embryos by SRY unless DAX1 is present in excess due to gene duplication (Morais da Silva et al., 1996; Swain et al., 1998). Thus, when DAX1 expression predominates over SRY expression (in wild-type XX gonads), *Sox9* transcription is re-

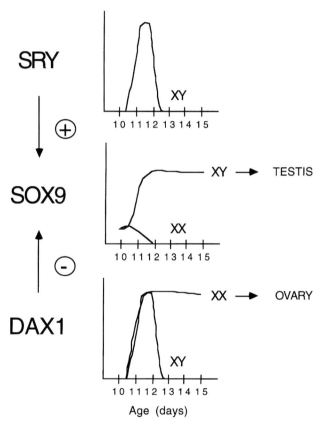

FIGURE 10-3. Proposed roles of SRY, SOX9, and DAX1 in mammalian sex determination. The relative levels of *Sry*, *Sox9*, and *Dax1* gene expression between days 10.5 and 15 of embryonic development in XX and XY mice are schematically illustrated. In this model, the predominance of SRY in XY gonads results in activation of *Sox9* transcription and testicular development, whereas the predominance of DAX1 in XX gonads results in repression of *Sox9* transcription and ovarian development. (Based on data from Morais da Silva et al., 1996; Swain et al., 1998.)

pressed and ovaries form; when SRY expression predominates over DAX1 expression (in wild-type XY gonads), *Sox9* transcription is activated and testes form (Fig. 10.3).

Sox9 is also expressed in developing chick cartilage and primordial testes, which is remarkable given the fact that, in contrast to mammals, birds utilize a ZZ (male)/ZW (female) system of sex determination and appear to lack SRY (Kent et al., 1996; Morais da Silva et al., 1996). Chicken SOX9 is 92% identical to human SOX9 over the amino-terminal half of the molecule containing the HMG domain and 96% identical in the carboxyl-terminal transactivation domain (Sudbeck et al., 1996). The appearance of SRY during mammalian evolution may have allowed the new XX/XY system of sex determination to utilize previously existing genetic pathways controlling testicular development that included SOX9. Further investigation of the avian and mammalian systems of testicular development are likely to provide even more fascinating insights into fundamental developmental and evolutionary processes. Analysis of 18 females with XY sex reversal without skeletal abnormalities (Swyer syndrome) revealed no evidence of mutations in *SOX9* (Meyer et al., 1997). Studies that determine the molecular basis for XY sex reversal in patients with deletions involving chromosomes 9p (Bennett et al., 1993) and 10q (Wilkie et al., 1993) may identify additional genes required for testicular development.

References

Bardoni, B., E. Zanaria, S. Guioli, G. Floridia, K. C. Worley, and G. Tonini. A dosage sensitive locus at chromosome Xp21 is involved in male to female sex reversal. *Nat. Genet.* 7:497–501, 1994.

Bennett, C. P., Z. Docherty, S. A. Robb, P. Ramani, J. R. Hawkins, D. Grant. Deletion 9p and sex reversal. *J. Med. Genet.* 30:518–520, 1993.

Berkovitz, G. D., P. Y. Fechner, S. M. Marcantonio, G. Bland, and G. Stetten. The role of the sex-determining region of the Y chromosome (SRY) in the etiology of 46, XX true hermaphroditism. *Hum. Genet.* 88:411–416, 1992.

Berta, P., J. R. Hawkins, A. H. Sinclair, A. Taylor, B. L. Griffiths, P. N. Goodfellow, and M. Fellous. Genetic evidence equating SRY and the testis-determining factor. *Nature* 348:448–450, 1990.

Dubin, R. A., and H. Ostrer. Sry is a transcriptional activator. *Mol. Endocrinol.* 8: 1182–1192, 1994.

Ferrari, S., V. R. Harley, A. Pontiggia, P. N. Goodfellow, R. Lovell-Badge, and M. E. Bianchi. SRY, like HMG 1, recognizes sharp angles in DNA. *EMBO J.* 11:4497–4506, 1992.

Foster, J. W., M. A. Dominguez-Steglich, S. Guioli, C. Kowk, P. A. Weller, M. Stevanovic, J. Weissenbach, S. Mansour, I. D. Young, P. N. Goodfellow, J. D. Brook, and A. Schafer. Campomelic dysplasia and autosomal sex reversal caused by mutations in an SRY-related gene. *Nature* 372:525–530, 1994.

Giese, K., J. Cox, and R Grosschedl. The HMG domain of lymphoid enhancer factor 1 bends DNA and facilitates assembly of functional nucleoprotein structures. *Cell* 69:185–195, 1992.

Goodfellow, P. N., and R. Lovell-Badge. SRY and sex determination in mammals. *Annu. Rev. Genet.* 27:71–92, 1993.

Grosschedl, R., K. Giese, and J. Pagel. HMG domain proteins: architectural elements in the assembly of nucleoprotein structures. *Trends Genet.* 10:94–100, 1994.

Gubbay, J., J. Collignon, P. Koopman, B. Capel, A. Economou, A. Munsterberg, N. Vivian, P. Goodfellow, and R. Lovell-Badge. A gene mapping to the sex-determining region of the mouse Y chromosome is a member of a novel family of embryonically expressed genes. *Nature* 346:245–250, 1990.

Hacker, A., B. Capel, P. N. Goodfellow, and R. Lovell-Badge. Expression of Sry, the mouse sex determining gene. *Development* 121:1603–1614, 1995.

Hall, B. D., and J. W. Spranger. Campomelic dysplasia: further elucidation of a distinct entity. *Am. J. Dis. Child.* 134:285–289, 1980.

Haqq, C. M., C. Y. King, P. K. Donahoe, and M. A. Weiss. SRY recognizes conserved DNA sites in sex-specific promoters. *Proc. Natl. Acad. Sci. U.S.A.* 90: 1097–1101, 1993.

Haqq, C. M., C.-Y. King, E. Ukiyama, S. Falsafi, T. N. Haqq, P. K. Donahoe, and M. A. Weiss. Molecular basis of mammalian sexual determination: activation of Mullerian inhibiting substance gene expression by SRY. *Science* 266:1494–1500, 1994.

Harley, V. R., D. I. Jackson, P. J. Hextall, J. R. Hawkins, G. D. Berkovitz, S. Sockanathan, R. Lovell-Badge, and P. N. Goodfellow. DNA-binding activity of recombinant SRY from normal males and XY females. *Science* 255:453–456, 1992.

Hawkins, J. R., A. Taylor, P. Berta, J. Levilliers, B. Van der Auwera, and P. N. Goodfellow. Mutational analysis of SRY: nonsense and missense mutations in XY sex reversal. *Hum. Genet.* 88:471–474, 1992.

Jager, R. J., M. Anvret, K. Hall, and G. Scherer. A human XY female with a frame shift mutation in the candidate testis-determining gene. *Nature* 348:452–454, 1990.

Jantzen, H.-M., A. Admon, S. P. Bell, and R. Tjian. Nucleolar transcription factor hUBF contains a DNA-binding motif with homology to HMG proteins. *Nature* 344:830–836, 1990.

Jeske, Y. W., J. Bowles, A. Greenfield, and P. Koopman. Expression of a linear Sry transcript in the mouse genital ridge. *Nat. Genet.* 10:480–482, 1995.

Jones, D. N., M. A. Searles, G. L. Shaw, M. E. Churchill, S. S. Ner, J. Keeler, A. A. Travers, and D. Neuhaus. The solution structure and dynamics of the DNA-binding domain of HMG-D from Drosophila melanogaster. *Structure* 2:609–627, 1994.

Kent, J., S. C. Theatley, J. E. Andrews, A. H. Sinclair, and P. Koopman. A male specific role for SOX9 in vertebrate sex determination. *Development* 122:2813–2822, 1996.

King, C. Y., and M. A. Weiss. The SRY high-mobility-group box recognizes DNA by partial intercalation in the minor groove: a topological mechanism of sequence specificity. *Proc. Natl. Acad. Sci. U.S.A.* 90:11990–11994, 1993.

Koopman, P., J. Gubbay, N. Vivian, P. Goodfellow, and R. Lovell-Badge. Male development of chromosomally female mice transgenic for Sry. *Nature* 351: 117–121, 1991.

Koopman, P., A. Munsterberg, B. Capel, N. Vivian, and R. Lovell-Badge. Expression of a candidate sex-determining gene during mouse testis differentiation. *Nature* 348:450–452, 1990.

Korinek, V., N. Barker, P. J. Morin, D. van Wichen, R. de Weger, K. W. Kinzler, B. Vogelstein, and H. Clevers. Constitutive transcriptional activation by a β-catenin-TCF complex in APC$^{-/-}$ colon carcinoma. *Science* 275:1784–1792, 1997.

Kwok, C., P. A. Weller, S. Guioli, J. W. Foster, S. Mansour, O. Zuffardi, H. H. Punnett, M. A. Dominguez-Steglich, J. D. Brook, I. D. Young, P. N. Goodfellow, and A. J. Schafer. Mutations in SOX9, the gene responsible for campomelic dysplasia and autosomal sex reversal. *Am. J. Hum. Genet.* 57:1028–1036, 1995.

Laudet, V., D. Stehelin, and H. Clevers. Ancestry and diversity of HMG box superfamily. *Nucleic Acids Res.* 21:2493–2501, 1993.

Lefebvre, V., W. D. Huang, V. R. Harley, P. N. Goodfellow, and B. De-Crombrugghe. SOX9 is a potent activator of the chondrocyte-specific enhancer of the pro-α1(II) collagen gene. *Mol. Cell. Biol.* 17:2336–2346, 1997.

Lovell-Badge, R., and A. Hacker. The molecular genetics of Sry and its role in mammalian sex determination. *Phil. Trans. R. Soc. Lond. B., Bio Sci.* 305:205–214, 1995.

Mansour, S., C. M. Hall, M. E. Pembrey, and I. D. Young. A clinical and genetic study of campomelic dysplasia. *J. Med. Genet.* 32:415–420, 1995.

Maroteaux, P., J. W. Spranger, J. M. Opitz, J. Kucera, R. B. Lowry, R. N. Schimke, and S. M. Kagan. Le syndrome campomelique. *Presse Med.* 22:1157–1162, 1971.

McElreavey, K. D., E. Vilain, C. Boucekkine, M. Vidaud, F. Jaubert, F. Richaud, and M. Fellous. XY sex reversal associated with a nonsense mutation in SRY. *Genomics* 13:838–840, 1992.

Meyer, J., P. Sudbeck, M. Held, T. Wagner, M. L. Schmitz, F. D. Bricarelli, E. Eggermont, U. Friedrich, O. A. Haas, A. Koblet, J. G. Leroy, L. Van Maldergem, E. Michel., B. Mitulla, R. A. Pfeiffer, A. Schinzel, H. Schmidt, and G. Scherer. Mutational analysis of the SOX9 gene in campomelic dysplasia and autosomal sex reversal: lack of genotype/phenotype correlations. *Hum. Mol. Genet.* 6:91–98, 1997.

Meyer, J., J. Wirth, M. Held, W. Schempp, and G. Scherer. SOX20, a new member of the SOX gene family, is located on chromosome 17p13. *Cytogenet. Cell Genet.* 72: 246–249, 1996.

Molenaar, M., M. van de Wetering, M. Oosterwegel, J. Peterson-Maduro, S. Godsave, V. Korinek, J. Roose, O. Destree, and H. Clevers. XTcf-3 transcription factor mediates β-catenin-induced axis formation in Xenopus embryos. *Cell* 86:391–399, 1996.

Morais da Silva, S., A. Hacker, V. Harley, P. Goodfellow, A. Swain, and R. Lovell-Badge. Sox9 expression during gonadal development implies a conserved role for the gene in testis differentiation in mammals and birds. *Nat. Genet.* 14:62–68, 1996.

Ng, L. J., S. Wheatley, G. E. O. Muscat, J. Conway-Campbell, J. Bowles, E. Wright,

D. M. Bell, P. L. P. Tam, K. S. E. Cheah, and P. Koopman. SOX9 binds DNA, activates transcription, and coexpresses with type II collagen during chondrogenesis in the mouse. *Dev. Biol.* 183:108–121, 1997.

Page, D. C., R. Mosher, E. M. Simpson, E. M. C. Fisher, G. Mardon, J. Pollack, B. McGillivray, A. de la Chapelle, and L. G. Brown. The sex-determining region of the human Y chromosome encodes a finger protein. *Cell* 51:1091–1104, 1987.

Pevny, L. H., and R. Lovell-Badge. Sox genes find their feet. *Curr. Opin. Genet. Dev.* 7:338–344, 1997.

Poulat, F., S. Soullier, C. Goze, F. Heitz, B. Calas, and P. Berta. Description and functional implications of a novel mutation in the sex-determining gene SRY. *Hum. Mutat.* 3:200–204, 1994.

Schmitt-Ney, M., H. Thiele, P. Kaltwasser, B. Bardoni, M. Cisternino, and G. Scherer. Two novel SRY missense mutations reducing DNA binding identified in XY females and their mosaic fathers. *Am. J. Hum. Genet.* 56:862–869, 1995.

Simpson, J. L., N. Blagowidow, and A. O. Martin. XY gonadal dysgenesis: genetic heterogeneity based on clinical observations, H-Y antigen status and segregation analysis. *Hum. Genet.* 58:91–97, 1981.

Sinclair, A. H., P. Berta, M. S. Palmer, J. R. Hawkins, B. L. Griffiths, M. J. Smith, J. W. Foster, A.-M. Frischauf, R. Lovell-Badge, and P. N. Goodfellow. A gene from the human sex-determining region encodes a protein with homology to a conserved DNA-binding motif. *Nature* 346:240–244, 1990.

Stevanovic, M., R. Lovell-Badge, J. Collignon, and P. N. Goodfellow. SOX3 is an X-linked gene related to SRY. *Hum. Mol. Genet.* 2:2013–2018, 1993.

Sudbeck, P., M. L. Schmitz, P. A. Baeuerle, and G. Scherer. Sex reversal by loss of the C-terminal transactivation domain of human SOX9. *Nat. Genet.* 13:230–232, 1996.

Swain, A., V. Narvaez, P. Burgoyne, G. Camerino, and R. Lovell-Badge. Dax1 antagonizes Sry action in mammalian sex determination. *Nature* 391:761–767, 1998.

Swain, A., E. Zanaria, A. Hacker, R. Lovell-Badge, and G. Camerino. Mouse Dax1 expression is consistent with a role in sex determination as well as in adrenal and hypothalamus function. *Nat. Genet.* 12:404–409, 1996.

Tommerup, N., W. Schempp, P. Meinecke, S. Pedersen, L. Bolund. C. Brandt, C. Goodpasture, P. Guldberg, K. R. Held, H. Reinwein, O. D. Saugstad, G Scherer, O. Skjeldal, R. Toder, J. Westvik, C. B. van der Hagen, and U. Wolf. Assignment of an autosomal sex reversal locus (SRA1) and campomelic dysplasia (CMPD1) to 17q24.3-q25.1. *Nat. Genet.* 4:170–174, 1993.

Turner, B., P. Y. Fechner, J. S. Fuqua, S. M. Marcantonio, E. J. Perlman, J. S. Vordermark, and G. D. Berkovitz. Combined Leydig cell and Sertoli cell dysfunction in 46,XX males lacking the sex determining region Y gene. *Am. J. Med. Genet.* 57:440–443, 1995.

Wagner, T., J. Wirth, J. Meyer, B. Zabel, M. Held, J. Zimmer, J. Pasantes, F. D. Bricarelli, J. Keutel, E. Hustert, U. Wolf, N. Tommerup, W. Schempp, and G. Scherer. Autosomal sex reversal and campomelic dysplasia are caused by mutations in and around the SRY-related gene SOX9. *Cell* 79:1111–1120, 1994.

Weir, H. M., P. J. Kraulis, C. S. Hill, A. R. Raine, E. D. Laue, and J. O. Thomas.

Structure of the HMG box motif in the B-domain of HMG1. *EMBO J.* 12: 1311–1319, 1993.

Whitfield, S., R. Lovell-Badge, and P. N. Goodfellow. Rapid sequence evolution of the sex determining gene SRY. *Nature* 364:713–715, 1993.

Wilkie, A. O., F. M. Campbell, P. Daubeney, D. B. Grant, R. J. Daniels, M. Mullarkey, N. A. Affara, M. Fitchett, and S. M. Huson. Complete and partial XY sex reversal associated with terminal deletion of 10q: report of 2 cases and literature review. *Am. J. Med. Genet.* 46:597–600, 1993.

Wright, E., M. R. Hargrave, J. Christiansen, L. Cooper, J. Kun, T. Evans, U. Gangadharan, A. Greenfield, and P. Koopman. The Sry-related gene Sox9 is expressed during chondrogenesis in mouse embryos. *Nat. Genet.* 9:15–20, 1995.

Wright, E. M., B. Snopek, and P. Koopman. Seven new members of the Sox gene family expressed during mouse development. *Nucleic Acids Res.* 21:744, 1993.

Young, I. D., J. M. Zuccollo, E. L. Maltby, and N. J. Broderick. Campomelic dysplasia associated with a de novo 2q;17q reciprocal translocation. *J. Med. Genet.* 29:251–252, 1992.

Zanaria, E., F. Muscatelli, B. Bardoni, T. M. Strom, S. Guioli, W. Guo, E. Lalli, C. Moser, A. P. Walker, E. R. B. McCabe, T. Meitinger, A. P. Monaco, P. Sassone-Corsi, and G. Camerino. An unusual member of the nuclear hormone receptor superfamily responsible for X-linked adrenal hypoplasia congenita. *Nature* 372:635–641, 1994.

POU Domain Proteins   **11**

Homeodomain transcription factors play essential roles in controlling embryonic development in all animal species studied. Within the super-family of homeodomain factors is the POU domain family, which was established on the basis of amino acid sequence homology between the transcription factors PIT1/GHF1, OCT1, OCT2, and UNC86 (hence the acronym POU, which is pronounced "pow") (Herr et al., 1988). PIT1/GHF (Bodner et al., 1988; Ingraham et al., 1988) controls transcription of the growth hormone and other pituitary-specific genes, OCT1 (Sturm et al., 1988) is ubiquitously expressed and activates transcription of histone H2B genes, OCT2 (Clerc et al., 1988; Ko et al., 1988) activates transcription of immunoglobulin genes in B lymphocytes, and UNC86 (Finney et al., 1988) determines neuroblast fate in *C. elegans*. Subsequently, over two dozen POU domain–containing proteins have been identified in *C. elegans, Drosophila*, and mammals (Verrijzer and Van der Vliet, 1993). A new system of genetic nomenclature has been devised so that the PIT1/GHF1, OCT1, OCT2, and BRN4/OCT9 proteins are encoded by *POU1F1, POU2F1, POU2F2,* and *POU3F4*, respectively (reviewed by Ezzell, 1996).

The defining characteristic of POU proteins is a bipartite DNA-binding domain of 150 to 160 amino acids that consists of a 60-amino-acid POU homeodomain (POU_{HD}) located just carboxyl-terminal to a POU-specific domain (POU_S) of 70 to 80 amino acids (Fig. 11.1). As described in Chapter 9, the homeodomain contains three α-helical regions so that helices 2 and 3 form a helix-turn-helix motif that is structurally similar to the DNA-binding domain of prokaryotic repressors, in which helix 3 contacts DNA in the major groove (Harrison and Aggarwal, 1990). The POU_S domain contains four α-helical regions so that helices 2 and 3 form a helix-turn-helix motif that is similar in its structure to the phage λ repressor DNA-binding domain (Assa-Munt et al., 1993).

POU_S

^{1}
EEPS DLEELEQFAKTFKQRRIKLGFTQGDVGLAMGKLYGNDFSQTTISRFEALNLSFKNMCKLKPLLEKWLNDAE ^{75}

LINKER

^{76}
NLSSDSSLSSPSALNSPGIEGLSR ^{99}

POU_{HD}

^{100}
RRKKRTSIETNIRVALEKSFLENQKPTSEEITMIADQLNMEKEVIRVWFCNRRQKEKRIN ^{159}

FIGURE 11-1. Structure of the POU domain. The amino acid sequences of the POU-specific domain (POU_S), linker, and POU-specific homeodomain (POU_{HD}) that constitute the OCT1 POU domain are shown with α-helical regions underscored. (Data from Klemm et al., 1994.)

As in the case of POU_{HD}, POU_S contacts DNA in the major groove via helix 3. The crystal structure of the POU domain of OCT1 bound to its octamer recognition sequence 5'-ATGCAAAT-3' revealed that POU_{HD} and POU_S represent structurally independent domains tethered by a flexible linker so that POU_S contacts the ATGC residues and POU_{HD} contacts the AAAT sequence in adjacent major grooves, and thus on opposite sides, of the double helix (Klemm et al., 1994). Despite the fact that the POU_{HD} domain is structurally similar to other homeodomains, it is not sufficient to mediate high-affinity sequence-specific DNA binding in the absence of the POU_S domain (Sturm and Herr, 1988) for reasons that are apparent from the crystallography results described above.

Thus far, two POU proteins have been linked to clinical disorders. Mutations in *POU1F1*, encoding PIT1/GHF1, and *POU3F4*, encoding BRN4/OCT9, have been identified as causes of hypopituitarism and deafness, respectively.

POU1F1/PIT1 and Hypopituitary Dwarfism

Pituitary Development, Dwarf Mice, and PIT1

Invagination of somatic ectoderm adjacent to the anterior neuropore on embryonic day 8.5 (E8.5) in the mouse ultimately results in the formation of Rathke's pouch, the primordium of the anterior pituitary. Organ commitment is first evident by the expression of αGSU, the common subunit of follicle-stimulating hormone (FSH), luteinizing hormone (LH), and thyroid stimulating hormone (TSH), in somatic ectoderm at E11 prior to formation of Rathke's pouch (Simmons et al., 1990). During subsequent organ development, five different anterior-pituitary cell types that are each characterized by the expression of a unique trophic hormone appear. Gonadotropes produce FSH and LH; corticotropes produce adrenocorticotropic hormone (ACTH); thyrotropes produce TSH; somatotropes produce growth hormone (GH); and lactotropes produce prolactin (PRL). A major step in cellular differentiation is the establishment, between E12 and E15, of two cell lineages, one that expresses PIT1 and gives rise to the somatotropes, thyrotropes, and lactotropes and another that does not express PIT1 and gives rise to the corticotropes and gonadotropes (Andersen and Rosenfeld, 1994).

Transient transfection analyses demonstrated that PIT1 activates transcription of the genes encoding GH, PRL, and TSHβ (Ingraham et al., 1988; Mangalam et al., 1989; Steinfelder et al., 1991) by recognizing binding sites with a consensus sequence of 5'-WTWATWCAT-3' (W = A or T) in which the 5' and 3' half-sites are recognized by the POU_{HD} and

POU$_S$ domains, respectively (Andersen and Rosenfeld, 1994). The temporospatial pattern of PIT1 expression in the developing pituitary correlated with the sites of target gene expression (Dolle et al., 1990; Simmons et al., 1990). In addition, the 5'-flanking region of the *PIT1* gene itself contains multiple PIT1 binding sites and *PIT1* transcription is activated by PIT1, suggesting an autoregulatory loop that assures continued *PIT1* expression (Chen et al., 1990; McCormick et al., 1990).

The essential role of PIT1 in the expression of GH, PRL, and TSHβ was demonstrated by the finding that the autosomal recessive Snell (*dw*) and Jackson (*dw^J*) dwarf mouse phenotypes were the result of homozygosity for mutations at the mouse *Pit1* locus (Li et al., 1990). The *dw^J* allele was due to deletion of *Pit1* sequences, whereas *dw* was due to a missense mutation (W261C) within the POU$_{HD}$ domain that disrupted DNA binding. These dwarf mice not only were deficient in GH and PRL production but also exhibited anterior pituitary hypoplasia, indicating that PIT1 was required for the proliferation and differentiation of the somatolactotrope lineage. When cell lines derived from pituitary tumors were treated with antisense oligonucleotides to inhibit PIT1 synthesis, marked decreases in GH and PRL expression and in cellular proliferation were observed (Castrillo et al., 1991).

PIT1 may affect cellular proliferation by several mechanisms. For example, binding of GH-releasing factor (GRF) to its receptor on somatotropes is essential for their proliferation, as evidenced by the demonstration that *little* mice, which are dwarfed due to a mutation in the GRF receptor, have 10-fold fewer somatotropes than wild-type mice (Godfrey et al., 1993; Lin et al., 1993). The GRF receptor is not expressed in Snell mice, suggesting that pituitary hypoplasia in these mice is caused, at least in part, by the absence of GRF receptor associated with PIT1 deficiency (Lin et al., 1992). Other growth factors would have to be similarly affected in thyrotropes and lactotropes to account for the hypoplasia of these cell types. PIT1 may also affect cellular proliferation at the level of DNA synthesis, as PIT1 (and other POU domain proteins) was shown to stimulate adenoviral DNA replication in vitro (Verrijzer et al., 1992).

The Ames dwarf (*df*) is a mouse mutant with a phenotype similar to that of the Jackson and Snell mutants, with anterior pituitary hypoplasia, but the mutation was linked to chromosome 11 rather than to the *Pit1* locus on chromosome 16 (Buckwalter et al., 1991). The *df* locus was shown to encode a (non-POU) homeodomain protein, which was designated PROP1 (<u>Pro</u>phet of <u>Pit</u>-1), and the mutation was a Ser-to-Pro substitution with helix 1 of the homeodomain, which is predicted to disrupt α helix formation and DNA binding (Sornson et al., 1996). In *df/df* mice, the initial determination of the PIT1-expressing cell lineage does not occur, resulting in absence of PIT1 expression and subsequent failure of somatotrope, thyrotrope, and lactotrope development, whereas the proliferation of corticotropes and gonadotropes is unaffected. Early *Pit1* gene expression, which is independent of the autoregulatory loop and which occurs normally in *dw/dw* mice, does not occur in *df/df* mice, suggesting that PROP1 may be responsible for the initial activation of *Pit1* transcription in pituitary progenitor cells. This mechanism is supported by the observation that *Prop1* expression declines coincident with the establishment of the *Pit1* autoregulatory loop (Sornson et al., 1996). In addition to PROP1, other homeodomain transcription factors are expressed in the developing anterior pituitary, including P-LIM, P-OTX, and RPX, and heterodimerization of RPX with PROP1 inhibits PROP1-dependent transcriptional activation, suggesting that combinatorial interactions of homeodomain factors may underlie pituitary differentiation (Sornson et al., 1996). The analysis of mouse mutants has thus facilitated the first steps in the delineation of the genetic regulatory cascade controlling anterior pituitary development.

Analysis of Patients with Combined Pituitary Hormone Deficiency

PIT1 mutations in human hypopituitary dwarfism have also been demonstrated (Pfaffle et al., 1992; Radovick et al, 1992; Tatsumi et al., 1992) (Fig. 11.2). The nonsense mutation R172X results in a truncated protein that cannot bind to DNA because it lacks the homeodomain (Tatsumi et al., 1992). This mutation was inherited from both parents, who were first cousins, resulting in homozygosity and complete PIT1 deficiency. In contrast, the missense mutation R271W within the homeodomain results in a mutant protein that can bind to DNA but cannot activate transcription, suggesting that in addition to its DNA-binding activity, the POU_{HD} domain may also be involved in protein-protein interactions (Radovick et al., 1992). The arginine residue that is substituted is conserved in all known POU_{HD} domains from humans to worms (Radovick et al., 1992; Verrijzer and van der Vliet, 1993). The R271W mutation occurred *de novo* in the affected individual and no other mutation could be detected, suggesting that this represented a dominant allele. Transfection experiments indicated that the mutant protein had a dominant-negative effect on the ability of the wild-type protein to activate transcription (Radovick et al., 1992). Homozygosity for an A158P missense mutation was demonstrated in two affected siblings (Pfaffle et al., 1992). The mutation introduces a proline residue into the first α-helical region of the POU_S domain. As in the case of the R271W mutation in the POU_{HD} domain, the A158P mutation in the POU_S domain did not affect DNA binding in vitro but pre-

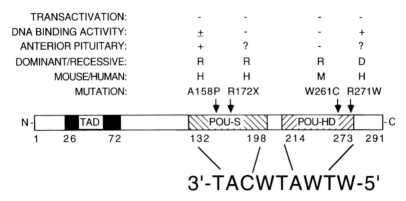

FIGURE 11-2. PIT1 mutations that cause combined pituitary hormone deficiency in humans and mice. The consensus binding site for PIT1 is shown at bottom (W = A or T) in reverse orientation in order to align sequences that are recognized by the POU$_S$ and POU$_{HD}$ domains. A transactivation domain (TAD) is present in the N-terminal region of the protein. In addition to the four point mutations shown, the autosomal recessive Jackson dwarf mutation (not shown) is due to deletion of *Pit1*.

vented transcriptional activation of target genes. Radiologic imaging of individuals homozygous for the A158P mutation suggested normal pituitary development. The A158P mutation therefore eliminated the ability of PIT1 to activate *GH* and *PRL* transcription without affecting its ability to direct the program of anterior pituitary cell proliferation and differentiation, suggesting that these functions reside in different domains of the PIT1 protein.

POU3F4/BRN4 and X-linked Deafness Type 3 (DFN3)

Hereditary congenital deafness is a common birth defect with an incidence of approximately 1 in 1000 live births (Morton, 1991). In 70% of cases, deafness occurs as an isolated (non-syndromic) defect (Bergstrom et al., 1971). Conductive, sensorineural, and mixed forms of deafness have been identified, each with multiple genetic etiologies. A review of OMIM at the time of this writing indicates that 13 autosomal and five X-linked loci for non-syndromic sensorineural deafness have already been mapped (see also review by Petit, 1996).

DFN3 (MIM 304400), the most common form of X-linked deafness, is a mixed form characterized by conductive hearing loss due to stapes fixation and a progressive sensorineural defect. In addition, operative mobilization of the stapes results in marked drainage of perilymph and cerebrospinal fluid (technically referred to as a "gusher") (Cremers et al., 1983). The *DFN3* locus was mapped to Xq21 by linkage studies and the identification of Xq21 deletions resulting in a contiguous gene syndrome that manifested as choroideremia, deafness, and mental retardation (Brunner et al., 1988; Nussbaum et al., 1987; Wallis et al., 1988). An 850-kb cosmid contig was constructed that allowed identification of patients with microdeletions that localized *DFN3* to a 500-kb region of Xq21.1 (Huber et al., 1994). The mouse *Brain 4 (Brn4)/Pou3f4* gene was mapped to a region showing conservation of synteny with human Xq13-q22 (Douville et al., 1994). In addition to being expressed in the brain, neural tube, and kidney, *Pou3f4* (formerly known as *Rhs2*) is also expressed in the otic vesicle between E15.5 and E17.5 of mouse development (de Kok et al., 1996; Le Moine and Young, 1992). Taken together, these data provided a strong case in support of *POU3F4* as a candidate gene for *DFN3*.

The search for mutations in DFN3 patients without large deletions was aided by the fact that *POU3F4*, like several other genes encoding POU domain proteins (Verrijzer and Van der Vliet, 1993), lacks introns so that the 1.4-kb cDNA sequence that was isolated was found to be colinear with the genomic DNA sequence (de Kok et al., 1995b). Point mutations and oligonucleotide deletions were identified in the *POU3F4* gene of affected males (Bitner-Glindzicz et al., 1995; de Kok et al., 1995b). Frameshifting deletions of 1 to 4 bp were identified in three patients that predict truncation of the protein prior to or within the POU_{HD} domain and two patients with missense mutations (L317W and K334E) involving conserved residues within the POU_{HD} domain were also characterized (de Kok et al., 1995b). The detection of large deletions and frameshift mutations in an X-linked gene causing disease only in hemizygous males suggests that the phenotype is caused by loss of function.

Among 23 DFN3 patients with characterized mutations, nine patients had missense or frameshift mutations, one patient had a duplication associated with a paracentric inversion, and 13 patients had microdeletions ranging in size from less than 10 kb to greater than 1 Mb (Bitner-Glindzicz et al., 1995 ; de Kok et al., 1995a, b, 1996). Ten of the 13 deletions did not appear to include *POU3F4* and the smallest region of overlap for these deletions was an 8-kb segment located 900 kb 5' to the known *POU3F4* coding sequences (de Kok et al., 1996). These results suggest the possible existence of a *cis*-acting regulatory element that is essential for *POU3F4* expression and is located almost a megabase away from the gene! It should be recalled that deletions located quite far from the *GLI3* (Chapter 6) and *PAX6* (Chapter 7) genes have also been associated with disease phenotypes. In the case of large deletions located 5' to the structural gene, it is usually not clear whether gene inactivation is the result of the loss of positive regulatory elements or the juxtaposition of negative regulatory elements (position effects). However, in the case of the DFN3, it seems unlikely that an 8-kb deletion located 900 kb away from the *POU3F4* gene (de Kok et al., 1996) could exert a significant position effect. Rather, the presence of a functionally essential enhancer element within the 8-kb region of deletion overlap seems most likely. The localization of potential transcriptional regulatory elements now provides the opportunity to identify regulators of the regulator and thus to further delineate genetic pathways involved in otic development.

References

Andersen, B., and M. G. Rosenfeld. Pit-1 determines cell types during development of the anterior pituitary gland: a model for transcriptional regulation of cell phenotypes in mammalian organogenesis. *J. Biol. Chem.* 269:29335–29338, 1994.

Assa-Munt, N., R. J. Mortshire-Smith, R. Aurora, W. Herr, and P. E. Wright. The solution structure of the Oct-1 POU-specific domain reveals a striking similarity to the bacteriophage λ repressor DNA-binding domain. *Cell* 73:193–205, 1993.

Bergstrom, L., W. G. Hemenway, and M. P. Downs. A high risk registry to find congenital deafness. *Otolaryngol. Clin. North Am.* 4:369–399, 1971.

Bitner-Glindzicz, M., P. Turnpenny, P. Hoglund, H. Kaariainen, E.-M. Sankila, S. M. van der Maarel, Y. J. M. de Kok, H.-H. Ropers, F. P. M. Cremers, M. Pembrey, and S. Malcolm. Further mutations in Brain 4 (POU3F4) clarify the phenotype in the X-linked deafness, DFN3. *Hum. Mol. Genet.* 4: 1467–1469, 1995.

Bodner, M., J.-L. Castrillo, L. E. Theill, T. Deerinck, M. Ellisman, and M. Karin. The pituitary-specific transcription factor GHF-1 is a homeobox-containing protein. *Cell* 55:505–518, 1988.

Brunner, H. G., C. A. van Bennekom, E. M. M. Lambermon, T. L. Oei, C. W. R. Cremers, B. Wieringa, and H.-H. Ropers. The gene for X-linked progressive mixed deafness with perilymphatic gusher during stapes surgery (DFN3) is linked to PGK. *Hum. Genet.* 80:337–340, 1988.

Buckwalter, M. S., R. W. Katz, and S. A. Camper. Localization of the panhypopituitary dwarf mutation (df) on mouse chromosome 11 in an intersubspecific backcross. *Genomics* 10:515–526, 1991.

Castrillo, J.-L., L. E. Theill, and M. Karin. Function of the homeodomain protein GHF1 in pituitary cell proliferation. *Science* 253:197–199, 1991.

Chen, R. P., H. A. Ingraham, M. N. Treacy, V. R. Albert, L. Wilson, and M. G. Rosenfeld. Autoregulation of pit-1 gene expression mediated by two cis-active promoter elements. *Nature* 346:583–536, 1990.

Clerc, R. G., L. M. Corcoran, J. H. LeBowitz, D. Baltimore, and P. A. Sharp. The B-cell-specific Oct-2 protein contains POU box- and homeo box-type domains. *Genes Dev.* 2:1570–1581, 1988.

Cremers, C. W. R. J., G. C. J. H. Gombergen, and R. T. R. Wentges. Perilymphatic gusher and stapes surgery: a predictable complication? *Clin. Otolaryngol.* 8: 235–240, 1983.

de Kok, Y. J. M., G. F. M. Merckx, S. M. van der Maarel, I. Huber, S. Malcolm, H.-H. Ropers, and F. P. M. Cremers. A duplication/paracentric inversion associated with familial X-linked deafness (DFN3) suggests the presence of a regulatory element more than 400 kb upstream of the POU3F4 gene. *Hum. Mol. Genet.* 4:2145–2150. 1995a.

de Kok, Y. J. M., S. M. van der Maarel, M. Bitner-Glindzicz, I. Huber, A. P. Monaco, S. Malcolm, M. E. Pembrey, H.-H. Ropers, and F. P. M. Cremers. Association between X-linked mixed deafness and mutations in the POU domain gene POU3F4. *Science* 267:685–688, 1995b.

de Kok, Y. J. M., E. R. Vossenaar, C. W. R. J. Cremers, N. Dahl, J. Laporte, L. J. hu, D. Lacombe, N. Fischel-Ghodsian, R. A. Friedman, L. S. Parnes, P. Thorpe, M. Bitner-Glindzicz, H.-J. Pander, H. Heilbronner, J. Graveline, J. T. den Dunnen, H. G. Brunner, H.-H. Ropers, and F. P. M. Cremers. Identification of a hotspot for microdeletions in patients with X-linked deafness type 3 (DFN3) 900 kb proximal to the DFN3 gene POU3F4. *Hum. Mol. Genet.* 5: 1229–1235, 1996.

Dolle, P., J. L. Castrillo, L. E. Theill, T. Deerinck, M. Ellisman, and M. Karin M. Expression of GHF-1 protein in mouse pituitaries correlates both temporally and spatially with the onset of growth hormone gene activity. *Cell* 60:809–820, 1990.

Douville, P. J., S. Atanasoski, A. Tobler, A. Fontana, and M. E. Schwab. The brain-specific POU-box gene Brn4 is a sex-linked transcription factor located on the human and mouse X chromosomes. *Mamm. Genome* 5:180–182, 1994.

Ezzell, C. Spotlight on the POU genes. *J. NIH Res.* 8:91–94, 1996.

Finney, M., G. Ruvkun, and H. R. Horvitz. The C. elegans cell lineage and differentiation gene unc-86 encodes a protein with a homeodomain and extended similarity to transcription factors. *Cell* 55:757–769, 1988.

Godfrey, P., J. O. Rahal, W. G. Beamer, N. G. Copeland, N. A. Jenkins, and K. E. Mayo. GHRH receptor of little mice contains a missense mutation in the extracellular domain that disrupts receptor function. *Nat. Genet.* 4:227–232, 1993.

Harrison, S. C., and A. K. Aggarwal. DNA recognition by proteins with the helix-turn-helix motif. *Annu. Rev. Biochem.* 59:933–969, 1990.

Herr, W., R. A. Sturm, R. G. Clerc, L. M. Corcoran, D. Baltimore, P. A. Sharp, H. A. Ingraham, M. G. Rosenfeld, M. Finney, G. Ruvkun, and H. R. Horvitz. The POU domain: a large conserved region in the mammalian pit-1, oct-1, oct-2, and Caenorhabditis elegans unc-86 gene products. *Genes Dev.* 2:1513–1516, 1988.

Huber, I., M. Bitner-Glindzicz, Y. J. M. de Kok, S. M. van der Maarel, Y. Ishikawa-Brush, A. P. Monaco, D. Robinson, S. Malcolm, M. E. Pembrey, H. G. Brunner, F. P. M. Cremers, and H.-H. Ropers. X-linked mixed deafness (DFN3): cloning and characterization of the critical region allows the identification of novel microdeletions. *Hum. Mol. Genet.* 3:1151–1154, 1994.

Ingraham, H. A., R. P. Chen, H. J. Mangalam, H. P. Elsholtz, S. E. Flynn, C. R. Lin, D. M. Simmons, L. Swanson, and M. G. Rosenfeld. A tissue-specific transcription factor containing a homeodomain specifies a pituitary phenotype. *Cell* 55:519–529, 1988.

Klemm, J. D., M. A. Rould, R. Aurora, W. Herr, and C. O. Pabo. Crystal structure of the Oct-1 POU domain bound to an octamer site: DNA recognition with tethered DNA-binding modules. *Cell* 77:21–32, 1994.

Ko, H. S., P. Fast, W. McBride, and L. M. Staudt. A human protein specific for the immunoglobulin octamer DNA motif contains a functional homeobox domain. *Cell* 55:135–144, 1988.

Le Moine, C., and W. S. Young III. RHS2, a POU domain-containing gene, and its expression in developing and adult rat. *Proc. Natl. Acad. Sci. U.S.A.* 89: 3285–3289, 1992.

Li, S., E. B. Crenshaw III, E. J. Rawson, D. M. Simmons, L. W. Swanson, and M. G. Rosenfeld. Dwarf locus mutants lacking three pituitary cell types result from mutations in the POU-domain gene pit-1. *Nature* 347:528–533, 1990.

Lin, C., S. C. Lin, C. P. Chang, and M. G. Rosenfeld. Pit-1-dependent expression of the receptor for growth hormone releasing factor mediates pituitary cell growth. *Nature* 360:765–768, 1992.

Lin, S. C., C. R. Lin, I. Gukovsky, A. J. Lusis, P. E. Sawchenko, M. G. Rosenfeld. Molecular basis of the little mouse phenotype and implications for cell type-specific growth. *Nature* 364:208–213, 1993.

Mangalam, H. J., V. R. Albert, H. A. Ingraham, M. Kapiloff, L. Wilson, C. Nelson, H. Elsholtz, and M. G. Rosenfeld. A pituitary POU domain protein, Pit-1, activates both growth hormone and prolactin promoters transcriptionally. *Genes Dev.* 3:946–958, 1989.

McCormick, A., H. Brady, L. E. Theill, and M. Karin. Regulation of the pituitary-specific homeobox gene GHF1 by cell-autonomous and environmental cues. *Nature* 345:829–832, 1990.

Morton, N. E. Genetic epidemiology of hearing impairment. *Ann. N.Y. Acad. Sci.* 630:16–31, 1991.

Nussbaum, R. L., J. G. Lesko, R. A. Lewis, S. A. Ledbetter, and D. A. Ledbetter. Isolation of anonymous DNA sequences from within a submicroscopic X chromosomal deletion in a patient with choroideremia, deafness and mental retardation. *Proc. Natl. Acad. Sci. U.S.A.* 84:6521–6525, 1987.

Petit, C. Genes responsible for human hereditary deafness: symphony of a thousand. *Nat. Genet.* 14: 385–391, 1996.

Pfaffle, R. W., G. E. DiMattia, J. S. Parks, M. R. Brown, J. M. Wit, M. Jansen, H. Van der Nat, J. L. Van den Brande, M. G. Rosenfeld, and H. A. Ingraham. Mutation of the POU-specific domain of Pit-1 and hypopituitarism without pituitary hypoplasia. *Science* 257:1118–1121, 1992.

Radovick, S., M. Nations, Y. Du, L. A. Berg, B. D. Weintraub, and F. E. Wondisford. A mutation in the POU-homeodomain of Pit-1 responsible for combined pituitary hormone deficiency. *Science* 257:1115–1118, 1992.

Simmons, D. M., J. W. Voss, H. A. Ingraham, J. M. Holloway, R. S. Broide, M. G. Rosenfeld, and L. W. Swanson. Pituitary cell phenotypes involve cell-specific Pit-1 mRNA translation and synergistic interactions with other classes of transcription factors. *Genes Dev.* 4:695–711, 1990.

Sornson, M. W., W. Wu, J. S. Dasen, S. E. Flynn, D. J. Norman, S. M. O'Connell, I. Gukovsky, C. Carriere, A. K. Ryan, A. P. Miller, L. Zuo, A. S. Gleiberman, B. Andersen, W. G. Beamer, and M. G. Rosenfeld. Pituitary lineage determination by the Prophet of Pit-1 homeodomain factor defective in Ames dwarfism. *Nature* 384:327–333, 1996.

Steinfelder, H. J., P. Hauser, Y. Nakayama, S. Radovick, J. H. McClaskey, T. Taylor, B. D. Weintraub, and F. E. Wondisford. Thyrotropin-releasing hormone regulation of human TSHB expression: role of a pituitary-specific transcription factor (Pit-1/GHF-1) and potential interaction with a thyroid hormone-inhibitory element. *Proc. Natl. Acad. Sci. U.S.A.* 88:3130–3134, 1991.

Sturm, R. A., G. Das, and W. Herr. The ubiquitous octamer-binding protein Oct-1 contains a POU domain with a homeo box subdomain. *Genes Dev.* 2:1582–1599, 1988.

Sturm, R. A., and W. Herr. The POU domain is a bipartite DNA-binding structure. *Nature* 336:601–604, 1988.

Tatsumi, K., K. Miyai, T. Notomi, K. Kaibe, N. Amino, Y. Mizuno, and H. Kohno. Cretinism with combined hormone deficiency caused by a mutation in the PIT1 gene. *Nat. Genet.* 1:56–58, 1992.

Verrijzer, C. P., M. Strating, Y. M. Mul, and P. C. van der Vliet. POU domain transcription factors from different subclasses stimulate adenovirus DNA replication. *Nucleic Acids Res.* 20:6369–6375, 1992.

Verrijzer, C. P., and P. C. Van der Vliet. POU domain transcription factors. *Biochim. Biophys. Acta* 1173:1–21, 1993.

Wallis, C., R. Ballo, G. Wallis, P. Beighton, and J. Goldblatt. X-linked mixed deafness with stapes fixation in a Mauritian kindred: linkage to Xq probe pDP34. *Genomics* 3:299–301, 1988.

12 Other Transcription Factor Families

In addition to the zinc finger, PAX, bHLH, homeodomain, HMG, and POU proteins described in the preceding seven chapters, other transcription factor families have been identified that utilize unique DNA-binding domains. Members of such families that have been implicated in genetic disorders, including the TBX and RFX family members, are described in this chapter. Finally, HNF-1α and HNF-4 are the homeodomain and nuclear receptor proteins, respectively. Because these two transcription factors interact genetically, both in normal development and in the pathogenesis of diabetes, they will be described together in this chapter.

Involvement of T-domain Transcription Factors in Limb Development

The first member of the T-domain family identified was the product of the *Brachyury (T)* gene (Herrmann et al., 1990). Mice that are heterozygous for loss-of-function *T* gene mutations have short tails and sacral malformations, whereas homozygous embryos die at E10 due to defects in mesoderm formation and notochord differentiation (reviewed by Herrmann and Kispert, 1994; Willison, 1990). The *T* gene encodes a transcription factor containing an amino-terminal DNA-binding domain and carboxyl-terminal activation and repression domains (Kispert et al., 1995). The T-protein DNA-binding domain showed remarkable amino acid sequence similarity to the product of the *Drosophila* gene *optomotor-blind (omb)*, which is required for optic lobe and wing development (Pflugfelder et al., 1992). The conserved DNA-binding motif and the genomic sequences encoding it were designated the T domain and T box, respectively, in analogy with the homeodomain/homeobox nomenclature. A total of eight genes in *Mus musculus (T, Tbx1, Tbx2, Tbx3, Tbx4,*

Tbx5, Tbx6, and *Tbr1*) and four genes in *Caenorhabditis elegans* have been identified that contain a T box (Agulnik et al., 1995; Bollag et al., 1994).

TBX5 and Holt-Oram Syndrome

Congenital heart disease represents a major category of birth defects, affecting 1% of all newborns (Hoffman, 1995). Atrial septal defects, ventricular septal defects, and tetralogy of Fallot each occur with an incidence of approximately 1 in 1000 live births. The high incidence of congenital defects reflects the complexity of cardiac morphogenesis and the many gene products required to successfully execute this essential developmental program. Only a few of the responsible genes have actually been identified (reviewed by Olson and Srivastava, 1996). Because many of these gene products are also expressed in noncardiac tissues, many genetic syndromes that include cardiac defects also manifest malformations in other systems.

An example of one of the many rare genetic disorders that contribute to the overall incidence of congenital heart disease is the Holt-Oram syndrome (Holt and Oram, 1960; MIM 142900), an autosomal dominant disorder with an incidence of 1 in 100,000 live births that is characterized by cardiac and skeletal defects (Basson et al., 1994). Atrial and ventricular septal defects are the most common cardiac malformations and conduction defects (sinus and atrioventricular node abnormalities) are also often present. The skeletal defects vary widely in severity, ranging from supernumerary carpal bones that are only detected radiographically to radial reduction defects and phocomelia. Most commonly, the thumb is either triphalangeal (Fig. 12.1) or absent (Temtany and McKusick, 1978).

Genetic analysis of seven families in which Holt-Oram syndrome was segregating revealed linkage of the phenotype to a locus on chromosome 12q2 in five of the seven families, indicating genetic heterogeneity (Terrett et al., 1994). The gene on chromosome 12q2 that is mutated in Holt-Oram syndrome was identified by two independent positional-cloning strategies. In one case, DNA from a patient with a complex chromosomal rearrangement involving chromosome 12q was utilized to identify exons near the translocation breakpoint (Li et al., 1997). In the second case, further linkage analysis localized the gene to a 1–cM interval, a DNA contig spanning the interval was constructed, and exons within it were identified (Basson et al., 1997). In both cases, the responsible gene was identified as *TBX5*, which encodes a 349–amino-acid protein that is a member of the T domain family of transcription factors.

Genomic analysis of the Holt-Oram syndrome locus revealed that *TBX5* was in close proximity to *TBX3* (Li et al., 1997), as previously

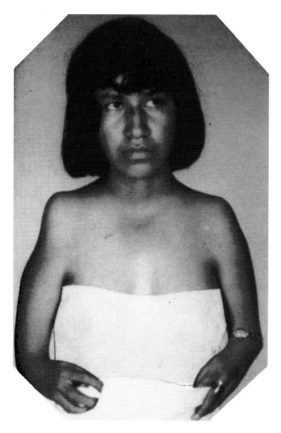

FIGURE 12-1. Limb defects in Holt-Oram syndrome. Note aplasia of thumbs, severe hypoplasia of radius and ulna (forearm), and reduction of the shoulder girdle. (Reproduced with permission from Jones, 1988.)

determined for the mouse homologues of these genes (Agulnik et al., 1996). However, disease-causing mutations were identified only in *TBX5* (Basson et al., 1997; Li et al., 1997). Seven point mutations were identified in DNA from affected individuals. Five nonsense, two frameshift, and one missense mutation were detected that each predicted either loss of transactivation function or DNA-binding activity. These results suggest that heterozygosity for a loss-of-function allele of the *TBX5* gene is sufficient to cause Holt-Oram syndrome, indicating a gene dosage (haploinsufficiency) mechanism of molecular pathophysiology, similar to what was described in previous chapters with respect to PAX (Chapter 7) and SOX (Chapter 10) genes. Once again, however, the identification of specific mutations does not provide a full explanation of the pathophysiology. Six individuals from three different families each inherited the same nonsense mutation yet displayed markedly different clinical phenotypes (Li et al., 1997). The limb phenotypes included triphalangeal thumbs, absent thumb and radius, and even shoulder joint involvement. The cardiac phenotypes included isolated electrocardiographic abnormalities, isolated ventricular septal defect, and atrial septal defect with multiple ventricular septal defects.

Analysis by *in situ* hybridization revealed the presence of TBX5 mRNA in human embryos between gestational days 26 and 52 (Li et al., 1997). *TBX5* expression was detected in the forelimbs and in the heart, including structures such as the atrial septum and atrioventricular endocardial cushions that are sites of malformation in Holt-Oram syndrome. High levels of expression were also detected in the anterior thoracic wall and eye, which are also sites of malformation in affected individuals. *TBX5* expression was also detected in the developing trachea and lungs, which are not affected in Holt-Oram syndrome, suggesting that there may be redundant expression of other TBX proteins in these tissues or that 50% of normal TBX5 activity is sufficient for proper pulmonary development. Both *Tbx4* and *Tbx5* are expressed in the developing murine heart (Chapman et al., 1996). Assuming a similar pattern of expression in humans, this result suggests that the products of these two genes have unique functions.

The T box of *TBX5* encodes amino acids 56–238, which are 97% identical to the T domain of mouse *Tbx5* and 62% identical to the T domain of *Drosophila* OMB (Basson et al., 1997). Loss-of-function mutations in *TBX5* and *omb* result in limb and wing malformations, respectively. Genetic analysis of wing development in *Drosophila* may identify signal transduction components (receptors, ligands, kinases) and other transcription factors whose mammalian homologues are required for proper limb and/or cardiac morphogenesis.

TBX3 and Ulnar-Mammary Syndrome

As in the case of Holt-Oram syndrome, a characteristic feature of the autosomal-dominant ulnar-mammary syndrome (MIM 181450) is upper limb malformations. Most affected individuals have defects involving the posterior (postaxial or ulnar) aspect of the limb, with extremely variable phenotypic severity ranging from hypoplasia of the distal fifth phalanx to aplasia of the entire forelimb (Fig. 12.2). The mammary defects in females are also of extremely variable severity ranging from decreased axillary hair and apocrine (sweat) glands to complete aplasia of the breasts, axillary hair follicles, and apocrine glands. Dental abnormalities

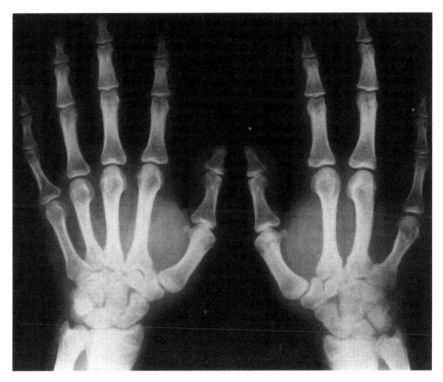

FIGURE 12-2. Hand radiograph of an individual with ulnar-mammary syndrome. The fourth digit on the right hand is absent. (Reproduced with permission from Bamshad et al., 1997.)

(hypoplasia or aplasia of the canine teeth) and genital abnormalities (micropenis, imperforate hymen) have also been reported. Linkage analysis of a large pedigree identified a locus on chromosome 12q23-24.1 in a 1-cM genetic interval that contained the *TBX3* and *TBX5* genes (Bamshad et al., 1995). In two isolated cases of ulnar-mammary syndrome, point mutations were identified in *TBX3* (Bamshad et al., 1997). An exon 1 frameshift mutation (227delT) and an intron 2 splice junction mutation (Int2:$G_1 \rightarrow C$) both were predicted to disrupt the protein coding sequence within the DNA-binding T domain. In both cases, the markedly truncated protein is unlikely to bind DNA, suggesting that the pathophysiology of ulnar-mammary syndrome involves haploinsufficiency for TBX3 (Bamshad et al., 1997).

The effects of mutations in the closely linked *TBX5* and *TBX3* genes are remarkably complementary in that decreased TBX5 expression results in defects of the anterior (radial) aspect of the forelimb, whereas decreased TBX3 expression results in defects of the posterior (ulnar) aspect of the forelimb. These results suggest that during evolution, the duplication of *TBX* genes and their subsequent structural and functional divergence may have contributed to the specialization of the mammalian forelimb. It is also of interest that TBX3 in particular is required for the development of structures (apocrine gland, limb, mammary gland, tooth, urogenital system) that form via epithelial-mesenchymal interactions. In this respect, TBX3 is similar to the homeodomain transcription factors MSX1 and MSX2 (Chapter 9), which are also required for inductive interactions both in developing craniofacial structures and in other tissues including the mammary glands. It will be interesting to learn how the TBX and homeodomain transcription factors interact during development.

The Bare Lymphocyte Immunodeficiency Syndrome

With the exception of several nuclear hormone receptors, mutations in genes encoding all of the transcription factors described in this and the preceding eight chapters result in malformation syndromes, providing dramatic clinical evidence for the crucial role of transcription factors in controlling human development. Here, another exception to this general rule is presented, involving genes with a highly specific role in immune system regulation.

The bare lymphocyte syndrome is an immunodeficiency disorder that results from defects in the regulation of class II genes of the major histocompatibility complex (MHC), which in humans is designated the HLA complex (Griscelli et al., 1989; reviewed by Reith et al., 1995). Genes encoding the α and β chains of the HLA-DR, HLA-DQ and HLA-DP class II MHC molecules, which are normally expressed specifically in antigen-presenting cells including B lymphocytes, dendritic cells, macrophages, activated T lymphocytes, and thymic epithelial cells, are not expressed in this disorder (De Preval et al., 1985, 1988; Griscelli et al., 1989; Lisowska-Grospierre et al., 1985). These molecules are required for the presentation of antigenic peptide fragments to CD4-positive helper T cells, and their absence prevents normal immune responses.

As one might expect from the loss of expression of multiple genes, genetic defects have been demonstrated involving *trans*-acting factors that are required for transcription of these genes (De Preval et al., 1985). Somatic cell hybridization studies utilizing Epstein-Barr virus–transformed B cells cultured from patients with the bare lymphocyte syndrome identified at least three different complementation groups, indicating the existence of at least three different *trans*-acting factors. In addition, mutagenesis of established B-lymphocyte cell lines (Gladstone and Pious, 1978) led to the identification of complementation group D (Benichou and Strominger, 1991). Thus far, the genes that are mutated in complementation groups A, C, and D have been identified, as described below.

CIITA

Complementation cDNA cloning revealed that cells from group A were deficient in CIITA, an 1130-amino-acid transcription factor with no significant homology to any other known protein (Steimle et al., 1993). Deletion of the amino-terminal acidic and proline/serine/threonine-rich region of the protein results in a dominant-negative form of CIITA that represses transcription of DR, DQ, and DP genes (Bontron et al., 1997), providing further evidence that the wild-type form of CIITA coordinately activates transcription of the MHC class II genes.

RFX5

Cells from complementation groups B and C lacked binding of a different nuclear factor, RFX, to the promoters of class II genes. Purification of RFX binding activity from wild-type cells yielded polypeptides of 36 and 75 kDa (Durand et al., 1994). Transfection of class C cells with a cDNA library from wild-type cells revealed that the class II defect could be corrected by a cDNA encoding a 616-amino-acid protein that corresponded to the 75-kDa subunit of purified RFX (Steimle et al., 1995). Database analysis revealed that the protein, RFX5, was the fifth member of a family of DNA-binding proteins that had previously been shown to bind to MHC class II promoter DNA sequences (Reith et al., 1994c). All five proteins share a conserved 75-amino-acid DNA-binding domain that is unique to these factors. Analysis of the RFX5 gene in DNA from the mutant cells used for complementation cloning revealed heterozygosity for a splice junction mutation, whereas the defect in the second allele was not determined although it did not give rise to full-length RFX5 mRNA (Steimle et al., 1995). RFX5 DNA from a second patient was homozygous for a nonsense mutation, again consistent with complete loss of RFX5 activity.

RFX5 corresponded to the 75-kDa subunit of the purified RFX protein, suggesting that the defect in complementation group B may involve the 36-kDa subunit of RFX (Steimle et al., 1995). Loss of RFX binding activity has a striking effect on class II promoters because binding of other factors that are present in the mutant cells does not occur in the absence of RFX (Kara and Glimcher, 1991a, 1991b, 1993). The reason for bare promoters in the bare lymphocyte syndrome (Kara and Glimcher, 1991a) is that RFX mediates cooperative binding of other transcription factors at adjacent DNA sites (Durand et al., 1994; Reith et al., 1994a, b). This important property of RFX demonstrates why the deficiency of RFX5 has such a devastating effect on class II gene transcription. An implication of these results is that neither RFX1, RFX2, RFX3, nor RFX4 can substitute for RFX5 in this role. In addition, the fact that the phenotype associated with RFX5 loss of function is limited to immunodeficiency indicates that the biological function of this factor is highly specialized, for it appears to play an essential role only in the regulation of class II MHC genes (Steimle et al., 1995).

RFXAP

In addition to cell lines derived from patients, an experimentally mutagenized B-lymphoid cell line, 6.1.6, was demonstrated to complement cells of groups A, B, and C, suggesting the presence of a genetically distinct mutation (Benichou and Strominger, 1991). The gene mutated in this cell line was recently shown to encode the 36-kDa subunit of RFX, which was designated RFXAP (RFX associated protein) because it interacts with RFX5 but is not a member of the RFX transcription-factor family as defined by the shared DNA-binding motif (Durand et al., 1997). The two *RFXAP* genes in 6.1.6 cells contained mutations that were 90 nucleotides apart in the mRNA sequence and that were both frameshift mutations due to the insertion of an extra guanine residue into a polyguanine tract. Analysis of DNA from an individual with MHC class II deficiency, who had not previously been classified by complementation analysis, revealed the presence of a single nucleotide deletion in all cDNA and genomic clones analyzed, suggesting homozygosity for the frameshift mutation, which was consistent with the fact that the patient's parents were first cousins (Durand et al., 1997).

The biochemical relationship between RFX5 and RFXAP is unclear because other RFX family members form either homodimers or heterodimers with each other (Emery et al., 1996). RFXAP and RFX5 could not be co-immunoprecipitated, although a physical interaction was detected in the yeast two-hybrid assay (Durand et al., 1997). Now that several of the players have been identified, critical studies can be undertaken to determine the molecular mechanisms by which CIITA, RFX5, RFXAP, and the factor encoded by the gene mutated in complementation group B interact to coordinately regulate transcription of the MHC class II genes.

CBFA1: Master Regulator of Osteoblast Differentiation

The bony skeleton in vertebrates serves several essential functions (reviewed by Rodan and Harada, 1997): It stockpiles calcium and phosphate; allows locomotion; protects the central nervous system; and both protects and participates in the function of the hematopoietic and respiratory systems. The intramembranous bone of the craniofacial skeleton is formed directly from osteoblasts that derive from the embryonic branchial arches of the embryo, whereas the endochondral bone that composes the remainder of the skeleton forms by replacement of a cartilaginous progenitor.

Osteoblasts are the cells responsible for both intramembranous and endochondral bone formation. Osteocalcin is a component of the extracellular matrix that is produced exclusively by osteoblasts and not by chondroblasts (cartilage progenitor cells), fibroblasts, or any other cell type known to produce extracellular matrix. Analysis of the promoter of the gene encoding Osteocalcin revealed the presence of a *cis*-acting DNA sequence element that could direct osteoblast-specific expression of a heterologous promoter and could bind nuclear factors present only in nuclear extracts prepared from osteoblasts (Ducy and Karsenty, 1995). The osteoblast-specific transcription factor was identified as OSF2, an alternatively spliced product of the previously described *Cbfa1* gene (Ducy et al., 1997). The *Cbfa* gene family consists of three genes, each of which has been given three different names: *Cbfa1/Pebp2αA/AML3*, *Cbfa2/ PEB2αB/AML1*, and *CBFA3/Pebp2αC/AML2* (reviewed by Rodan and Harada, 1997). Each of these genes encodes a protein containing a 128-amino-acid DNA-binding domain that is homologous to the product of the *runt* gene of *Drosophila melanogaster* (Kagoshima et al., 1993). In the case of CBFA2, dimerization with a structurally unrelated protein, CBFB, is required for DNA-binding activity (Wang et al., 1993).

Expression of the OSF2 isoform of CBFA1 mRNA was detected during the first morphologically identifiable step of skeletal development, mesenchymal cell condensation, at E12.5 of mouse development (Ducy et al., 1997). OSF2/CBFA1 mRNA was expressed in the anlage of all endochondral and intramembranous bones. Transfection of *Osf2/Cbfa1* antisense oligonucleotides into cultured osteoblastic cells resulted in markedly decreased levels of mRNAs encoding α1(I) Collagen, Osteopontin, and Osteocalcin. Forced expression of OSF2/CBFA1 in nonosteoblastic cells resulted in *Osteocalcin* gene expression (Ducy et al., 1997).

These data were consistent with the hypothesis that OSF2/CBFA1 played an important role in the regulation of osteoblast differentiation. This hypothesis was confirmed by the analysis of mice homozygous for targeted mutations at the *Cbfa1* locus (Komori et al., 1997; Otto et al., 1997). These mice died shortly after birth because of respiratory insufficiency. The reason that they could not breathe was apparent by x-ray: neither the ribs nor any other part of the skeleton was ossified. Analysis at E18.5 revealed that osteoblasts in control embryos expressed the *Osteonectin, Osteopontin,* and *Osteocalcin* genes, whereas the few osteoblasts identified in the homozygous-mutant embryos expressed *Osteonectin,* weakly expressed *Osteopontin,* and did not express *Osteocalcin,* indicating arrest at an early stage of osteoblast differentiation (Komori et al., 1997)

The heterozygous-mutant mice exhibited hypoplastic clavicles and nasal bones, and decreased ossification of the parietal, interparietal, and supraoccipital bones of the skull. Multiple wormian bones, which represent abnormal ossification of the calvarium, were also detected (Otto et al., 1997). These findings are similar to those described in the autosomal-dominant human malformation syndrome cleidocranial dysplasia (MIM 119600). A mouse model of cleidocranial dysplasia previously shown to result from γ-irradiation (Sillence et al., 1987) was associated with a heterozygous deletion of the *Cbfa1* locus (Otto et al., 1997).

Insertion, deletion, and missense mutations in the human *CBFA1* gene were demonstrated in patients with cleidocranial dysplasia. Most of these mutations were predicted to result in protein truncation either within the DNA-binding domain or the carboxyl-terminal transactivation domain (Mundlos et al., 1997). Identification of affected individuals in which the entire *CBFA1* gene was deleted indicated that the disease results from haploinsufficiency. Two missense mutations, M175R and S191N, involved residues within the DNA-binding domain that are conserved in human, *Drosophila,* and sea urchin proteins containing a RUNT domain and resulted in a loss of DNA-binding activity (Lee et al., 1997). Perhaps the most interesting mutation was a 30-bp insertion that increased the length of a polyalanine sequence in the protein from A_{17} to A_{27} (Mundlos et al., 1997). Individuals heterozygous for this mutation had an unusual phenotype: the craniofacial manifestations of cleidocranial dysplasia were mild and, in addition, the patients manifested brachdactyly. This mutation is strikingly similar to the insertion in the *HOXD13* gene associated with synpolydactyly, in which the mutant protein is believed to have a dominant-negative effect (see Chapter 9).

The story of CBFA1 and cleidocranial dysplasia is instructive in several respects. First, the analysis of mice homozygous for a loss-of-function mutation in *Cbfa1* provided an understanding of its function that could not be appreciated by analysis of humans that were heterozygous for similar mutations. Second, the phenotype of the heterozygous knockout mice immediately identified the candidate gene for mutational analysis in the human condition. Third, the analysis of CBFA1 function in cultured cells provided some understanding of the molecular basis for CBFA1 control of osteogenesis by the identification of *cis*-acting elements within target genes expressed specifically within osteoblasts. The synergistic effects of these clinical and basic science research strategies explain in part the remarkable acceleration of progress in our understanding of the molecular bases of inherited human malformation syndromes.

HNF-1α, HNF-4α, and Maturity-Onset Diabetes of the Young

In general, the specific genetic disorders that have been described in this book are individually quite rare, with most having an incidence of 1 in 100,000 live births, give or take an order of magnitude. Their importance lies in what they tell us about more general processes of broad clinical relevance. Thus, whereas mutations in *TBX5* occur with an incidence of only 1 in 100,000, analyzing the effects of these mutations on cardiac morphogenesis will provide important insights toward a general understanding congenital heart disease that occurs with an overall incidence of 1 in 100 newborns.

One of the most common disorders of adulthood is non–insulin-dependent (type 2) diabetes mellitus (NIDDM), which affects 1 in 50 individuals and is characterized by hyperglycemia (high blood glucose) and hypoinsulinemia (insulin deficiency) (reviewed by Polonsky, 1995; Polonsky et al., 1996). As in the case of congenital heart disease, NIDDM represents a collection of many different disorders with different etiologies. Between 2% and 5% of individuals with NIDDM have a clinical subtype designated maturity-onset diabetes of the young (MODY), which is characterized by its early onset (before age 25 years and often in childhood) and autosomal-dominant inheritance pattern (reviewed by Fajans, 1989). Genetic linkage analysis of families in which MODY was segregating localized genes (*MODY1*, *MODY2*, and *MODY3*) involved in disease pathogenesis to chromosomes 20, 7, and 12, respectively (Bell et al., 1991; Froguel et al., 1993; Vaxillaire et al., 1995). Whereas the *MODY2* locus on chromosome 7 was shown to encode the glycolytic enzyme glucokinase (Froguel et al., 1993), the *MODY3* and *MODY1* loci were found to encode transcription factors (Yamagata et al., 1996a, b).

MODY3 and HNF-1α

Genetic and physical mapping data localized *MODY3* to chromosome band 12q24.2 in a region containing at least 26 candidate genes. Mutations that segregated with MODY were found exclusively within the gene encoding hepatocyte nuclear factor–1α (HNF-1α) (Yamagata et al., 1996b). Dimerization, DNA binding, and transactivation domains have been localized to amino acid residues 1–32, 150–280, and 281–631, respectively (reviewed by Tronche and Yaniv, 1992). Seven different frame-shift, missense, and splice site mutations were identified, all of which would result in the synthesis of a mutant protein containing an intact dimerization domain but lacking either an intact DNA-binding or transactivation domain. These results suggest the possibility that a dominant-negative mechanism may account for the dominant inheritance of the disease phenotype, although haploinsufficiency cannot be ruled out by these data.

HNF-1α is expressed in liver, kidney, intestine, pancreas, and stomach, and mice homozygous for a null allele resulting in complete deficiency of HNF-1α were liveborn but died of a progressive wasting syndrome before reaching maturity, with hepatic dysfunction, phenylketonuria, and renal tubular dysfunction with massive urinary loss of glucose (Pontoglio et al., 1996). These animals had no evidence of diabetes mellitus although the glucosuria may have prevented hyperglycemia and/or they may not have survived long enough to manifest this aspect of the phenotype. These findings are also consistent with the hypothesis that dominant-negative mutations, which might interfere with HNF-1β as well as HNF-1α function, are required for the MODY phenotype. An analysis of heterozygous HNF-1α-null mice and similar mice that also expressed an HNF-1α transgene containing one of the MODY mutations would be highly informative in this regard.

Although HNF-1α is known to control expression of several hepatocyte-specific genes including those encoding albumin, α1-antitrypsin, α-fibrinogen, β-fibrinogen, and phenylalanine hydroxylase (Pontoglio et al., 1996, and references therein), it is not known what genes are activated by HNF-1α in β cells of the pancreatic islets. The gene encoding glucokinase is a reasonable candidate given the fact that mutations at that locus also cause MODY. In addition, HNF-1α expression has been detected in a hamster insulinoma and shown to transactivate the rat insulin I gene (Emens et al., 1992).

MODY1 and HNF-4α

Genetic analysis of a single pedigree that included 360 individuals spanning six generations allowed mapping of *MODY1* to a 13-cM interval of chromosome 20 (Yamagata et al., 1996a). This localization corresponded to approximately 7 Mb of DNA, which would be expected to encompass dozens of genes. However, included within this interval was the *TCF14* gene, which encodes HNF-4α. Because of the involvement of HNF-1α in *MODY3*, and the fact that HNF-4α was known to be required for HNF-1α expression, *TCF14* became an immediate candidate gene for *MODY1*. A nonsense mutation, Q268X, was identified in DNA from affected family members. Unlike HNF-1α, which contains a homeodomain, HNF-4α is a member of the zinc finger nuclear-receptor superfamily, representing one of the so-called orphan receptors (see Chapter 5). The Q268X mutation in HNF-4α would result in the synthesis of a truncated protein that could not dimerize and thus could not bind to DNA or activate transcription, suggesting that in this case haploinsufficiency is the basis for the disease phenotype. Given the fact that HNF-1α is a downstream target of HNF-4α, it is possible that the mutations affecting HNF-1α (described above) also result in simple loss of function.

Like HNF-1α, HNF-4α is expressed in the liver, kidney, intestines, and pancreas, but known targets have been identified only in the liver and include genes encoding proteins involved in glucose, cholesterol, and fatty acid metabolism (reviewed by Yamagata et al., 1996a). Mice homozygous for a null allele resulting in complete deficiency of HNF-4α suffer embryonic lethality due to defective gastrulation (Chen et al., 1994). As in the case of the HNF-1α-deficient mice, mice that are heterozygous for the HNF-4α null allele have not been carefully studied for evidence of an NIDDM-like phenotype. These results clearly implicate a genetic pathway that includes HNF-1α and HNF-4α in the pathogenesis of MODY. Thus, MODY may represent a disorder in which normal genetic responses to hyperglycemia do not occur in pancreatic β cells either because of decreased expression of transcriptional activators (HNF-1α and HNF-4α) or because of mutations in their target genes.

References

Agulnik, S. I., R. J. Bollag, and L. M. Silver. Conservation of the T-box gene family from Mus musculus to Caenorhabditis elegans. *Genomics* 25:214–219, 1995.

Agulnik, S. I., et al. Evolution of mouse T-box genes by tandem duplication and cluster dispersion. *Genetics* 144:249–254, 1996.

Bamshad, M. P. A. Krakowiak, W. S. Watkins, S. Root, J. C. Carey, and L. B. Jorde. A gene for ulnar-mammary syndrome maps to 12q23-q24.1. *Hum. Mol. Genet.* 4: 1973–1977, 1995.

Bamshad, M. R. C. Lin, D. J. Law, W. S. Watkins, P. A. Krakowiak, M. E. Moore, P. Franceschini, R. Lala, L. B. Holmes, T. C. Gebuhr, B. G. Bruneau, A. Schinzel, J. G. Seidman, C. E. Seidman, and L. B. Jorde. Mutations in human TBX3 alter limb, apocrine and genital development in ulnar-mammary syndrome. *Nat. Genet.* 16: 311–315, 1997.

Basson, C. T., D. R. Bachinsky, R. C. Lin, T. Levi, J. A. Elkins, J. Soults, D. Grayzel, E. Kroumpouzou, T. A. Traill, J. Leblanc-Straceski, B. Renault, R. Kucherlapati, J. G. Seidman, and C. E. Seidman. Mutations in human cause limb and cardiac malformation in Holt-Oram syndrome. *Nat. Genet.* 15:30–35, 1997.

Basson, C. T., G. S. Cowley, S. D. Solomon, B. Weissman, A. K. Poznanski, T. Traill, J. G. Seidman, and C. E. Seidman. The clinical and genetic spectrum of the Holt-Oram syndrome (heart-hand syndrome). *N. Engl. J. Med.* 330: 885–891, 1994.

Bell, G. I., K. S. Xiang, M. V. Newman, S. H. Wu, L. G. Wright, S. S. Fajans, R. S. Spielman, and N. J. Cox. Gene for non-insulin-dependent diabetes mellitus (maturity-onset diabetes of the young subtype) is linked to DNA polymorphism on human chromosome 20q. *Proc. Natl. Acad. Sci. U. S. A.* 88:1484–1488, 1991.

Benichou, B., and J. L. Strominger. Class II-antigen-negative patient and mutant B-cell lines represent at least three, and probably four, distinct genetic defects defined by complementation analysis. *Proc. Natl. Acad. Sci. U.S.A.* 88:4285–4288, 1991.

Bollag, R. J., Z. Siegfried, J. A. Cebra-Thomas, N. Garvey, E. M. Davison, and L. M. Silver. An ancient family of embryonically expressed mouse genes sharing a conserved protein motif with the T locus. *Nat. Genet.* 7:383–389, 1994.

Bontron, S., C. Ucla, B. Mach, and V. Steimle. Efficient repression of endogenous major histocompatibility complex class II expression through dominant negative CIITA mutants isolated by a functional selection strategy. *Mol. Cell. Biol.* 17:4249–4258, 1997.

Chapman, D. L., N. Garvey, S. Hancock, M. Alexiou, S. I. Agulnik, J. J. Gibson-Brown, J. Cebra-Thomas, R. J. Bollag, L. M. Silver, and V. E. Papaioannou. Expression of the T-box family genes, Tbx1-Tbx5, during early mouse development. *Dev. Dyn.* 206:379–390, 1996

Chen, W. S., K. Manova, D. C. Weinstein, S. A. Duncan, A. S. Plump, V. R. Prezioso, R. F. Bachvarova, and J. E. Darnell, Jr. Disruption of the HNF-4 gene, expressed in visceral endoderm, leads to cell death in embryonic ectoderm and impaired gastrulation of mouse embryos. *Genes Dev.* 8:2466–2477, 1994.

De Preval, C., M. R. Hadam, and B. Mach. Regulation of genes for HLA class II antigens in cell lines from patients with severe combined immunodeficiency. *N. Engl. J. Med.* 318:1295–1300, 1988.

De Preval, C., B. Lisowska-Grospierre, M. Loche, C. Griscelli, and B. Mach. A trans-acting class II regulatory gene unlinked to the MHC controls expression of HLH class II genes. *Nature* 318:292–293, 1985.

Ducy, P., and G. Karsenty. Two distinct osteoblast-specific cis-acting elements control expression of a mouse osteocalcin gene. *Mol. Cell. Biol.* 15:1858–1869, 1995.

Ducy, P., R. Zhang, V. Geoffroy, A. L. Ridall, and G. Karsenty. Osf2/Cbfa1: a transcriptional activator of osteoblast differentiation. *Cell* 89:747–754, 1997.

Durand, B., M. Kobr, W. Reith, and B. Mach. Functional complementation of major histocompatibility complex class II regulatory mutants by the purified X-box-binding protein RFX. *Mol. Cell. Biol.* 14:6839–6847, 1994.

Durand, B., P. Sperisen, P. Emery, E. Barras, M. Zufferey, B. Mach, and W. Reith. RFXAP, a novel subunit of the RFX DNA binding complex is mutated in MHC class II deficiency. *EMBO J.* 16:1045–1055, 1997.

Emens, L.A., D. W. Landers, and L. G. Moss. Hepatocyte nuclear factor 1 alpha is expressed in a hamster insulinoma line and transactivates the rat insulin I gene. *Proc. Natl. Acad. Sci. U. S. A.* 89:7300–7304, 1992.

Emery, P., B. Durand, B. Mach, and W. Reith. RFX proteins, a novel family of DNA binding proteins conserved in the eukaryotic kingdom. *Nucleic Acids Res.* 24:803–807, 1996.

Fajans, S. S. Maturity-onset diabetes of the young (MODY). *Diabetes Metab. Rev.* 5:579–606, 1989.

Froguel, P., H. Zouali, N. Vionnet, G. Velho, M. Vaxillaire, F. Sun, S. Lesage, M. Stoffel, J. Takeda, P. Passa, M. A. Permutt, J. S. Beckmann, G. I. Bell, and D. Cohen. Familial hyperglycemia due to mutations in glucokinase: definition of a subtype of diabetes mellitus. *N. Engl. J. Med.* 328:697–702, 1993.

Gladstone, P., and C. Pious. Stable variants affecting B cell alloantigens in human lymphoid cells. *Nature* 271:459–461, 1978.

Griscelli, C., B. Lisowska-Grospierre, F. Le Deist, A. Durandy, A. Marcadet, A. Fisher, C. De Preval, and B. Mach. Combined immunodeficiency with abnormal expression in MHC class II genes. *Clin. Immunol. Immunopathol.* 50: S140–S148, 1989.

Herrmann, B. G., and A. Kispert. The T genes in embryogenesis. *Trends Genet.* 10:280–286, 1994.

Herrmann, B. G., S. Labeit, A. Poustka, T. R. King, and H. Lehrach. Cloning of the T gene required in mesoderm formation in the mouse. *Nature* 343:617–622, 1990.

Hoffman, J. I. E. Incidence of congenital heart disease: I. Postnatal incidence. *Pediatr. Cardiol.* 16:103–113, 1995.

Holt, M., and S. Oram. Familial heart disease with skeletal malformations. *Br. Heart J.* 22:236–242, 1960.

Jones, K. L. *Smith's Recognizable Patterns of Human Malformation.* 4th ed. Philadelphia: W. B. Saunders Company, p. 272, 1988,

Kagoshima, H., K. Shigesada, M. Satake, Y. Ito, H. Miyoshi, M. Ohki, M. Pepling, and P. Gergen. The Runt domain identifies a new family of heteromeric transcriptional regulators. *Trends Genet.* 9:338–341, 1993.

Kara, C. J., and L. H. Glimcher. In vivo footprinting of MHC class II genes: bare promoters in the bare lymphocyte syndrome. *Science* 252:709–712, 1991a.

Kara, C. J., and L. H. Glimcher. Regulation of MHC class II gene transcription. *Curr. Opin. Immunol.* 3:16–21, 1991b.

Kara, C. J., and L. H. Glimcher. Three in vivo promoter phenotypes in MHC class II deficient combined immunodeficiency. *Immunogenetics* 37:227–230, 1993.

Kispert, A., B. Koschorz, and B. G. Herrmann. The T protein encoded by Brachyury is a tissue-specific transcription factor. *EMBO J.* 14:4763–4772, 1995.

Komori, T., H. Yagi, S. Nomura, A. Yamaguchi, K. Sasaki, K. Deguchi, Y. Shimizu, R. T. Bronson, Y.-H. Gao, M. Inada, M. Sato, R. Okamoto, Y. Kitamura, S. Yoshiki, and T. Kishimoto. Targeted disruption of Cbfa1 results in a complete lack of bone formation owing to maturational arrest of osteoblasts. *Cell* 89:755–764, 1997.

Lee, B., K. Thirunavukkarasu, L. Zhou, L. Pastore, A. Baldini, J. Hecht, V. Geoffroy, P. Ducy, and G. Karsenty. Missense mutations abolishing DNA binding of the osteoblast–specific transcription factor OSF2/CBFA1 in cleidocranial dysplasia. *Nat. Genet.* 16:307–310, 1997.

Li, Q. Y., R. A. Newbury-Ecob, J. A. Terrett, D. I. Wilson, A. R. J. Curtis, C. H. Yi, T. Gebuhr, P. J. Bullen, S. C. Robson, T. Strachan, D. Bonnet, S. Lyonnet, I. D. Young, J. A. Raeburn, A. J. Buckler, D. J. Law, J. D. Brook. Holt-Oram syndrome is caused by mutations in TBX5, a member of the Brachyury (T) gene family. *Nat. Genet.* 15:21–29, 1997.

Lisowska-Grospierre, B., D. Charron, C. De Preval, A. Durandy, C. Griscelli, and B. Mach. A defect in regulation of major histocompatibility complex class II gene expression in human HLA-DR negative lymphocytes from patients with combined immunodeficiency syndrome. *J. Clin. Invest.* 76:381–385, 1985.

Mundlos, S., F. Otto, C. Mundlos, J. B. Mulliken, A. S. Aylsworth, S. Albright, D. Lindhout, W. G. Cole, W. Henn, J. H. M. Knoll, M. J. Owen, R. Mertels-mann, B. U. Zabel, and B. R. Olsen. Mutations involving the transcription factor CBFA1 cause cleidocranial dysplasia. *Cell* 89:773–779, 1997.

Olson, E. N., and D. Srivastava. Molecular pathways controlling heart development. *Science* 272:671–676, 1996.

Otto, F., A. P. Thornell, T. Crompton, A. Denzel, K. C. Gilmour, J. R. Rosewell, G. W. H. Stamp, R. S. P. Beddington, S. Mundlos, B. R. Olsen, P. B. Selby, and M. J. Owen. Cbfa1, a candidate gene for cleidocranial dysplasia syndrome, is essential for osteoblast differentiation and bone development. *Cell* 89:765–771, 1997.

Pflugfelder, G. O., H. Roth, and B. Poeck. A homology domain shared between Drosophila optomotor-blind and mouse Brachyury is involved in DNA binding. *Biochem. Biophys. Res. Commun.* 186:918–925, 1992.

Polonsky, K. S. Lilly Lecture 1994: The beta-cell in diabetes: from molecular genetics to clinical research. *Diabetes* 44:705–717, 1995.

Polonsky, K. S., J. Sturis, and G. I. Bell. Non-insulin-dependent diabetes mellitus—a genetically programmed failure of the beta cell to compensate for insulin resistance. *N. Engl. J. Med.* 334:777–783, 1996.

Pontoglio, M., J. Barra, M. Hadchouel, A. Doyen, C. Kress, J. P. Bach, C. Babinet, and M. Yaniv. Hepatocyte nuclear factor 1 inactivation results in hepatic dysfunction, phenylketonuria, and renal Fanconi syndrome. *Cell* 84:575–585, 1996.

Reith, W., V. Steimle, and B. Mach. Molecular defects in the bare lymphocyte syndrome and regulation of MHC class II genes. *Immunol. Today* 16:539–546, 1995.

Reith, W., M. Kobr, P. Emery, B. Durand, C. A. Siegrist, and B. Mach. Cooperative binding between factors RFX and X2b to the X and X2 boxes of MHC class II promoters. *J. Biol. Chem.* 269:20020–20025, 1994a.

Reith, W., C. A. Siegrist, B. Durand, E. Barras, and B. Mach. Function of major histocompatibility complex class II promoters requires cooperative binding between factors RFX and NF-Y. *Proc. Natl. Acad. Sci. U.S.A.* 91:554–558, 1994b.

Reith, W., C. Ucla, E. Barras, A. Gaud, B. Durand, C. Herrero Sanchez, M. Kobr, and B. Mach. RFX1, a transactivator of hepatitis B virus enhancer I, belongs to a novel family of homodimeric and heterodimeric DNA-binding proteins. *Mol. Cell. Biol.* 14:1230–1244, 1994c.

Rodan, G. A., and S.-I. Harada. The missing bone. *Cell* 89:677–680, 1997.

Sillence, D. O., H. E. Ritchie, and P. B. Selby. Animal model: skeletal anomalies in mice with cleidocranial dysplasia. *Am. J. Med. Genet.* 27:75–85, 1987.

Steimle, V., B. Durand, E. Barras, M. Zufferey, M. R. Hadam, B. Mach, and W. Reith. A novel DNA-binding regulatory factor is mutated in primary MHC class II deficiency (bare lymphocyte syndrome). *Genes Dev.* 9:1021–1032, 1995.

Steimle, V., L. A. Otten, M. Zufferey, and B. Mach. Complementation cloning of an MHC class II transactivator mutated in hereditary MHC class II deficiency (or bare lymphocyte syndrome). *Cell* 75:135–146, 1993.

Temtamy, S. A., and V. A. McKusick. *The Genetics of Hand Malformations.* New York: Alan R. Liss, pp. 117–133, 1978.

Terrett, J. A., R. Newbury-Ecob, G. S. Cross, I. Fenton, J. A. Raeburn, I. D. Young, and J. D. Brook, J. D. Holt-Oram syndrome is a genetically heterogeneous disease with one locus mapping to human chromosome 12q. *Nat. Genet.* 6: 401–404, 1994.

Tronche, F., and M. Yaniv. HNF1, a homeoprotein member of the hepatic transcription regulatory network. *Bioessays* 14:579–587, 1992.

Vaxillaire, M., V. Boccio, A. Philippi, C. Vigouroux, J. Terwilliger, P. Passa, J. S. Beckmann, G. Velho, G. M. Lathrop, and P. Froguel. A gene for maturity onset diabetes of the young (MODY) maps to chromosome 12q. *Nat. Genet.* 9:418–423, 1995.

Wang, S., Q. Wang, B. E. Crute, I. N. Melnikova, S. R. Keller, and N. A. Speck. Cloning and characterization of subunits of the T-cell receptor and murine leukemai virus enhancer core-binding factor. *Mol. Cell. Biol.* 13:3324–3339, 1993.

Willison, K. The mouse Brachyury and mesoderm formation. *Trends Genet.* 6: 104–105, 1990.

Yamagata, K., H. Furata, N. Oda, P. J. Kaisaki, S. Menzel, N. J. Cox, S. S. Fajans, S. Signorini, M. Stoffel, and G. I. Bell. Mutations in the hepatocyte nuclear factor-4α gene in maturity-onset diabetes of the young (MODY). *Nature* 384: 458–460, 1996a.

Yamagata, K., N. Oda, P. J. Kaisaki, S. Menzel, H. Furata, M. Vaxillaire, L. Southam, R. D. Cox, G. M. Lathrop, V. V. Boriraj, X. Chen, N. J. Cox, Y. Oda, H. Yano, M. M. Le Beau, S. Yamada, H. Nishigori, J. Takeda, S. S. Fajans, A. T. Hattersley, N. Iwasaki, T. Hansen, O. Pedersen, K. S. Polonsky, R. C. Turner, G. Velho, J.-C. Chevre, P. Froguel, and G. I. Bell. Mutations in the hepatocyte nuclear factor-1α gene in maturity-onset diabetes of the young (MODY). *Nature* 384:455–458, 1996b.

Coactivators   13

In contrast to Chapters 5 through 12, which described genetic defects involving *trans*-acting factors that directly bind to DNA and either activate or repress the transcription of target genes, this chapter will focus on disorders involving mutations in genes encoding coactivators, proteins that exert their effects on transcription strictly via protein-protein interactions (see Chapter 3). Coactivators function by establishing physical interactions between sequence-specific DNA-binding proteins and the transcription initiation complex containing Pol II and associated general transcription factors. In addition, many coactivators contain catalytic domains involved in the enzymatic modification of other regulatory proteins or chromatin.

Both DNA-binding proteins and coactivators share in common the characteristic that they each regulate only a subset of the Pol II–transcribed sequences in the genome. Whereas the specificity of DNA-binding proteins is based on the presence of high-affinity binding-site sequences in proximity to target genes, the specificity of coactivator function must be based in turn on the nature of the DNA-binding proteins that have assembled at regulatory sequences. Because multiple, relatively low-affinity interactions may be involved in determining coactivator interactions, the rules defining coactivator specificity may be more difficult to delineate than those determining DNA-binding activity. On the other hand, it is likely that some high-affinity DNA-binding sites are functionally irrelevant because they are not in a context that allows coactivator recruitment, which is essential to link the DNA-binding activators to the transcriptional machinery. Because coactivators appear to participate in the regulation of genes by interacting with many different DNA-binding proteins, it appears (based on the two examples provided below), that deficiencies of these proteins may have even more global effects on development than the loss of any one of the DNA-binding proteins with which they interact.

X-Linked α-Thalassemia and Mental Retardation (ATR-X) Syndrome

Genetic defects that manifest X-linked inheritance are the most common cause of mental retardation in males, occurring with an incidence of 2 to 3 per 1000 individuals and including over 50 different syndromes (Gibbons et al., 1995c; Neri et al., 1994). Among these, the most common cause is the fragile X syndrome (see Chapter 4). A much less common cause of X-linked mental retardation, associated with α-thalassemia as well as facial and genital malformations (Table 13.1), has been designated the ATR-X syndrome (MIM 301040) (Gibbons et al., 1995a, 1995b; Weatherall et al., 1981; Wilkie et al., 1990). In this disorder, synthesis of α-globin in erythroid precursors is reduced by approximately one half, resulting in the presence of hemoglobin H (β-globin tetramer) precipitates in circulating erythrocytes (Wilkie et al., 1990). Because the genes encoding α-globin are located on chromosome 16, these results suggested the possibility that mutation in an X-linked *trans*-acting factor might have an adverse effect on the expression of α-globin and other gene products. Linkage analysis localized *ATR-X* to a 1.4-cM region of Xq13, and a 2-kb deletion that disrupted a previously identified gene designated *XNP* or *XH2* was identified in a single patient (Gibbons et al., 1995c). Although detected at low levels in many tissues, XH2/XNP mRNA was highly expressed in developing human and mouse brain, and was down-regulated following neuronal differentiation, leading to the suggestion that it might represent a candidate locus for X-linked mental retardation

TABLE 13.1. Clinical manifestations of ATR-X syndrome

Feature	% Individuals
Mental retardation	100
Genital abnormalities	96
Dysmorphic facies	93
Neonatal hypotonia	92
Skeletal abnormalities	91
Short stature	76
Microcephaly	71
Seizures	40

Data from Gibbons et al., 1995.

syndromes (Gecz et al., 1994; Stayton et al., 1994). Missense and nonsense mutations were then identified in *XH2/XNP* in a large number of males with ATR-X (Gibbons et al., 1995c; Picketts et al., 1996).

The 2-kb deletion reduced XH2/XNP mRNA to less than 1% of normal levels, suggesting that ATR-X syndrome results from loss-of-function mutations (Gibbons et al., 1995c). However, the fact that several splicing mutations result in up to 30% of normal levels of XH2/XNP mRNA indicates considerable sensitivity to reduction from wild-type expression levels (Picketts et al., 1996). Two first cousins with classic ATR-X syndrome were found to have a mutation that prevented normal splicing (Villard et al., 1996). In contrast, a distant cousin with dysmorphic facies and mental retardation but without evidence of α-thalassemia, was found to have 30% of normal mRNA levels, despite the same *ATRX* mutation. These results suggested, first, that differences in genetic background affected the ability to utilize the mutant splice site and, second, that a greater reduction in XH2/XNP levels was required to result in α-thalassemia as compared to mental retardation. More severe genital malformations also appear to be associated with complete loss-of-function *ATRX* alleles (Picketts et al., 1996). In one family the genital abnormalities were so severe that three out of four of the affected 46,XY individuals were reared as females (McPherson et al., 1995). In another family, *XH2* mutation was associated with 46,XY gonadal dysgenesis, dysmorphic facies, and mental retardation in the absence of α-thalassemia (Ion et al., 1996). In this family, a 4-bp deletion at an intron/exon boundary caused abnormal splicing that resulted in an 8-bp deletion in the XH2 mRNA, which generated a frameshift. The fact that α-globin synthesis was reduced only 15% suggests that the truncated protein still had residual activity with respect to *α-globin* gene transcription.

Sequence analysis of XH2/XNP (Gibbons et al., 1995c; Picketts et al., 1996; Stayton et al., 1994) revealed similarity to SNF2, a yeast coactivator protein containing DNA-dependent ATPase and DNA helicase domains that is believed to participate in transcription-associated chromatin remodeling (Hirschhorn et al., 1992; Peterson and Tamkun, 1995) (see Chapter 3). Analysis of alternatively spliced cDNA sequences and genomic DNA revealed that the human *ATRX* gene, consisting of 36 exons encompassing 300 kb, encodes proteins of 2288, 2337, and 2375 amino acids (Picketts et al., 1996). The central region of the proteins contains the helicase domains, whereas the amino-terminal half contains a putative nuclear localization signal and a sequence of 21 consecutive glutamic acid residues, and the carboxyl terminus is rich in glutamine residues and contains a 15-amino-acid sequence with similarity to family members (including SNF2) that are transcriptional regulators (Picketts et al.,

1996). Taken together with the finding of decreased α-globin expression in affected individuals, these results suggest that XH2/XNP may also be a transcriptional regulator. In contrast to other disorders involving mutations in genes encoding helicases of the SNF2 superfamily, the ATR-X syndrome is not associated with increased risk of malignancy, sensitivity to ultraviolet light, or chromosomal breakage, suggesting that XH2/XNP is not required for DNA repair, despite the fact that the helicase domain shows greatest similarity to the RAD54 DNA-repair protein (Stayton et al., 1994).

ATRX mutations in XH2 identified thus far are clustered in four regions of the gene encoding a zinc finger–like motif, the Glu_{21} region, the helicase domain, and the 15-amino-acid sequence that is found in other members of the SNF2 family (Fig. 13.1) (Gibbons et al., 1997). The zinc finger–like motif contains a Cys_4-His-Cys_3 structure that has been designated the PHD finger, which is composed of 50–80 amino acids and has been identified in over 40 proteins, including factors implicated in transcription-associated chromatin remodeling (Aasland et al., 1995).

α-thalassemia indicates that ATRX mutations affect expression of α-globin but not of β-globin, implying different mechanisms of transcriptional regulation for these two genes, which have been shown to employ the same battery of erythroid-specific transcriptional activators, EKLF, GATA-1, and NF-E2. However, the chromatin environment of the two gene clusters appears to differ significantly. Whereas the α-globin locus is in a constitutively "open" chromatin configuration (Vyas et al., 1992), the β-globin locus assumes an open chromatin configuration only in erythroid cells under the direction of the cis-acting locus control region (see Chapter 2). Furthermore, whereas the locus control region determines long-range chromatin structure and chromatin accessibility at the promoters of the β-globin locus (Forrester et al., 1990), the HS-40 enhancer of the α-globin locus does not have these properties (Craddock et al., 1995). Thus, chromatin remodeling may be performed by LCR-

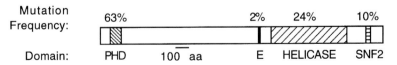

FIGURE 13-1. Mutations in XH2 in ATR-X syndrome. The protein is shown with PHD finger, polyglutamate (E), helicase, and SNF2 homology domains indicated at bottom with frequency of ATRX mutations identified in each domain indicated at top. (Data from Gibbons et al., 1997.)

associated factors at the β-globin locus, and by XH2/XNP (and other associated factors) at the α-globin locus. It will thus be of great interest to compare the chromatin structure of the α-globin locus in wild-type erythroid cells and cells lacking XH2/XNP.

Female carriers of *ATRX* mutations have significantly skewed X-inactivation patterns in tissues derived from mesoderm (blood), endoderm (buccal mucosa), and ectoderm (hair root) (Gibbons et al., 1992), indicating that there is a powerful negative selection against cells in which the wild-type allele has been inactivated by Lyonization. These results suggest that expression levels of XH2/XNP have a major impact on overall cellular growth rates, providing further evidence for a global role in transcriptional regulation. Establishing the many other genes that are regulated by XH2/XNP will be an important goal of future studies.

Rubinstein-Taybi Syndrome

Rubinstein and Taybi (1963) described a malformation syndrome (MIM 180849) characterized by broad thumbs and toes, dysmorphic facial features (including downslanting palpebral fissures, epicanthal folds, strabismus, maxillary hypoplasia, low-set and/or malformed ears, and beaked nose), mental retardation, and growth retardation (Fig. 13.2). Genital (male) and renal defects are also observed in at least half and cardiac defects are found in over one third of all patients (Stevens and Bhakta, 1995). The degree of mental retardation is significant, with most patients having an I.Q. of 40 to 50 (Jones, 1988). Among 243 children with Rubinstein-Taybi syndrome there were only two affected siblings (Simpson and Brissenden, 1973), thus giving a recurrence risk of approximately 1%, which although less than expected for a syndrome with Mendelian inheritance is substantially greater than the estimated general population incidence of 1 per 125,000 live births (Hennekam et al., 1990). Prior to molecular genetic analysis, Rubinstein-Taybi syndrome was listed in MIM as a recessive disorder (MIM 26860; McKusick, 1986), based perhaps on the report of an affected brother and sister from mating of consanguineous parents (Der Kaloustian et al., 1972), although the diagnosis of Rubinstein-Taybi syndrome in those children was questionable based on the clinical description.

The inheritance and genetic basis of Rubinstein-Taybi syndrome remained obscure until the identification of a patient with a *de novo* t(2; 16)(p13.3;p13.3) reciprocal translocation (Imaizumi and Kuroki, 1991). However, in the presence of a single case, it was impossible to determine whether the 2p13.3 or 16p13.3 chromosomal region might contain a gene for Rubinstein-Taybi syndrome. The subsequent identification of a pa-

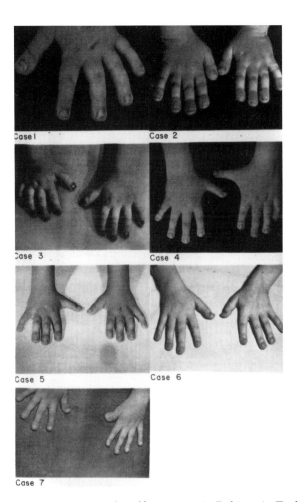

FIGURE 13-2. Digital malformations in Rubinstein-Taybi syndrome. Hands of the original patients reported by Rubenstein and Taybi are shown. Note the broad, radially deviated thumbs. (Reprinted with permission from Rubenstein and Taybi, 1963. Copyright ©1963 by the American Medical Association.)

tient with a *de novo* t(7;16)(q34;p13.3) reciprocal translocation strongly suggested that chromosome 16p13.3 contained the relevant locus (Tommerup et al., 1992). Using probes that were derived from the 16p13.3 region to which the two translocation breakpoints mapped, fluorescence *in situ* hybridization (FISH) revealed submicroscopic deletions on one copy of chromosome 16 in six of 24 patients (Bruening et al., 1993; Hennekam et al., 1993).

Although the presence of microdeletions and the complexity of the

Rubinstein-Taybi syndrome phenotype suggested the possibility of a contiguous gene syndrome, the fact that both translocation breakpoints mapped adjacent to a marker that was deleted in 25% of patients suggested that a single gene defect was responsible, with the remaining 75% of cases due to inactivating point mutations (Breuning et al., 1993). This prediction was validated by the identification of point mutations within the gene encoding the coactivator CBP (CREB [cyclic AMP response element binding protein] binding protein) (Petrij et al., 1995). Specifically, a protein truncation test was used to identify two nonsense mutations, Q136X and W357X. The resulting truncated proteins lack the majority of the 2441-amino-acid protein. Several of the microdeletions appeared to involve the entire CBP coding sequence. These results suggest that haploinsufficiency for CBP is the pathogenetic mechanism.

As described in Chapter 3, CBP has been implicated as coactivator for a number of essential transcriptional activators with known roles in cellular growth control, including CREB, CFOS, CJUN, CMYB, SAP1/ELK1, and nuclear hormone receptors (reviewed by Janknecht and Hunter, 1996). Furthermore, injection of anti-CBP antibodies into cells prevents mitogen-activated gene transcription (Arias et al., 1994). CBP can bind to transcriptional activators as well as to TFIIB (Kwok et al., 1994), thus providing a physical connection between sequence-specific DNA-binding proteins and general transcription factors of the transcription initiation complex. Despite the structural and functional similarities between CBP and the related protein P300 (see Chapter 3), the association of Rubinstein-Taybi syndrome with heterozygous loss-of-function mutations in *CBP* suggests that there are some functions that are unique to CBP.

Most individuals with Rubinstein-Taybi syndrome represent isolated cases. Although the demonstration of *de novo* mutations accounts for the absence of affected siblings, it does not account for the absence of affected offspring. There is no reported effect of the mutation on fertility and despite the presence of mental retardation, it is likely that some patients have offspring, yet parent-to-child transmission has not been reported. Furthermore, apparent monozygotic twins only one of whom was affected have been reported (reviewed by McKusick, 1986). Taken together with the tremendous clinical variability among affected individuals (Jones, 1988), these observations suggest the possibility that Rubinstein-Taybi syndrome may result from somatic (post-zygotic) mutations and that mutations that are transmitted through the germline result in embryonic lethality. However, monozygotic twins concordant for Rubinstein-Taybi syndrome have also been reported (Preis and Majewski, 1995; Robinson et al., 1993), arguing against this hypothesis. Analysis of mice in which one or both alleles of the *Cbp* gene have been inactivated by homologous recombination in embryonic stem cells will help to clarify the pathophysiology and genetics of Rubinstein-Taybi syndrome.

References

Aasland, R., T. J. Gibson, and A. F. Stewart. The PHD finger: implications for chromatin-mediated transcriptional regulation. *Trends Biochem. Sci.* 20:56–59, 1995.

Arias, J., A. S. Alberts, P. Brindle, F. X. Claret, T. Smeal, M. Karin, J. Feramisco, and M. Montminy. Activation of cAMP and mitogen responsive genes relies on a common nuclear factor. *Nature* 370:226–229, 1994.

Bruening, M. H., H. G. Dauwerse, G. Fugazza, J. J. Saris, L. Spruit, H. Wijnen, N. Tommerup, C. B. van der Hagen, K. Imaizumi, Y. Kuroki, M.-J. van den Boogaard, J. M. de Pater, E. C. M. Mariman, B. C. J. Hamel, H. Himmelbauer, A.-M. Frischauf, R. L. Stallings, G. C. Beverstock, G.-J. van Ommen, and R. C. M. Hennekam. Rubinstein-Taybi syndrome caused by submicroscopic deletions within 16p13. *Am. J. Hum. Genet.* 52:249–254, 1993.

Craddock, C. F., P. Vyas, J. A. Sharpe, H. Ayyub, W. G. Wood, and D. R. Higgs. Contrasting effects of alpha and beta-globin regulatory elements on chromatin structure may be related to their different chromosomal environments. *EMBO J.* 14:1718–1726, 1995.

Der Kaloustian, V. M., A. K. Afifi, A. A. Sinno, and J. Mire. The Rubinstein-Taybi syndrome: clinical and muscle electron microscopic study. *Am. J. Dis. Child.* 124:897–902, 1972.

Forrester, W. C., E. Epner, M. C. Driscoll, T. Enver, M. Brice, T. Papayannopoulou, and M. Groudine. A deletion of the human β-globin locus activation region causes a major alteration in chromatin structure and replication across the entire β-globin locus. *Genes Dev.* 4:1637–1649, 1990.

Gecz, J., H. Pollard, G. G. Consalez, L. Villard, C. Stayton, P. Millasseau, M. Khrestchatisky, and M. Fontes. Cloning and expression of the murine homologue of a putative human X-linked nuclear protein gene closely linked to PGK1 in Xq13.3. *Hum. Mol. Genet.* 3:39–44, 1994.

Gibbons, R. J., S. Bachoo, D. J. Picketts, S. Aftimos, B Asenbauer, J. Bergoffen, S. A. Berry, N. Dahl, A. Fryer, K. Keppler, K. Kurosawa, M. L. Levin, M. Masuno, G. Neri, M. E. Pierpont, S. F. Slaney, and D. R. Higgs. Mutations in a transcriptional regulator (hATRX) establish the functional signficance of a PHD-like domain. *Nat. Genet.* 17:146–148, 1997.

Gibbons, R. J., L. Brueton, V. J. Buckle, J. Burn, J. Clayton-Smith, B. C. Davison, R. J. Gardner, T. Homfray, L. Kearney, H. M. Kingston, R. Newbury-Ecob, M. E. P. Porteous, A. O. M. Wilkie, and D. R. Higgs. Clinical and hematologic aspects of the X-linked alpha-thalassemia/mental retardation syndrome (ATR-X). *Am. J. Med. Genet.* 55:288–299, 1995a.

Gibbons, R. J., D. J. Picketts, and D. R. Higgs. Syndromal mental retardation due to mutations in a regulator of gene expression. *Hum. Mol. Genet.* 4 Supplement:1705–1709, 1995b.

Gibbons, R. J., D. J. Picketts, L. Villard, and D. R. Higgs. Mutations in a putative global transcriptional regulator cause X-linked mental retardation with α-thalassemia (ATR-X syndrome). *Cell* 80:837–845, 1995c.

Gibbons, R. J., G. K. Suthers, A. O. M. Wilkie, V. J. Buckle, and D. R. Higgs. X-linked α thalassemia/mental retardation (ATR-X) syndrome: localisation to Xq12-21.31 by X-inactivation and linkage analysis. *Am. J. Hum. Genet.* 51: 1136–1149, 1992.

Hennekam, R. C. M., C. A. Stevens, and J. J. P. Van de Kamp. Etiology and recurrence risk in Rubinstein-Taybi syndrome. *Am. J. Med. Genet.* 6 (suppl.): 56–64, 1990.

Hennekam, R. C. M., M. Tilanus, B. C. J. Hamel, H. Voshart-van Heeren, E. C. M. Mariman, S. E. C. van Beeresum, M.-J. H. van den Boogaard, and M. H. Breuning. Deletion at chromosome 16p13.3 as a cause of Rubinstein-Taybi syndrome: clinical aspects. *Am. J. Hum. Genet.* 52:255–262, 1993.

Hirschhorn, J. N., S. A. Brown, C. D. Clark, and F. Winston. Evidence that SNF2/SWI2 and SNF5 activate transcription in yeast by altering chromatin structure. *Genes Dev.* 6:2288–2298, 1992.

Imaizumi, K., and Y. Kuroki. Rubinstein-Taybi syndrome with de novo reciprocal translocation t(2;16)(p13.3;p13.3). *Am. J. Med. Genet.* 38:636–639, 1991.

Ion, A., L. Telvi, J. L. Chaussain, F. Galacteros, J. Valayer, M. Fellous, and K. McElreavey. A novel mutation in the putative DNA helicase XH2 is responsible for male-to-female sex reversal associated with an atypical form of the ATR-X syndrome. *Am. J. Hum. Genet.* 58:1185–1191, 1996.

Janknecht, R., and T. Hunter. Transcriptional control: versatile molecular glue. *Curr. Biol.* 6:951–954, 1996.

Jones, K. L. *Smith's Recognizable Patterns of Human Malformation, 4th ed.* Philadelphia: W. B. Saunders Co., 1988.

Kwok, R. P. S., J. R. Lundblad, J. C. Chrivia, J. P. Richards, H. P. Bachinger, R. G. Brennan, S. G. E. Roberts, M. R. Green, and R. H. Goodman. Nuclear protein CBP is a coactivator for the transcription factor CREB. *Nature* 370: 223–226, 1994.

McKusick, V. A. *Mendelian Inheritance in Man: Catalogs of Autosomal Dominant, Autosomal Recessive, and X-linked Phenotypes, 7th ed.* Baltimore: The Johns Hopkins University Press, 1986.

McPherson, E. W., M. M. Clemens, R. J. Gibbons, and D. R. Higgs. X-linked alpha-thalassemia/mental retardation (ATR-X) syndrome: a new kindred with severe genital anomalies and mild hematologic expression. *Am. J. Med. Genet.* 55: 302–306, 1995.

Neri, G., P. Chiurazzi, J. F. Arena, and H. A. Lubs. XLMR genes: update 1994. *Am. J. Med. Genet.* 51:542–549, 1994.

Peterson, C. L., and J. W. Tamkun. The SWI-SNF complex: a chromatin remodeling machine? *Trends Biochem. Sci.* 20:143–146, 1995.

Petrij, F., R. H. Giles, H. G. Dauwerse, J. J. Saris, R. C. M. Hennekam, M. Masuno, N. Tommerup, G.-J. B. van Ommen, R. H. Goodman, D. J. M. Peters, and M. H. Breuning. Rubinstein-Taybi syndrome caused by mutations in the transcriptional co-activator CBP. *Nature* 376:348–351, 1995.

Picketts, D. J., D. R. Higgs, S. Bachoo, D. J. Blake, O. W. J. Quarrell, and R. J. Gibbons. *ATRX* encodes a novel member of the SNF2 family of proteins: mutations point to a common mechanism underlying the ATR-X syndrome. *Hum. Mol. Genet.* 5:1899–1907, 1996.

Preis, S., and F. Majewski. Monozygotic twins concordant for Rubinstein-Taybi syndrome: changing phenotype during infancy. *Clin. Genet.* 48:72–75, 1995.

Robinson, T. W., D. L. Stewart, and J. H. Hersh. Monozygotic twins concordant for Rubinstein-Taybi syndrome and implications for genetic counseling. *Am. J. Med. Genet.* 45:671–673, 1993.

Rubinstein, J. H., and H. Taybi. Broad thumbs and toes and facial abnormalities: a possible mental retardation syndrome. *Am. J. Dis. Child.* 105:588–608, 1963.

Simpson, N. E., and J. E. Brissenden. The Rubinstein-Taybi syndrome: familial and dermatoglyphic data. *Am. J. Hum. Genet.* 25:225–229, 1973.

Stayton, C. L., B. Dabovic, M. Gulisano, J. Gecz, V. Broccoli, S. Giovanazzi, M. Bossolasco, L. Monaco, S. Rastan, E. Boncinelli, M. E. Bianchi, and G. G. Consalez. Cloning and characterization of a new human Xq13 gene, encoding a putative helicase. *Hum. Mol. Genet.* 3:1957–1964, 1994.

Stevens, C. A., and M. G. Bhakta. Cardiac abnormalities in the Rubinstein-Taybi syndrome. *Am. J. Med. Genet.* 59:346–348, 1995.

Tommerup, N., C. B. van der Hagen, and A. Heiberg. Tentative assignment of a locus for Rubinstein-Taybi syndrome to 16p13.3 by a de novo reciprocal translocation t(7;16)(q34;p13.3). *Am. J. Med. Genet.* 44:237–241, 1992.

Villard, L., A. Toutain, A.-M. Lossi, J. Gecz, C. Houdayer, C. Moraine, and M. Fontes. Splicing mutation in the ATR-X gene can lead to dysmorphic mental retardation phenotype without α-thalassemia. *Am. J. Hum. Genet.* 58:499–505, 1996.

Vyas, P., M. A. Vickers, D. L. Simmons, H. Ayyub, C. F. Craddock, and D. R. Higgs. Cis-acting sequences regulating expression of the human α-globin cluster lie within constitutively open chromatin. *Cell* 69:781–793, 1992.

Weatherall, D J. , D. R. Higgs, C. Bunch, J. M. Old, D. M. Hunt, L. Pressley, J. B. Clegg, N. C. Bethlenfalvay, S. Sjolin, R. D. Koler, E. Magenis, J. L. Francis, and D. Bebbington. Hemoglobin H disease and mental retardation: a new syndrome or a remarkable coincidence? *N. Engl. J. Med.* 305:607–612, 1981.

Wilkie, A. O. M., H. C. Zeitlin, R. H. Lindenbaum, V. J. Buckle, N. Fischel-Ghodsian, D. H. K. Chui, D. Gardner-Medwin, M. H. MacGillivray, D. J. Weatherall, and D. R. Higgs. Clinical features and molecular analysis of the α thalassemia/mental retardation syndromes II. Cases without detectable abnormality of the α-globin complex. *Am. J. Hum. Genet.* 46:1127–1140, 1990.

General Transcription Factors **14**

As described in Chapter 1, formation of the transcription initiation complex is required for Pol II transcription of protein-coding genes. This complex contains, in addition to the multiple subunits of Pol II, a set of general transcription factors that includes TFIIA, TFIIB, TFIID, TFIIE, TFIIF, and TFIIH (Table 14.1). These factors are involved in DNA-protein interactions (TFIID only); protein-protein interactions with Pol II, DNA-binding transcriptional activators, and activator-bound coactivators; and enzymatic activities (DNA-dependent ATPase, DNA helicase, and protein kinase). In addition, TFIIH appears to play an essential role in both Pol II transcription and DNA repair processes (reviewed by Drapkin et al., 1994). (A complete description of DNA repair is beyond the scope of this book and interested readers should consult an authoritative text by Friedberg et al. [1995].) Among the many genes that encode components of the transcription initiation complex, germline mutations affecting only subunits of TFIIH have been identified as being responsible for heritable human disorders.

Disorders of Transcription and DNA Repair

Xeroderma pigmentosum, Cockayne syndrome, and trichothiodystrophy are three rare human disorders that demonstrate autosomal recessive inheritance and are associated with defects in nucleotide excision repair of DNA damaged by exposure either to ultraviolet light, resulting in the formation of pyrimidine dimers, or to certain chemical mutagens that form DNA adducts (reviewed by Aso et al., 1996; Cleaver and Kraemer, 1995). Xeroderma pigmentosum (MIM 278700) is characterized by extreme sensitivity of the skin to the ultraviolet rays of sunlight, pigmentation abnormalities, marked predisposition to skin cancer (2000–fold in-

TABLE 14.1. The general transcription factors of the transcription initiation complex (TIC)

Factor	Subunit Structure	Composition	Functional Properties
TFIIA	Heterodimer	14 kDa, 32 kDa	Interactions with TBP and activators
TFIIB	Monomer	35 kDa	Interactions with Pol II, TFIID, activators, and coactivators
TFIID	Multimer	TBP, TAFs	DNA binding, interactions with Pol II, TFIIB, activators, and coactivators
TFIIE	Heterodimer	34 kDa, 58 kDa	Required for promoter clearance
TFIIF	Heterodimer	30 kDa, 74 kDa	May help TFIIB recruit Pol II to TIC; phosphorylated by $TAF_{II}250$
TFIIH	Multimer	8 subunits	Required for promoter clearance
	XPB/ERCC3	89 kDa	DNA-dependent ATPase/DNA helicase
	XPD/ERCC2	80 kDa	DNA-dependent ATPase/DNA helicase
	P62	62 kDa	Not determined
	P44	44 kDa	Not determined; zinc finger protein; interacts with CSA
	P52	52 kDa	Not determined
	MO15/CDK7	38 kDa	Phosphorylation of Pol II CTD; CDK-activating kinase
	CYCLIN H	34 kDa	Regulation of CDK7 activity
	P34	34 kDa	Not determined; zinc finger protein

Adapted from Aso et al., 1996.

creased risk relative to the general population), and in some patients, neurological abnormalities. Genetic complementation analyses by somatic cell hybridization using fibroblasts from affected individuals have identified seven distinct complementation groups (XP-A through XP-G).

The prominent features of Cockayne syndrome (MIM 216400) are photosensitivity, dwarfism, microcephaly with severe mental retardation, deafness, pigmentary retinal degeneration and optic atrophy, skeletal abnormalities (disproportionately long extremities with flexion contractures), a wizened, precociously aged appearance, and premature death at a mean age of 12 years (Nance and Berry, 1992). Two complementation groups (CS-A and CS-B) have been identified. DNA repair of transcribed genes in wild-type cells has been shown to occur specifically on the DNA strand that is used as the mRNA template (Mellon et al., 1987), an observation that provided one of the first connections between DNA repair and transcription. The genetic defect in Cockayne syndrome has been proposed to eliminate the preferential repair of actively transcribed DNA sequences, based on the observation that in CS cells, UV-induced pyrimidine dimers within two actively transcribed genes were not repaired, whereas nucleotide excision repair in bulk DNA appeared to be normal (Venema et al., 1990).

Trichothiodystrophy is characterized by ichthyosis, sulfur-deficient brittle hair, dysmorphic facial features, and mental retardation. Cells from most patients with trichothiodystrophy were unable to complement XP-D cells (Stefanini et al., 1986). In addition to these three disorders, several patients with xeroderma pigmentosum (complementation groups XP-B, XP-D, and XP-G) also manifested features of Cockayne syndrome or trichothiodystrophy or both (reviewed by Aso et al., 1996; Wood, 1991).

Disease in Humans, Yeast, and Flies: *ERCC3/XPB, RAD25,* and *haywire*

In addition to studying defects in nucleotide excision repair in cells from patients, mutant UV-sensitive Chinese hamster ovary cell lines were identified and eight complementation groups established (Busch et al., 1989). The mutant cells have been screened for human DNA sequences capable of complementation, resulting in the identification of human *ERCC* (excision repair cross-complementing) genes. Furthermore, the *ERCC2, ERCC3,* and *ERCC4* genes were shown to correct the sensitivity to UV radiation and defective nucleotide excision repair in xeroderma pigmentosum cells of complementation groups XP-D, XP-B, and XP-F cells, respectively (Flejter et al., 1992; Sijbers et al., 1996; Weeda et al., 1990).

A splice junction mutation was identified in the *ERCC3* gene of the sole patient of the XP-B complementation group, who manifested features of both xeroderma pigmentosum and Cockayne syndrome (Weeda et al., 1990). The other *ERCC3* allele was not detectably expressed and the mutation responsible for its loss of expression was not identified. Analysis of the open reading frame in the wild-type *ERCC3* cDNA sequence revealed that it encoded a 782-amino-acid protein with a calculated molecular mass of 89 kDa. Database comparisons of the amino acid sequence revealed putative nucleotide binding and DNA helicase domains with homology to the *RAD3* gene product, which (as described below) is required for nucleotide excision repair in yeast and has known ATPase and DNA helicase activities (Weeda et al., 1990).

Subsequently, two siblings with xeroderma pigmentosum of the XP-B complementation group were identified. These siblings manifested a relatively mild phenotype consisting of mild cutaneous symptoms, no skin tumors even beyond the age of 40 years, late onset of neurological impairment, and no evidence of Cockayne syndrome (Vermeulen et al., 1994). As in the patient described above, only a single *ERCC3* allele was expressed, and it was found to contain a missense mutation within a domain conserved in *Drosophila*, mouse, and yeast homologues of ERCC3 (see below). Nucleotide excision repair activity was virtually absent in cells from the patient, a surprising finding given the mild cutaneous manifestations of defective DNA repair, suggesting that factors other than, or in addition to, nucleotide excision repair activity determine the frequency of skin cancer in XP patients (Vermeulen et al., 1994).

In contrast to the two mutations in *ERCC3/XPB* described above that result in xeroderma pigmentosum and Cockayne syndrome, two siblings from a consanguineous mating who were affected with trichothiodystrophy were found to be either homozygous or hemizygous for a T119P missense mutation in *ERCC3/XPB* (Weeda et al., 1997). Compared to other XP-B cells, fibroblasts from these individuals had much higher levels of DNA repair activity and resistance to ultraviolet light exposure, which presumably accounted for the absence of a xeroderma pigmentosum phenotype in these patients.

The *RAD25/SSL2* gene product, which is required for nucleotide excision repair and cell viability, was identified as the yeast homologue of ERCC3 based on a remarkable 55% amino acid identity (Gulyas and Donahue, 1992; Park et al., 1992). RAD25 was shown to possess single-stranded DNA-dependent ATPase and DNA helicase activities (Guzder et al., 1994). A temperature-sensitive mutant, *rad25-ts24*, exhibited a thermolabile transcriptional defect that could be corrected by addition of RAD25 protein, confirming its role as a general transcription factor (Guzder et al., 1994). Another mutant, *rad25-799am*, was defective in DNA repair but not in transcription, suggesting that the repair and transcriptional activities involve different domains of the protein. A lethal mutation in the ATP-binding domain was associated with transcription defects, suggesting that the ATPase/helicase activity of RAD25 may be essential for unwinding DNA at the transcription initiation site (Guzder et al., 1994; Park et al., 1992).

Purification of an 89-kDa subunit of human TFIIH revealed that its amino acid sequence was identical to that of the *ERCC3* gene product, indicating that the ERCC3 protein is a common factor for two important nuclear functions, nucleotide excision repair and transcription (Schaeffer et al., 1993). This conclusion was consistent with the genetic and biochemical analysis of *RAD25* mutants, which demonstrated that the yeast homologue of ERCC3 was required for both transcription and repair (Guzder et al., 1994; Park et al., 1992). In considering the phenotype of the XP-B patient in whom the first *ERCC3* mutation was identified, the sensitivity to UV light and predisposition to skin cancer are likely to reflect the defect in DNA repair, whereas the malformations associated with Cockayne syndrome are likely to reflect defects in gene expression.

The *haywire* gene of *Drosophila melanogaster* encodes a protein with 66% amino acid identity to ERCC3 and 50% identity to RAD25 (Mounkes et al., 1992). Although many *haywire* alleles result in autosomal recessive lethality, viable alleles are associated with sensitivity to UV irradiation in both the hemizygous and heterozygous state, and progeny of females carrying a maternal effect allele manifested central nervous system defects (hence, *haywire*). The observation that most *haywire* alleles were lethal in the homozygous state points to the essential nature of the gene product and may explain in part why xeroderma pigmentosum, Cockayne syndrome, and trichothiodystrophy are such rare human disorders, each having a population incidence of less than 1 in 100,000. The structural and functional similarities between the *ERCC3*, *haywire,* and *RAD25* gene products suggest that the role of this protein in DNA repair and transcription, and thus the biochemical pathways in which it participates, have been highly conserved over the billion years of eukaryotic evolution.

ERCC2/XPD

The *ERCC2* gene product was shown to correct the sensitivity to ultraviolet irradiation and defective nucleotide excision repair activity of XP-D cells (Flejter et al., 1992). As described above, the *Saccharomyces cerevisiae RAD3* gene product contains DNA-dependent ATPase and DNA helicase activity and was identified as the yeast homologue of ERCC2 (Sung et al., 1993; reviewed by Friedberg et al., 1992). Furthermore, expression of the human *ERCC2/XPD* gene in yeast rescued the lethal phenotype associated with mutations in *RAD3* (Sung et al., 1993). Biochemical analysis of yeast Pol II initiation factor b, a pentameric complex that is functionally analagous to mammalian TFIIH, revealed that the amino acid sequence of one subunit was identical to the polypeptide encoded by the open reading frame of the *RAD3* gene (Feaver et al., 1993). Furthermore, factor b interacted specifically with SSL2, the protein product of the *RAD25* gene that is homologous to the human ERCC3/XPB protein.

RAD3 is an essential yeast gene, but nonlethal mutations have been identified. *rad3-21* mutant cells have markedly increased sensitivity to ultraviolet radiation, indicating defective nucleotide excision repair, due to the substitution of glutamic acid for a conserved lysine residue within the putative nucleotide-binding domain. However, factor b transcriptional activity was normal in *rad3-21* mutant cell extracts (Feaver et al., 1993). Taken together these results suggest that (1) the essential requirement for RAD3 may not be related to its involvement in nucleotide excision repair, but may instead reflect its involvement in transcription, and (2) the transcriptional activity of RAD3 may not require its ATPase/ DNA helicase activity. These results thus stand in contrast to the mutation in the ATP-binding domain of RAD25 described above, which was associated with lethality and transcriptional defects. These results suggest that the helicase activities of RAD3 and RAD25 may be specialized for use in nucleotide excision repair and transcription, respectively.

ERCC6/CSB and CSA

As described above, fibroblasts from patients with Cockayne syndrome were shown to be specifically defective in the preferential repair of transcribed DNA (Venema et al., 1990; van Hoffen et al., 1993). The 1493-amino-acid product of the *ERCC6* gene, another protein that contains a putative DNA helicase domain, was shown to functionally complement the repair defect in CS-B cells that was due to mutations in the *ERCC6* gene (Troelstra al., 1992). Examination of the sequence of ERCC6 also revealed extensive similarity with the yeast SNF2 family of coactivators (see Chapter 3), suggesting that ERCC6 may also have a direct role in transcription.

   Identification of a gene that complemented the defect of CS-A cells revealed that it encoded a 396-amino-acid WD-repeat protein (Henning et al., 1995). In CS-A cell lines derived from two affected siblings, 279-bp and 81-bp deletions were identified within the coding region of c-DNAs presumably derived from the two *CSA* alleles. However, because these children were the products of a consanguineous mating and therefore likely to be homozygous for a single mutation (identity by descent), and because both deletions had the same 3' endpoint, it was proposed that a splice site mutation might result in mRNA missing either one (81 bp) or two (279 bp) upstream exons (Henning et al., 1995). In several other recessive disorders, compound heterozygosity has been reported in affected offspring of consanguineous matings; thus, analysis of genomic DNA sequences is required to resolve this issue. CSA protein was shown to physically interact with CSB, both in vitro and in cotransfected tissue culture cells. CSA also physically interacted with P44, the 44-kDa subunit of human TFIIH. The amino-terminal 146 amino acids of CSA, containing the first two of five WD repeats, were sufficient for interaction with CSB or P44 (Henning et al., 1995). This result is consistent with the observation that WD repeat proteins are often components of multiprotein complexes (Neer et al., 1994). Furthermore, the *Drosophila* coactivator dTAF$_{II}$80, which interacts with TFIID, and the yeast TUP1 transcriptional repressor, are also WD repeat proteins (Dynlacht et al., 1993; Keleher et al., 1992).

Taken together, these studies again suggest that mutations that result in Cockayne syndrome may have direct effects on transcription. One possibility that is suggested by the homology of CSB with SNF2 is that CSA and CSB are involved in modulating chromatin structure during transcription and repair (Christians and Hanawalt, 1994; Henning et al., 1995). Transcription of reporter genes transfected into CS-A or CS-B cells was reported to be decreased (Henning et al., 1995), which is not consistent with a chromatin effect, because in this case transcription presumably occurs from naked DNA rather than a chromatin template. However, nuclear proteins may associate with the transfected DNA, and DNA helicase activity would likely be required to transcribe RNA from the supercoiled plasmid DNA. In any case, these results provide further support that the CSA and CSB proteins are required for optimal Pol II transcription.

As described above, some xeroderma pigmentosum patients in groups XP-B, XP-D, and XP-G manifest clinical signs of Cockayne syndrome. *XPB* and *XPD* mutations affect subunits of TFIIH and thus affect basal transcription. XPB/ERCC3, XPD/ERCC2, and P44 all interact with each other (Iyer et al., 1996) and P44 interacts with CSA (Henning et al., 1995). Furthermore, the XPG protein has been shown to physically interact with CSB (which interacts with CSA) and with multiple subunits of TFIIH (Iyer et al., 1996), providing a link between XPG and transcription. These results suggest the existence of a large multiprotein complex containing CSA, CSB, and XPG, which associates with TFIIH (including XPB/ERCC3 and XPD/ERCC2) both physically and functionally in order to couple transcription and DNA repair. One hypothesis to explain the coupling of transcription and repair is that the CSA-CSB-XPG complex displaces stalled Pol II at sites of DNA damage and recruits the ERCC/XP proteins involved in nucleotide excision repair (Drapkin et al., 1994). During this process, components of "holoTFIIH" such as XPB/ERCC3 and XPD/ERCC2 may dissociate from the transcriptional apparatus and reassociate with components of the nucleotide excision "repairosome" (Svejstrup et al., 1995).

Deletion of a Gene Encoding P44 in Patients with Spinal Muscular Atrophy

Spinal muscular atrophy is a lethal autosomal recessive disorder characterized by degeneration of anterior horn cells of the spinal cord, resulting in skeletal muscle denervation and paralysis. In type I spinal muscular atrophy, or Werdnig-Hoffmann disease, onset of symptoms occurs within the first 3 months of life, with death by age 2 years. Large-scale deletions of DNA at chromosome 5q13.3 have been identified in these patients (Melki et al., 1994). Two genes have been identified in the deletion interval: *NAIP*, which encodes the neuronal apoptosis inhibitory protein, and *SMN*, the survival motor neuron gene (Lefebvre et al., 1995; Roy et al., 1995). However, the presence or absence of these two genes does not appear sufficient to determine the phenotype, suggesting the presence of other genes in the deletion interval. This hypothesis was confirmed by the identification of not one but two genes encoding the P44 subunit of TFIIH within the deletion interval (Burglen et al., 1997). The proteins encoded by the telomeric (*P44T*) and centromeric (*P44C*) genes differ by three amino acids and *P44T* is deleted in patients with Werdnig-Hoffman disease. However, TFIIH composition, transcription, and DNA repair activities appear to be normal in lymphoblasts from affected individuals (Burglen et al., 1997). These results suggest that a single *P44* gene may be sufficient for normal TFIIH function and that deletion of *P44T* may not contribute to the pathogenesis of Werdnig-Hoffman disease, although the possibility of specific effects within anterior horn cells cannot be excluded.

Transcription and Repair Are Linked in All Species

The studies described in this chapter suggest an intimate relationship between transcription and repair that has been maintained throughout the course of eukaryotic evolution. DNA damage, such as the formation of a pyrimidine dimer, is known to have an inhibitory effect on transcription by preventing Pol II progression and thus blocking elongation of nascent RNA transcripts (Sauerbier and Hercules, 1978). Blocked transcription of essential genes may interfere with the viability of quiescent cells, and DNA damage may also interfere with DNA replication in dividing cells (Drapkin et al., 1994). However, as described above for RAD3 and RAD25, there appears to be a strong association specifically between transcriptional activity and viability. Pyrimidine dimers in the actively transcribed *DHFR* gene of Chinese hamster ovary cells were repaired with fivefold greater efficiency relative to the genome as a whole (Bohr et al., 1985) and preferential repair was limited to the transcription template strand (Mellon et al., 1987). Similar observations were made in *E. coli* (Mellon and Hanawalt, 1989), indicating that the connection between transcription and repair is universal (Drapkin et al., 1994).

References

Aso, T., A. Shilatifard, J. W. Conaway, and R. C. Conaway. Transcription syndromes and the role of RNA polymerase II general transcription factors in human disease. *J. Clin. Invest.* 97:1561–1569, 1996.

Bohr, V. A., C. A. Smith, D. S. Okumoto, and P. C. Hanawalt. DNA repair in an active gene: removal of pyrimidine dimers from the DHFR gene of CHO cells is much more efficient than in the genome overall. *Cell* 40:359–369, 1985.

Burglen, L., T. Seroz, P. Miniou, S. Lefebvre, P. Burlet, A. Munnich, E. V. Pequignot, J.-M. Egly, and J. Melki. The gene encoding p44, a subunit of the transcription factor TFIIH, is involved in large-scale deletions associated with Werdnig-Hoffmann disease. *Am. J. Hum. Genet.* 60:72–79, 1997.

Busch, D., C. Greiner, K. Lewis, R. Ford, G. Adair, and L. H. Thompson. Summary of complementation groups of UV-sensitive CHO cell mutants isolated by large-scale screening. *Mutagenesis* 4:349–354, 1989.

Christians, F. C., and P. C. Hanawalt. Repair in ribosomal RNA genes is deficient in xeroderma pigmentosum group C and Cockayne's syndrome cells. *Mutat. Res.* 323:179–187, 1994.

Cleaver, J. E., and K. H. Kraemer. Xeroderma pigmentosum and Cockayne syndrome. In: *The Metabolic and Molecular Bases of Inherited Disease*, C. R. Scriver, A. L. Beaudet, W. S. Sly, and D. Valle, eds. New York: McGraw-Hill, pp. 4393–4419, 1995.

Drapkin, R., A. Sancar, and D. Reinberg. Where transcription meets repair. *Cell* 77:9–12, 1994.

Dynlacht, B. D., R. O. J. Werinzieri, A. Admon, and R. Tjian. The dTAF$_{II}$80 subunit of Drosophila TFIID contains β-transducin repeats. *Nature* 363:176–179, 1993.

Feaver, W. J., J. Q. Svejstrup, L. Bardwell, A. J. Bardwell, S. Buratowski, K. D. Gulyas, T. F. Donahue, E. C. Friedberg, and R. D. Kornberg. Dual roles of a multiprotein complex from S. cerevisiae in transcription and DNA repair. *Cell* 75:1379–1387, 1993.

Flejter, W. L., L. D. McDaniel, D. Johns, E. C. Friedberg, and R. A. Schultz. Correction of xeroderma pigmentosum complementation group D mutant cell phenotypes by chromosome and gene transfer: involvement of the human ERCC2 DNA repair gene. *Proc. Natl. Acad. Sci. U.S.A.* 89:261–265, 1992.

Friedberg, E. C. Xeroderma pigmentosum, Cockayne's syndrome, helicases, and DNA repair: what's the relationship? *Cell* 71:887–889, 1992.

Friedberg, E. C., G. C. Walker, and W. Siede. *DNA Repair and Mutagenesis*. Washington D.C.: American Society for Microbiology, pp. 655–658, 1995.

Gulyas, K. D., and T. F. Donahue. SSL2, a suppressor of a stem-loop mutation in the HIS4 leader encodes the yeast homolog of human ERCC-3. *Cell* 69:1031–1042, 1992.

Guzder, S. N., P. Sung, V. Bailly, L. Prakash, and S. Prakash. RAD25 is a DNA helicase required for DNA repair and RNA polymerase II transcription. *Nature* 369:578–581, 1994.

Henning, K. A., L. Li, N. Iyer, L. D. McDaniel, M. S. Reagan, R. Legerski, R. A. Schultz, M. Stefanini, A. R. Lehmann, L. V. Mayne, and E. C. Friedberg. The Cockayne syndrome group A gene encodes a WD repeat protein that interacts with CSB protein and a subunit of RNA polymerase II TFIIH. *Cell* 82: 555–564, 1995.

Iyer, N., M. S. Reagan, K. J. Wu, B. Canagarajah, and E. C. Friedberg. Interactions involving the human RNA polymerase II transcription/nucleotide excision repair complex TFIIH, the nucleotide excision repair protein XPG, and Cockayne syndrome group B (CSB) protein. *Biochemistry* 35:2157–2167, 1996.

Keleher, C. A., M. J. Redd, J. Schultz, M. Carlson, and A. D. Johnson. Ssn6–Tup1 is a general repressor of transcription in yeast. *Cell* 68:709–719, 1992.

Lefebvre, S., L. Burglen, S. Reboullet, O. Clermont, P. Burlet, L. Viollet, B. Benichou, C. Cruaud, P. Millasseau, M. Zeviani, D. Le Paslier, J. Frezal, D. Cohen, J. Weissenbach, A. Munnich, and J. Melki. Identification and characterization of a spinal muscular atrophy-determining gene. *Cell* 80:155–165, 1995.

Melkie, J., S. Lefebvre, L. Burglen, P. Burlet, O. Clearmont, P. Millasseau, S. Reboullet, B. Benichou, M. Zeviani, D. Le Paslier, D. Cohen, J. Weissenbach, and A. Munnich. De novo and inherited deletions of the 5q13 region in spinal muscular atrophies. *Science* 264:1474–1477, 1994.

Mellon, I., and P. C. Hanawalt. Induction of the Escherichia coli lactose operon selectively increases repair of its transcribed DNA strand. *Nature* 342:95–98, 1989.

Mellon, I., G. Spivak, and P. C. Hanawalt. Selective removal of transcription-blocking DNA damage from the transcribed strand of the mammalian DHFR gene. *Cell* 51:241–248, 1987.

Mounkes, L. C., R. S. Jones, B.-C. Liang, W. Gelbart, and M. T. Fuller. A Drosophila model for xeroderma pigmentosum and Cockayne's syndrome: haywire encodes the fly homolog of ERCC3, a human excision repair gene. *Cell* 71:925–937, 1992.

Nance, M. A., and S. A. Berry. Cockayne syndrome: review of 140 cases. *Am. J. Med. Genet.* 42:68–84, 1992.

Neer, E. J., C. J. Schmidt, R. Nambudripad, and T. F. Smith. The ancient regulatory-protein family of WD-repeat proteins. *Nature* 371:297–300, 1994.

Park, E., S. N. Guzder, M. H. Koken, I. Jaspers-Dekker, G. Weeda, J. H. Hoeijmakers, S. Prakash, and L. Prakash. RAD25 (SSL2), the yeast homolog of the human xeroderma pigmentosum group B DNA repair gene, is essential for viability. *Proc. Natl. Acad. Sci. U. S. A.* 89:11416–11420, 1992.

Roy, N., M. S. Mahadevan, M. McLean, G. Shutler, Z. Yaraghi, R. Farahani, S. Baird, A. Besner-Johnston, C. Lefebvre, X. Kang, M. Salih, H. Aubry, K. Tamai, X. Guan, P. Ioannou, T. O. Crawford, P. J. De Jong, L. Surh, J.-E Ikeda, R. E. Korneluk, and A. MacKenzie. The gene for neuronal apoptosis inhibitory protein is partially deleted in individuals with spinal muscular atrophy. *Cell* 80:167–178, 1995.

Sauerbier, W., and K. Hercules. Gene and transcription unit mapping by radiation effects. *Annu. Rev. Genet.* 12:329–262, 1978.

Schaeffer, L., R. Roy, S. Humbert, V. Moncollin, W. Vermeulen, J. H. J. Hoeijmakers, P. Chambon, and J.-M. Egly. DNA repair helicase: a component of BTF2 (TFIIH) basic transcription factor. *Science* 260:58–63, 1993.

Sijbers, A. M., W. L. de Laat, R. R. Ariza, M. Biggerstaff, Y.-F. Wei, J. G. Moggs, K.C. Carter, B. K. Shell, E. Evans, M. C. de Jong, S. Rademakers, J. de Rooij, N. G. Jaspers, J. H. J. Hoeijmakers, and R. D. Wood. Xeroderma pigmentosum group F caused by a defect in a structure-specific DNA repair endonuclease. *Cell* 86:811–822, 1996.

Stefanini, M., P. Lagomarsini, C. F. Arlett, S. Marinoni, C. Borrone, F. Crovato, G. Trevisan, G. Cordone, and F. Nuzzo. Xeroderma pigmentosum (complementation group D) mutation is present in patients affected by trichothiodystrophy with photosensitivity. *Hum. Genet.* 74:107–112, 1986.

Sung, P., V. Bailly, C. Weber, L. H. Thompson, L. Prakash, and S. Prakash. Human xeroderma pigmentosum group D gene encodes a DNA helicase. *Nature* 365:852–855, 1993.

Svejstrup, J. Q., Z. Wang, W. J. Feaver, X Wu, T. F Donahue, E. C. Friedberg, and R. D. Kornberg. Different forms of RNA polymerase transcription factor IIH (TFIIH) for transcription and DNA repair: holoTFIIH and a nucleotide repair repairosome. *Cell* 80:21–28, 1995.

Troelstra, C., A. van Gool, J. de Wit, W. Vermeulen, D. Bootsma, and J. H. J. Hoeijmakers. ERCC6, a member of a subfamily of putative helicases, is involved in Cockayne's syndrome and preferential repair of active genes. *Cell* 71: 939–953, 1992.

van Hoffen, A., A. T. Natarajan, L. V. Mayne, A. A. van Zeeland, L. H. F. Mullenders, and J. Venema. Deficient repair of the transcribed strand of active genes in Cockayne's syndrome. *Nucleic Acids Res.* 21:5890–5895, 1993.

Venema, J., L. H. F. Mullenders, A. T. Natarajan, A. A. van Zeeland, and L. V. Mayne. The genetic defect in Cockayne syndrome is associated with a defect in repair of UV-induced DNA damage in transcriptionally active DNA. *Proc. Natl. Acad. Sci. U.S.A.* 87:4707–4711, 1990.

Vermeulen, W., R. J. Scott, S. Rodgers, H. J. Muller, J. Cole, C. F. Arlett, W. J. Kleijer, D. Bootsma, J. H. Hoeijmakers, and G. Weeda. Clinical heterogeneity within xeroderma pigmentosum associated with mutations in the DNA repair and transcription gene ERCC3. *Am. J. Hum. Genet.* 54:191–200, 1994.

Weeda, G., E. Eveno, I. Donker, W. Vermeulen, O. Chevallier-Lagente, A. Taieb, A. Stary, J. H. J. Hoeijmakers, M. Mezzina, and A. Sarasin. A mutation in the *XPB/ERCC3* DNA repair transcription gene, associated with trichothiodystrophy. *Am. J. Hum. Genet.* 60:320–329, 1997.

Weeda, G., R. C. A. van Ham, W. Vermeulen, D. Bootsma, A. J. van der Eb, and J. H. J. Hoeijmakers. A presumed DNA helicase encoded by ERCC-3 is involved in the human repair disorders xeroderma pigmentosum and Cockayne's syndrome. *Cell* 62:777–791, 1990.

Wood, R. D. Seven genes for three diseases. *Nature* 350:190, 1991.

15 Somatic Cell Genetic Disease: Cancer

The molecular pathophysiology of carcinogenesis is based to a great extent on somatic mutation. Through a process of clonal selection, tumor cells accumulate mutations that increase their ability to proliferate. These mutations are of two general types: (1) activating mutations in growth-promoting genes known as oncogenes and (2) inactivating mutations in growth-restricting genes known as tumor suppressor genes. The vast majority of these mutations occur within the tumor cells only, either spontaneously or in response to an environmental mutagen. In the case of the tumor suppressor genes, however, rare germline loss-of-function mutations can result in a hereditary predisposition to cancer, as described for the *WT1* gene in the WAGR syndrome (see Chapter 6). In these cases, the affected individual is heterozygous for an inactivating mutation in all cells of the body. When a somatic mutation occurs on the second allele within a target cell, both alleles have been inactivated and the process of oncogenesis is initiated, in accordance with the "two-hit" model originally proposed by Knudson (1971; Knudson et al., 1975). For these affected individuals, the risk of developing a cancer (such as Wilms tumor in patients heterozygous for deletion of *WT1*) is greatly increased, approaching 100% in some cases. In addition to an extremely high incidence of tumorigenesis, the tumors appear at an earlier age, are bilateral in paired organs, and multifocal. In unaffected individuals, the presence of an inactivating somatic mutation in a single *WT1* allele in one or more cells is of no consequence; it is only in the rare case where somatic mutations have inactivated both alleles in a single cell that a Wilms tumor will develop. In contrast, in WAGR syndrome patients, any somatic mutation that inactivates the remaining *WT1* allele will result in tumorigenesis.

Germline mutations have also been identified in two other tumor suppressor genes that encode transcription factors, *RB* and *TP53*. Hereditary cancer predisposition syndromes involving mutations in these genes will be described below, followed by a discussion of some of the somatic mutations in tumors that involve genes encoding transcription factors. It should be noted that many oncogenes and tumor suppressor genes do not encode transcription factors, although in many cases they do encode signaling molecules such as growth factor receptors and kinases that regulate the expression of transcription factors that are required for cellular proliferation. The discussion presented in this chapter, however, will be limited to an illustrative (rather than comprehensive) discussion of the role of transcription factors in cancer. (In keeping with the genetic nomenclature utilized throughout the text, proteins will be designated by capital letters, so that the more familiar p16, p21, p53, etc. will instead be presented as P16, P21, P53, etc.)

Germline and Somatic Mutations in Tumor Suppressor Genes Encoding Transcription Factors

RB

Predisposition to retinoblastoma can also be inherited as an autosomal dominant trait (MIM 180200), due to a germline deletion of one copy of the *RB* tumor supressor gene (Friend et al., 1987). In addition to retinoblastoma, affected heterozygotes also have a 500-fold increased risk of osteogenic sarcoma. In contrast, mice that are heterozygous for a null allele at the *Rb* locus develop pituitary and thyroid tumors (Hu et al., 1994; Jacks et al., 1992; Williams et al., 1994). The limited tumor types seen in humans and mice lacking RB may reflect functional redundancy in most cells between RB and the structurally related proteins P130 and P107.

The *RB* gene product has several important qualities. First, RB and related proteins (P130 and P107) appear to play a key role in regulating the cell cycle, and thus cellular proliferation, in all cells. Second, RB is a transcription factor that does not bind to DNA but instead exerts its biological effects by binding to and regulating the activity of other transcription factors (see Chapter 3). Third, RB is a target for the transforming proteins of several tumor viruses, including E7 of human papilloma virus (HPV) (Dyson et al., 1989), T antigen of simian virus 40 (SV40) (DeCaprio et al., 1988), and E1A of adenovirus (Whyte et al., 1988).

The principal target of RB appears to be E2F, a family of heterodimeric transcription factors that bind to the sequence 5'-TTTTCGCG-3' present in promoter or enhancer elements of genes whose protein products are required for cell division such as C-MYC, CDC2, cyclin A, cyclin D, cyclin E, dihydrofolate reductase, DNA polymerase α, proliferating cell nuclear antigen, ribonucleotide reductase, thymidine kinase, thymidylate synthetase, and E2F-1 itself (Chellappan et al., 1991; reviewed by Sherr, 1996; Slansky and Farnham, 1996). RB inhibits the ability of E2F to activate transcription (Hiebert et al., 1992) and actively represses transcription of genes to which E2F has bound (Weintraub et al., 1992, 1995). Recent studies indicate that interaction of RB with HBRM/BRG-1, a component of the SWI/SNF complex (see Chapter 3), is required for transcriptional repression of genes containing binding sites for E2F1 (Trouche et al., 1997). The demonstration that binding of RB protects E2F1 from proteolytic degradation (Hofmann et al., 1996; Hateboer et al., 1996) provides further evidence that active transcriptional repression by the E2F1-RB complex is important for proper cell cycle control. RB that has been phosphorylated by the cyclin D_1-CDK4 (cyclin-dependent kinase) complex is no longer capable of binding to E2F; the latter can then activate transcription of genes necessary for S phase initiation and progression (reviewed by Weinberg, 1995). Cell cycle progression is therefore determined by the phosphorylation status of RB, which is dependent on CDK4 activity, which, in turn, is dependent on the balance between its positive regulator, cyclin D, and the CDK inhibitors, P16 and P21 (see Fig. 15.1).

Whereas germline mutations in *RB* are rare, somatic mutations in CDK4, cyclin D_1, P16, or RB have been detected in almost every human cancer that has been analyzed (reviewed by Levine, 1997). Thus, RB function can be inactivated by several different mechanisms: (1) germline *RB* mutation/deletion; (2) somatic *RB* mutation/deletion; (3) overexpression of CDK4 or cyclin D by gene amplification; (4) loss of P16 expression; (5) expression of E1A, T antigen, or E7 (in cells infected by adenovirus, SV40, or HPV, respectively). In addition to germline mutations that eliminate or inactivate the RB coding sequence, mutations in the *RB* promoter have also been described that may prevent the binding of factors required for transcription of the gene (Sakai et al., 1991) and thus (to belabor the nomenclature established in Chapters 1 through 4) represent examples of a *cis*-acting mutation affecting expression of a *trans*-acting factor.

The results presented above suggest that E2F functions as a growth-promoting oncogene. However, mice homozygous for a null mutation in the *E2f1* gene develop atrophy in some tissues and abnormal cellular proliferation and tumor formation in other tissues, indicating that *E2f1* functions both as an oncogene and a tumor suppressor gene (Field et al., 1996; Yamasaki et al., 1996). This is not surprising considering the fact that E2F-1 activates or represses transcription depending on whether or

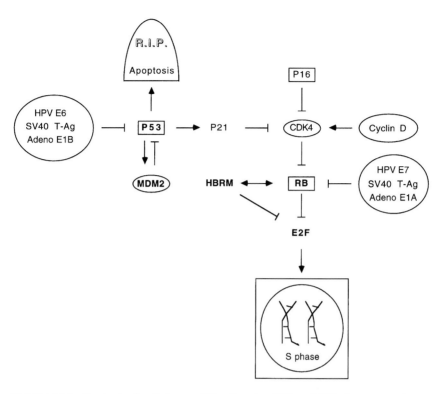

FIGURE 15-1. Control of cellular proliferation by P53 and RB. Arrows and perpendicular lines indicate positive and negative regulation, respectively. Known oncogenes and tumor suppressor genes are indicated by ovals and rectangles, respectively. Transcription factors are shown in bold type. Three outcomes are possible: apoptosis, cell cycle arrest (not shown), and progression to S phase. Only selected components of the pathways are shown.

not RB is bound. These data once again suggest that the phosphorylation status of RB plays an essential role in determining the biological function of E2F and the level of cellular proliferation in a given tissue.

P53

Germline mutations: Li-Fraumeni syndrome. Heterozygous germline mutations of the *TP53* gene have been identified in patients with the rare Li-Fraumeni syndrome, which is characterized by a predisposition to multiple tumor types, including adrenocortical carcinoma, breast carcinoma, leukemia, osteosarcoma, and soft tissue sarcoma (Li and Fraumeni, 1969; Malkin et al., 1990; reviewed by Malkin, 1994). Affected individuals may develop multiple primary tumors while still in childhood (Strong et al., 1987). The penetrance of the mutant allele is very high: over 90% of obligate heterozygotes develop cancer by age 70 years (Malkin, 1994). Mice that are homozygous for a null allele at the *p53* locus also have a greatly increased incidence of tumor formation (Donehower et al., 1992). The range of tumor types that develop in *p53*$^{-/-}$ mice is strongly influenced by genetic background (Table 15.1). As in the case of WT1 and RB, P53 functions as a tumor suppressor. However, whereas WT1 and RB function as transcriptional repressor and corepressor, respectively, P53 appears to function as a transcriptional activator (reviewed by Vogelstein and Kinzler, 1992).

Somatic mutations. As in the case of *RB*, germline mutations in *TP53* are rare, but somatic mutations in cancers are exceedingly common. Indeed, *TP53* is the most highly mutated gene in human cancers, with mutations present in approximately 50% of tumors analyzed (Hollstein et al., 1991; Levine et al., 1991). Furthermore, transfection of a P53 expression vector into a P53-deficient tumor cell line resulted in growth suppression (Chen et al., 1990). A database of *TP53* somatic mutations has been established that, as of January 1997, contained more than 6000 mutations affecting over 250 codons of the *TP53* gene from more than 50 different tumor types (Hainaut et al., 1997). Point mutations most commonly affect P53

TABLE 15.1. Tumor types in *p53*$^{-/-}$ mice as a function of genetic background

Tumor Type	Strain		
	129/Sv	C57BL/6 x 129/Sv	CD-1
Lymphoma	65%	75%	36%
Testicular cancer	35%	9%	2%
Hemangiosarcoma	8%	23%	—
Osteosarcoma	8%	5%	36%
Undifferentiated sarcoma	—	7%	—
Meningioma	4%	—	—
Mammary adenocarcinoma	4%	2%	—
Rhabdomyosarcoma	4%	—	8%
Leiomyosarcoma	4%	—	—
Medulloblastoma	—	2%	—
Schwannoma	—	2%	—
Glioblastoma	—	2%	—
Lung adenocarcinoma	—	—	56%
Skin cancer	—	—	8%
Neuroblastoma	—	—	2%

From Malkin, 1994.

DNA-binding activity (Bargonetti et al., 1991; Kern et al., 1991, 1992; Lin et al., 1995). As in the case of RB, tumor viruses also inactivate P53: SV40 T antigen and adenovirus 55-kDa E1B target the P53 DNA-binding and transactivation domains, respectively, whereas HPV E6 promotes P53 degradation (reviewed by Ko and Prives, 1996; Levine, 1997).

P53 function. A major function of P53 is to preserve the integrity of the cell's genomic DNA. When DNA damage occurs as a result of γ- or ultraviolet irradiation or exposure to a chemical clastogen, the steady-state levels of P53 protein increase dramatically, leading to the transcriptional activation of genes containing P53 binding sites, particularly *P21*, which encodes an inhibitor of cyclin-dependent kinases (El-Deiry et al., 1993; Harper et al., 1993; Xiong et al., 1993) (Fig. 15.1). Expression of P21 results in cell cycle arrest at the G_1/S transition, allowing DNA repair prior to the next round of synthesis. Although γ- and ultraviolet irradiation cause other types of DNA damage, DNA strand breakage in particular appears to be the signal for induction of P53 expression by these agents (Lu and Lane, 1993; Nelson and Kastan, 1994). In addition to responding to DNA strand breakage, P53 is induced by depletion of cellular ribonucleotide pools, which are required for DNA synthesis (Linke et al., 1996). P53 is also induced when cells are subjected to severe hypoxia ($\leq 0.02\%$ O_2), but it is not known whether this is a direct effect or secondary to hypoxia-induced DNA damage, and P53-deficient cells still arrest in G_1 when subjected to hypoxia (Graeber et al., 1994). In tumor cells, expression of wild-type P53 is associated with apoptosis (Fig. 15.1) rather than G_1 arrest under hypoxic conditions and loss of P53 expression results in resistance to apoptosis (Graeber et al., 1996). Hypoxia is commonly found within tumors because of their abnormal vasculature (reviewed by Vaupel et al., 1989) and may thus contribute to the selection of P53-deficient cells during tumorigenesis.

In addition to its roles in mediating G_1 arrest and apoptosis, P53 may also play a role at the G_2/M transition to prevent entry into S phase prior to mitosis and thus polyploidization (Cross et al., 1995). Finally, P53 function is also required to maintain centrosome number and ensure proper chromosome segregation at mitosis (Fukusawa et al., 1996). It is apparent from these observations that loss of P53 function must have profoundly adverse effects on genomic stability.

P53 structure. P53 is a protein of 393 amino acid residues that is composed of four structural and functional domains as follows (Fig. 15.2): (1) transactivation domain (amino acids 1–44); (2) sequence-specific DNA-binding domain (amino acids 102–292); (3) oligomerization domain

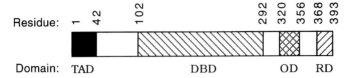

FIGURE 15-2. Functional domains of P53. The transactivation domain (TAD), sequence-specific DNA-binding domain (DBD), oligomerization domain (OD) and regulatory domain (RD), encompassing the indicated amino acid residues are shown.

(amino acids 320–356); and (4) DNA-binding regulatory domain (amino acids 368–393). Each of these domains has been analyzed extensively, as described below.

Transactivation domain. Transcriptional activation by P53 is dependent on amino acid residues 1–42, and substitution of residues Phe-19, Leu-22, or Trp-23 results in loss of transactivation and loss of binding to the TBP-associated factors hTAF$_{II}$70 and hTAF$_{II}$31 (Lin et al., 1995; Lu and Levine, 1995; Thut et al., 1995). MDM2, which was identified as the product of an amplified oncogene in human sarcomas, binds to the P53 transactivation domain and inhibits its ability to activate transcription (Momand et al., 1992; Oliner et al., 1992). Analysis of the crystal structure of the MDM2-P53 transactivation-domain complex revealed that the same residues of P53 that contact TAFs also contact MDM2 (Kussie et al., 1996) confirming that MDM2 conceals the P53 transactivation domain (Oliner et al., 1993). The *MDM2* gene is a target for transcriptional activation by P53, indicating that MDM2 serves as a feedback mechanism to down-regulate P53 expression after its biological functions have been performed. The complexity of this feedback relationship was increased by the discovery that binding of MDM2 to P53 also targets the protein for degradation (Haupt et al., 1997; Kubbutat et al., 1997). Two general characteristics of P53 mutations in cancer are that they result in a loss of P53 transcriptional activity and increased stability of the mutant protein. These recent findings suggest that it is the specific loss of *MDM2* transcription that is responsible for the increased accumulation of transcriptionally inactive P53 protein.

DNA binding domain. Over 90% of *TP53* missense mutations identified in tumors affect the DNA binding domain (Levine, 1997). P53 does not contain a previously identified DNA-binding motif such as the bHLH, bZIP, homeodomain, or zinc finger (see Chapter 3). The crystal structure of P53 amino acid residues 102–292 complexed with a DNA binding-site oligonucleotide revealed that two antiparallel β sheets (a "β sandwich") serve as a scaffold for the DNA binding surface, which is composed of two large loops (the conformation of which is maintained by a tetrahedrally coordinated zinc atom) and a loop-β sheet-α helix motif (Cho et al., 1994). The loop-sheet-helix contacts the major groove of the DNA double helix and an arginine residue in one of the loops contacts the minor groove. P53 inserts an α helix into the major groove in a manner that is similar to the other DNA-binding motifs described above. The majority of *TP53* missense mutations identified in tumors result in amino acid substitutions within highly conserved residues that compose the loop-sheet-helix motif or one of the loops. These mutations prevent binding of the protein to DNA either by eliminating critical DNA contact residues or by destabilizing the loops and/or loop-sheet-helix motif (Cho et al., 1994). Based on the sequence of *bona fide* P53 binding sites and the properties of the protein in solution, P53 was proposed to bind DNA as a homotetramer in which each monomer recognizes DNA of consensus sequence 5'-RRRCW-3' (R, A or G; W, A or T). Modeling based on crystal structure analysis supported the hypothesis that P53 binds to DNA as a tetramer (Fig. 15.3A).

Oligomerization domain. Oligomerization is required for the biological activity of P53 as a tumor suppressor because mutant P53 that could not oligomerize could not suppress the growth of $TP53^{-/-}$ cells (Pietenpol et al., 1994). Crystal structure analysis of a peptide containing P53 amino acids 320–356 revealed that a monomer, consisting of a β strand and an α helix, associates with a second monomer via antiparallel β-sheet and helix-helix interfaces to form a dimer, which associates with another dimer via a separate, parallel helix-helix interface to form the tetramer (Jeffrey et al., 1995) (Fig. 15.3B). Less than 1% of *TP53* mutations are within the oligomerization domain (Greenblatt et al., 1994), which is consistent with the hypothesis that many *TP53* mutations result in the production of a dominant-negative protein that can oligomerize with wild-type P53 to form inactive tetramers (Milner and Medcalf, 1991; Shaulian et al., 1992). An alternative but not mutually exclusive explanation is that there are only a few amino acid residues that are absolutely required for dimerization (Jeffrey et al., 1995). Although oligomerization is required for DNA binding and tumor suppression, replacement of the oligomerization domain with the dimerization domain of the yeast transcription factor GCN4 resulted in a chimeric protein that was still capable of growth suppression when expressed in $TP53^{-/-}$ cells (Pietenpol et al.,

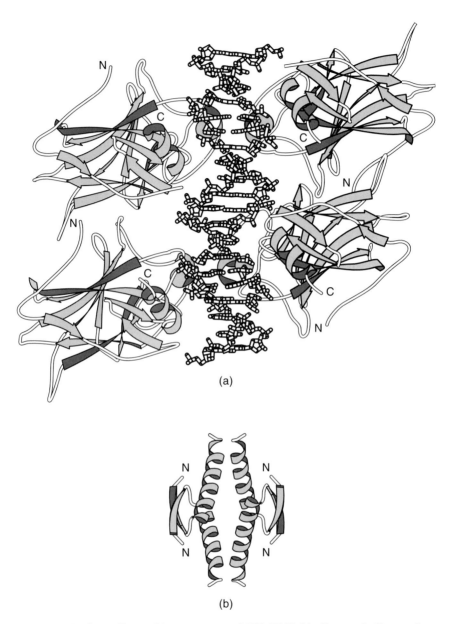

(a)

(b)

FIGURE 15-3. Crystallographic structures of P53 DNA-binding and oligomerization domains. (A) P53 DNA-binding-domain tetramer complexed with a pentameric DNA binding-site oligonucleotide. The amino (N) and carboxyl (C) terminus of each monomer is indicated. Note the present of α helices in the major
groove. (Reproduced with permission from Cho et al., 1994.) (B) Tetramer formation by the oligomerization domain. (Reproduced with permission from Jeffrey et al., 1995. Copyright ©1995 by the American Association for the Advancement of Science.)

1994). These results suggest that the oligomerization domain has no additional functions and that dimerization is sufficient for P53 function.

Regulatory domain. P53, via its carboxyl terminal 26 residues (amino acids 368–393), can also bind to DNA containing insertion/deletion mismatches (Lee et al., 1995). These results suggest that P53 may directly detect DNA damage and perhaps recruit proteins that both activate P53 sequence-specific DNA-binding activity and repair DNA. Several different alterations of the C-terminal domain have been shown to activate DNA binding mediated by amino acids 102–292: (1) complete deletion; (2) phosphorylation of Ser-378 by protein kinase C or Ser-392 by casein kinase II; (3) binding of monoclonal antibody PAb421 to amino acids 370–378; and (4) binding of short (e.g., 40 nucleotides) single-stranded DNA molecules (Hupp and Lane, 1994; Jayaraman and Prives, 1995). The regulation of the sequence-specific DNA-binding domain by C-terminal sequences may therefore represent an essential aspect of P53 biology. Most recently, the coactivator protein P300 (see Chapters 3 and 13) was shown to acetylate lysine residues 370, 373, 373, 381, and 382 within the regulatory domain, which dramatically increased sequence-specific DNA binding of P53 (Gu and Roeder, 1997). This remarkable result thus provides a novel mechanism for regulation of transcription factor activity and indicates that histones are not the sole substrate for the acetyltransferase reaction catalyzed by coactivator proteins.

Mechanisms of P53 inactivation in tumor cells. As described above, mutations that affect P53 DNA-binding activity are commonly detected in human cancer cells. Many of these mutations also result in stabilization of the mutant protein. In heterozygous cells, mutant protein will predominate over wild-type protein and most tetramers will therefore contain one or more mutant subunits, which may have a dominant-negative effect on P53 function. However, most commonly, tumors are found to contain one missense mutation and one deleted allele at the *TP53* locus, suggesting that the dominant-negative effect is not sufficient to functionally inactivate the wild-type gene product.

In many tumors that do not have mutations at the *TP53* locus, P53 function is nonetheless disrupted by a variety of mechanisms, including the following: (1) inactivation by complex formation with SV40 T-antigen (Mietz et al., 1992), adenovirus E1B (Yew and Berk, 1992), or hepatitis B virus X (Ueda et al., 1995; Wang et al., 1994) proteins; (2) increased degradation targeted by binding of human papilloma virus E6 protein (Scheffner et al., 1990); (3) inhibition of transactivation domain function by overexpression of MDM2 due to gene amplification (Momand et al.,

1992; Oliner et al., 1992); and (4) cytoplasmic sequestration of P53 by an undetermined mechanism (Moll et al., 1992, 1995).

P53 and chemotherapy. Not only does P53 play a key role in tumorigenesis, but the presence or absence of wild-type P53 also determines whether chemotherapeutic agents will induce apoptosis of certain cancer cell types (Lowe et al., 1993a, b; reviewed by Levine, 1997). All human testicular teratocarcinomas analyzed contain wild-type P53 and chemotherapy with cisplatin, which induces tumor cell apoptosis, results in a cure rate of >90%. Acute lymphoblastic leukemia is also associated with wild-type P53 expression, an excellent apoptotic response to chemotherapy, and a high cure rate. In contrast, chemotherapy-resistant relapses are often associated with new *TP53* mutations. In breast cancers, new *TP53* mutations are also correlated with acquisition of doxorubicin resistance (Aas et al., 1996).

Inactivation of Tumor Suppressor Genes by Aberrant Methylation

In addition to gene deletions, frameshift, missense, and nonsense mutations, another mechanism by which the expression of tumor suppressor genes can be eliminated is by tumor-specific hypermethylation of the locus, which results in transcriptional inactivation (reviewed by Laird and Jaenisch, 1994; Versteeg, 1997). Hypermethylation has been reported for an increasing number of tumor suppressor genes, including those encoding RB (Greger et al., 1994), the cyclin-dependent kinase inhibitors p15[INK4B] and p16[INK4A] (Gonzalez-Zulueta et al., 1995; Herman et al., 1997; Merlo et al., 1995; Swafford et al., 1997), and the VHL protein (Herman et al., 1994; Prowse et al., 1997) which may be involved in the regulation of transcription elongation (Duan et al., 1995; Kibel et al., 1995; reviewed by Krumm and Groudine, 1995), mRNA stability (Gnarra et al., 1996; Iliopoulos et al., 1996), and/or protein stability (Pause et al., 1997). These recent studies suggest that transcriptional silencing by hypermethylation represents an important means by which tumor suppressor gene expression is eliminated in tumor cells. Further investigation will be required to determine whether the altered methylation is due to mutations in *cis*-acting sequences, or *trans*-acting factors, or both.

Translocations and Transcriptional Pathophysiology in Cancer Cells

Functional alterations in transcription factors represent a common component of multistep tumorigenesis, which represents a process of selection whereby cells incur genomic alterations (such as deletion, gene amplification, point mutation, and translocation) that result in increased cellular proliferation. Thus, transcription factors that function in cell cycle pathways to restrict proliferation, such as the tumor suppressors P53, RB, and WT1, are inactivated, whereas proto-oncogene transcription factors that normally function to stimulate cell cycle progression are activated. Activation can be achieved either by altering the *cis*-acting regulatory elements that control transcription of the gene encoding the transcription factor, or by altering the protein sequence to impart novel biological properties to the transcription factor.

Chromosomal translocations, which are common in cancer cells, can achieve transcription factor dysregulation by either of the two mechanisms described above (reviewed by Cleary, 1991; Rabbitts, 1994). Indeed, many forms of cancer and, in particular, leukemia are characterized by specific and unique chromosome translocations within the tumor cells, indicating that the alteration of gene expression resulting from the genomic alteration is a crucial aspect of the disease pathogenesis. It should be emphasized that these translocations (1) occur in tumor cells and are absent from the patient's germline and (2) often, but by no means always, involve genes encoding transcription factors. Translocations are most commonly detected in leukemia and lymphoma but can be identified at a lower frequency in solid tumors as well.

Burkitt's Lymphoma

Leukemia and lymphoma represent the clonal expansion of hematopoietic precursor cells that are arrested at a proliferative stage of development. In B and T lymphocytes, the immunoglobulin and T-cell receptor genes, respectively, undergo a process of DNA rearrangement that is required for their normal expression. These cells are therefore at increased risk for aberrant chromosomal rearrangement and the tumor-specific rearrangements often involve either one of the immunoglobulin or T-cell receptor loci, as exemplified by Burkitt's lymphoma, a disease of B cells. In approximately 90% of Burkitt's lymphoma patients, the lymphoma cells have undergone a t(8;14)(q24;q32) translocation that juxtaposes the *IGH* locus, encoding immunoglobulin heavy chains, to the *CMYC* locus, encoding a bHLH-ZIP transcription factor that is induced in cells that have been subjected to growth factor stimulation (see Chapter 3). One of the targets of C-MYC transactivation is the *CDC25A* gene, which encodes a protein phosphatase that activates CDK2, a cyclin-dependent kinase that phosphorylates RB at the G1/S cell-cycle transition (Galaktionov et al., 1996). In the other 10% of cases of Burkitt's lymphoma, a t(2;8) or t(8;22) translocation juxtaposes the *CMYC* locus to the locus encoding the immunoglobulin κ or λ light chains, respectively (reviewed by Rabbitts, 1994). These translocations, which do not alter the C-MYC amino-acid coding sequence, place the *CMYC* transcriptional unit under the control of the immunoglobulin locus enhancer element, resulting in constitutive high-level expression of C-MYC within the tumor cells. The translocation breakpoint can be as much as 140 kilobases 3' to the *CMYC* transcriptional unit (reviewed by Spencer and Groudine, 1991), demonstrating the powerful long-range effects of immunoglobulin enhancer elements on gene transcription.

Acute Promyelocytic Leukemia

Acute promyelocytic leukemia (APL) is characterized by three important clinical observations: (1) all APL cells are arrested at the promyelocytic stage of hematopoietic differentiation; (2) most APL cells carry a t(15; 17)(q22;q21) translocation; and (3) treatment of patients with high doses of retinoic acid can in many cases induce remission (Castaigne et al., 1990; Huang et al., 1988; Mitelman, 1988). These observations were unified by the discovery that the APL translocation creates a fusion gene between the *RARA* gene on chromosome 17q21, and the *PML* gene on chromosome 15q22 (Kakizuka et al., 1991; de The et al., 1991). The *RARA* gene encodes the retinoic acid receptor α (RARα), a member of the nuclear receptor superfamily of zinc-finger transcription factors (see Chapter 5) which binds all-*trans* retinoic acid, a vitamin A derivative that has been shown to play an important role in cellular differentiation and morphogenesis in a variety of vertebrate species including humans (reviewed by Brockes, 1990; Lammer et al., 1985) (see Chapter 16). *PML* also encodes a putative transcription factor with potential zinc finger and leucine zipper motifs (de The et al., 1991). Expression of a *PML/RARA* fusion gene in transgenic mice was associated with impaired neutrophil maturation that progressed in a small percentage of mice to APL; in these mice, as in humans with APL, retinoic acid administration resulted in leukemic cell differentiation and clinical remission (Brown et al., 1997).

Despite variation in the location of the translocation breakpoint, all translocation-derived fusion genes encode a chimeric PML-RARα transcription factor that contains the RARα ligand- and DNA-binding domains (Fig. 15.4) but manifests altered transactivation properties compared to RARα (de The et al., 1991; Diverio et al., 1992; Nervi et al., 1992; Pandolfi et al., 1991). Expression of the fusion gene inhibits differentiation and apoptosis of myeloid progenitor cells at low retinoic acid concentrations, whereas at high concentrations of retinoic acid the

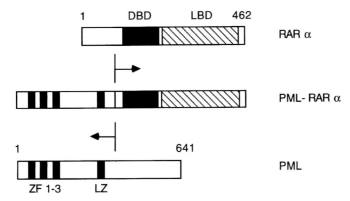

FIGURE 15-4. Structure of RARα, PML, and the RARα-PML fusion protein expressed in acute promyelocytic leukemia cells carrying a t(15;17) translocation. The DNA-binding domain (DBD) and ligand-binding domain (LBD) of RARα and the zinc finger (ZF1-3) and leucine zipper (LZ) domains of PML are indicated.

expression of PML-RARα actually increases the frequency with which myeloid progenitor cells differentiate in vitro (Grignani et al., 1993). The retinoic acid concentration–dependent behavior of the fusion protein suggests that its tumorigenic effects may be mediated by the PML moiety at low (physiologic) retinoic acid concentrations (10^{-9} M), whereas the differentiation effects are mediated through the RARα moiety at high (pharmacologic) concentrations of retinoic acid (10^{-6} M). These studies have thus provided insight into the pathogenesis of APL as well as the molecular mechanisms of normal myelopoiesis.

Pre-B-Cell Acute Lymphoblastic Leukemia

In 20% to 25% of children with pre-B-cell acute lymphoblastic leukemia (ALL), which accounts for approximately 5% of all children with ALL (Hunger, 1996), the tumor cells carry a t(1;19)(q23; p13) translocation that fuses sequences from the *E2A* and *PBX1* genes (Hunger et al., 1991; Kamps et al., 1990; Mellentin et al., 1989a; Monica et al., 1991; Nourse et al., 1990). The *E2A* breakpoints all occur within the 3.5-kb intron 13 and, because all fusion mRNAs contain identical PBX1 sequences, the *PBX1* breakpoints also appear to localize to a single intron that is at least 50 kb in size (Mellentin et al., 1990). Based on these findings, the translocation can be reliably identified by blot hybridization of DNA from leukemia cells using an *E2A* cDNA probe, which may be a more sensitive test than karyotype analysis (Mellentin et al., 1990; Hunger, 1996). RT-

PCR can also be used to detect the fusion mRNA in leukemic cells and, because of the sensitivity of the technique, can detect subclinical disease in treated patients (Hunger et al., 1991). Accurate diagnosis has clinical implications because t(1;19)-positive ALL is more aggressive than other types of ALL and requires more intensive therapy to induce remission (Hunger, 1996).

The *E2A* gene encodes (by alternative splicing) the E2A proteins E12, E47, and E2-5, which are class I basic helix-loop-helix (bHLH) proteins that can either homodimerize or heterodimerize with class II bHLH proteins (see Chapter 3). Despite *E2A* expression in most tissues, E2A homodimers capable of binding to DNA are found only in B lymphocytes, apparently because of the presence of an intermolecular disulfide bond that is catalyzed specifically in B cells and that can be disrupted by incubating B-cell with non-B-cell nuclear extracts (Benezra, 1994). Loss of *E2A* expression by gene targeting in knockout mice has no apparent effect on general development but arrests maturation of B lymphoid progenitors at an early stage (Bain et al., 1994; Zhuang et al., 1994). Heterozygous null mice contained about half as many B lymphocytes as wild-type mice, suggesting that the level of E2A expression determines the proliferative rate of B lymphoid progenitor cells (Zhuang et al., 1994).

PBX1 encodes a homeodomain protein that is homologous to the product of the *Drosophila melanogaster extradenticle (exd)* gene. Certain *Drosophila* homeodomain proteins, such as the products of the *abdominal-A* and *ultrabithorax* genes, bind to DNA cooperatively with EXD (see Chapter 3), whereas other homeodomain proteins such as the products of the *antennapedia* and *abdominal-B* genes do not, suggesting that EXD is important for the determination of homeodomain binding-site selection *in vivo* (Chan et al., 1994; Van Dijk and Murre, 1994). PBX1 was subsequently shown to bind cooperatively with HOXA5, HOXB7, HOXB8, or HOXC8 to DNA containing both a canonical HOX binding site, 5'-TCAATTAA-3', and a PBX1 binding site, 5'-ATCAATCAA-3' (Lu et al., 1995), thus demonstrating functional as well as structural homology between *Drosophila* EXD and mammalian PBX1.

The chimeric gene created by the translocation consists of the 5' half of the *E2A* gene, encoding two amino-terminal transactivation domains but lacking the bHLH domain required for dimerization and DNA binding, fused to the 3' half of *PBX1* encoding the carboxyl-terminal homeodomain (Fig. 15.5). Expression of E2A-PBX1 coding sequences under the control of immunoglobulin heavy chain promoter and enhancer (E_μ) elements in transgenic mice resulted in the development of malignant lymphomas, demonstrating that the fusion protein is oncogenic in lymphoid cells (Dedera et al., 1993). Curiously however, all the tumors were

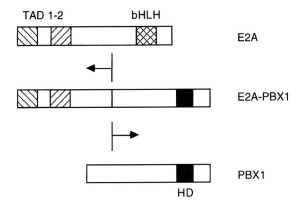

FIGURE 15-5. Structure of E2A, PBX1, and the E2A-PBX1 fusion protein expressed in pre-B-cell acute lymphoblastic leukemia cells carrying a t(1;19) translocation. The transactivation domains (TAD 1-2) and basic helix-loop-helix domain (bHLH) of E2A and the homeodomain (HD) of PBX1 are indicated.

composed of T lymphoid cells, in contrast to mice expressing an E_μ-*CMYC* transgene, which developed tumors that were exclusively of B cell origin (Adams et al., 1985). This outcome may have resulted from preferential expression of the E_μ-*E2A-PBX1* transgene in T cells or perhaps reflects increased susceptibility of these cells to transformation by E2A-PBX1. Introduction of a large genomic fragment (e.g., a yeast or bacterial artificial chromosome) encompassing the *E2A-PBX1* fusion gene into the mouse germline would allow transcriptional regulation analagous to that occurring in human leukemic cells and may provide a more definitive animal model of pre–B-cell ALL. Expression of E2A-PBX1 in mouse bone marrow progenitor cells resulted in acute myeloid leukemia (Kamps and Baltimore, 1993). This development of myeloid, rather than lymphoid, leukemia may reflect the expression of the fusion gene in a cell population in which the translocation does not otherwise occur.

PBX1 is normally expressed in all tissues other than B and T lymphocytes (Monica et al., 1991; Nourse et al., 1990), suggesting that the translocation may function to activate transcription of PBX1 sequences, as described for C-MYC in Burkitt's lymphoma. Forced expression of E2A-PBX1, but not PBX1, transformed NIH 3T3 cells, suggesting that the E2A sequences were in fact required for transformation (Monica et al., 1994), possibly by activating transcription of genes containing PBX1 binding sites. However, a mutant E2A-PBX1 protein lacking the homeodomain was still able to transform fibroblasts and, when expressed from the immunoglobulin promoter and enhancer elements described above, induced malignant lymphomas in transgenic mice (Monica et al., 1994). Because the deletion of the homeodomain eliminates E2A-PBX1 DNA-binding activity, these results suggest that PBX1 may associate with other homeodomain proteins and thus target the fusion protein to certain promoters in the absence of direct DNA binding, as has been demonstrated for EXD (Van Dijk and Murre, 1994). If this hypothesis is correct, then further analysis of the PBX1 sequences required for transformation should identify the amino acid residues that are required for interaction of E2A-PBX1 with other DNA-binding transcription factors. These PBX1 sequences could then be used as bait to pull out interacting proteins in a yeast two-hybrid assay. Of interest is the fact that overexpression of HOXA1, HOXA5, HOXA7, HOXB7, or HOXC8 results in transformation of NIH 3T3 cells (Maulbecker and Gruss, 1993a) and expression of HOXB8 in myeloid progenitors results in their continuous proliferation in the presence of growth factors (Perkins and Cory, 1993). Thus, the oncogenic effect of E2A-PBX1 may be mediated in part by increased transcription of HOX-regulated genes, and an important goal of future research will be to identify genes whose transcription in pre-B lymphocytes is altered by the presence of E2A-PBX1.

Pro-B-cell Acute Lymphoblastic Leukemia

In approximately 1% of children with B-lymphoid ALL, a t(17;19)(q22; p13) translocation is present within the genome of leukemic cells (Raimondi et al., 1991). As might be predicted from the presence of a chromosome 19p13 breakpoint, the *E2A* gene forms the 5' end of a fusion gene created by the translocation and the 3' end is formed by the chromosome 17q22 gene, *HLF*, which encodes a basic leucine zipper (bZIP; see Chapter 3) transcription factor (Hunger et al., 1992; Inaba et al., 1992). As in the case of the t(1;19) fusion gene of pre-B ALL, the fusion gene resulting from t(17;19) in pro-B ALL encodes a chimeric protein consisting of the amino-terminal activation domains of E2A and the carboxylterminal bZIP DNA-binding domain of HLF (Fig. 15.6). The t(17;19) breakpoints are heterogeneous in different cases of pro-B ALL, with *E2A* disrupted either within intron 12 or 13, whereas the chromosome 17 breakpoint is located within intron 3 of *HLF* (Hunger et al., 1994b). The biological properties of the resulting fusion proteins appear to be identical (Hunger et al., 1994a).

The *HLF* gene is normally expressed at high levels in the liver, at lower levels in lung and kidney, and, as in the case of *PBX1*, expression of *HLF* cannot be detected in hematopoietic (including lymphoid) cells (Hunger et al., 1992; Inaba et al., 1992). Expression of full-length E2A-

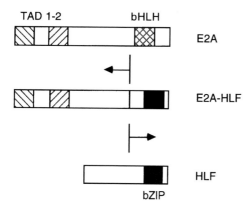

FIGURE 15-6. Structure of E2A, HLF, and E2A-HLF fusion protein expressed in pro-B-cell acute lymphoblastic leukemia cells carrying a t(17;19). The transactivation domains (TAD 1-2) and bHLH domain of E2A and the basic leucine zipper domain (bZIP) of HLF are indicated.

HLF induces cellular transformation of tissue culture cells and deletion of either the E2A transactivation domains or the HLF bZIP domain results in loss of transformation (Yoshihara et al., 1995). These results suggest that the transcriptional activation of genes containing binding sites for HLF or related bZIP proteins may result in leukemogenesis in E2A-HLF–expressing cells. E4BP4 is another bZIP protein that demonstrates similar DNA-binding specificity to that of HLF, is expressed in B-lymphoid cells (including leukemias), and functions as a transcriptional repressor (Cowell et al., 1992). Transcriptional activation by E2A-HLF of genes normally repressed by E4BP4 may contribute to the leukemic phenotype (reviewed by Hunger, 1996).

The biological activity of the E2A-HLF fusion protein was experimentally inhibited by overexpression of a dominant-negative (dn) protein that lacked the first transactivation domain of E2A and contained mutations in the basic domain of HLF, so that E2A-HLF(dn) could dimerize with E2A-HLF but the resulting heterodimer could not bind to DNA or activate transcription (Inaba et al., 1996). Expression of E2A-HLF(dn) induced apoptosis (programmed cell death) in a human pro-B-cell leukemia line carrying the t(17;19) translocation but had no effect on the viability of pre-B or T cell leukemia lines that lacked t(17;19). Conversely, expression of E2A-HLF in a murine pro-B-cell line prevented apoptosis in response to growth factor withdrawal or ionizing radiation. Taken together, these results suggest that E2A-HLF contributes to leukemogenesis by preventing the death of pro-B cells (Inaba et al., 1996).

Remarkably, HLF has significant amino acid identity with CES-2, a bZIP transcription factor that regulates apoptosis in *C. elegans*. Because HLF is not normally expressed in hematopoietic cells, it is possible that E2A-HLF competes with CES-2 homologues that normally regulate apoptosis in pro-B cells (Inaba et al., 1996).

T-Cell Acute Lymphocytic Leukemia

In approximately 30% of T-cell ALL cases, a genomic rearrangement within tumor cells results in dysregulated expression of a bHLH transcription factor (reviewed by Hunger, 1996). In 3% to 5% of cases of T-cell ALL, transcription of the *TAL1* (also known as *SCL* and *TCL5*) gene is activated by a translocation that juxtaposes TAL1 coding sequences on chromosome 1p34 with one of the loci encoding T-cell receptor subunits on chromosomes 7q35 and 14q11 (Bernard et al., 1991; Brown et al., 1990; Finger et al., 1989; Fitzgerald et al., 1991). In an additional 25% to 30% of T-cell ALL cases, a deletion of approximately 90 kb, which is not cytogenetically visible, results in the juxtaposition of *TAL1* and the enhancer of an upstream gene, resulting in *TAL1* expression in leukemic cells (Aplan et al., 1992; Bernard et al., 1991; Brown et al., 1990; reviewed by Hunger, 1996). Two other translocations observed in a small number of T-cell ALL cases, t(7;19)(q34;p13) and t(7;9)(q34;q32) involve juxtaposition of the T-cell receptor-β gene locus on chromosome 7 with the *LYL1* and *TAL2* genes, respectively, which encode bHLH factors that have extensive sequence similarity with TAL1 (Mellentin et al., 1989b; Xia et al., 1991). In addition, heterodimers consisting of E2A and either TAL1 or LYL1 displayed similar DNA binding specificities in vitro, suggesting that these two factors may be able to regulate a common set of target genes in vivo (Miyamoto et al., 1996).

TAL1 is expressed during early hematopoiesis (Begley et al., 1989) and mice homozygous for a null mutation in the *Tal1* gene manifest profound defects in hematopoiesis, most notably a complete absence of erythrocytes (Shivdasani et al., 1995). TAL1 may therefore play an important role in the proliferation of hematopoietic precursors and its persistent expression under the control of a T-cell receptor gene enhancer may result in T-lymphoid progenitor cells remaining in an undifferentiated, proliferative state. These results underscore the important role of E2A-containing bHLH heterodimers in normal hematopoiesis and leukemogenesis.

CBF and M2 Acute Myeloid Leukemia

In addition to the bHLH factors described above, dysregulated expression of core-binding factor (CBF; also known as polyoma enhancer binding protein 2 [PEBP2]), another transcription factor that plays an essential role in normal hematopoiesis, has been demonstrated in leukemia cells. Alterations of genes encoding subunits of CBF represent the most frequent genomic rearrangements identified in human leukemias (Castilla et al., 1996). CBF has been implicated in the transcriptional regulation of a battery of genes whose products play essential roles in hematopoiesis, including colony-stimulating factor-1 receptor, granulocyte-macrophage colony-stimulating factor (GM-CSF), interleukin-3, macrophage colony-stimulating factor (M-CSF), myeloperoxidase, neutrophil elastase, T cell receptor (TCR) α, and TCR β (Cameron et al., 1994; Frank et al., 1995; Nuchprayoon et al., 1994; Prosser et al., 1992; Takahashi et al., 1995; Zhang et al., 1996). CBF is a heterodimer consisting of CBFα, which is the DNA-binding subunit, and CBFβ, which does not bind to DNA but increases the DNA-binding affinity of CBFα (Ogawa et al., 1993; Wang et al., 1993).

CBFα subunits are heterogeneous products of three different genes, *CBFA1* (also known as *PEBP2αA*), *CBFA2* (also known as *AML1* or *PEBP2αB*), and *CBFA3* (also known as *PEBP2αC*) (Bae et al., 1993, 1995; Levanon et al., 1994). The *CBFA2* locus, which maps to human chromosome 21, is rearranged as a result of translocations: t(8;21) in the M2 subtype of acute myeloid leukemia, t(12;21) in childhood acute lymphoblastic leukemia, and t(3;21) in chronic myeloid leukemia (Golub et al., 1995; Mitani et al., 1994; Miyoshi et al., 1991; Romana et al., 1995). All of the the translocations generate a chimeric gene encoding all or part of CBFα, including the DNA-binding domain, fused to protein sequences encoded by a gene on another chromosome (reviewed by Wang et al., 1996b). The t(8;21) chimeric gene encodes a fusion between amino acids 1–177 of the 250-amino-acid CBFα (AML1) and 575 amino acids of a 604-amino-acid putative zinc finger transcription factor known as ETO or MTG8 (Erickson et al., 1992; Miyoshi et al., 1993; Nisson et al., 1992) (Fig. 15.7). CBFα (AML1) contains a 117-amino-acid region with significant sequence similarity to the product of the *Drosophila* segmentation gene *runt*. This RUNT-homology domain mediates both protein dimerization and DNA binding and is included within the AML1–ETO fusion protein (Meyers et al., 1993). Expression of AML1–ETO has been shown to repress AML1–dependent transcription, suggesting that the fusion protein may have a dominant negative effect on AML1 function in vivo (Frank et al., 1995; Meyers et al., 1995).

CBFβ subunits are encoded by a single gene, *CBFB* (Ogawa et al., 1993; Wang et al., 1993). Acute myeloid leukemia subtype M4Eo is characterized by an inversion of chromosome 16, inv(16)(p13;q22), that creates a fusion gene between *CBFB*, which is located on chromosome 16q, and *MYH11*, which is located on 16p and encodes SMMHC, the smooth

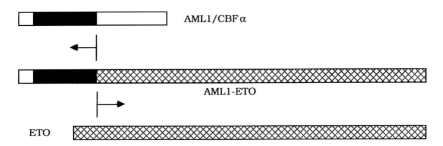

FIGURE 15-7. Structure of AML1/CBFA2, ETO, and AML1-ETO fusion protein expressed in M2 subtype of acute myeloid leukemia cells carrying a t(8;21). The RUNT-homology DNA-binding domain of AML1/CBFA2 is indicated by the solid box.

muscle myosin heavy chain (Liu et al., 1993). Less commonly, the *CBFB-MYH11* fusion gene is created by a t(16;16)(p13;q22) translocation (Shurtleff et al., 1995). The *CBFB-MYH11* fusion gene encodes most (amino acids 1–165) of CBFβ and the carboxyl-terminal tail of the myosin polypeptide, which forms an α-helical rod. The CBFβ-SMMHC protein can, like CBFβ, dimerize with CBFα and the resulting dimers retain CBF DNA-binding activity (Liu et al., 1994), suggesting that the fusion protein may interfere with normal CBF function. Additionally, unlike CBFβ, CBFβ-SMMHC can also undergo homodimerization, which is presumably mediated by the myosin tail (Liu et al., 1994; Wijmenga et al., 1996).

The important role of CBF in normal hematopoiesis has been demonstrated by the analysis of knockout mice deficient for either CBFα or CBFβ. Mice homozygous for a null mutation in the *Cbfa2* or *Cbfb* gene have normal primitive erythropoiesis in the yolk sac but severely impaired definitive hematopoiesis in the yolk sac and fetal liver involving all cell lineages and resulting in embryonic lethality at midgestation (Okuda et al., 1996; Wang et al., 1996a, b). These results indicate that in the absence of CBF, the developmental program responsible for establishing definitive erythropoiesis cannot be successfully carried out, perhaps because of an inability to generate the appropriate stem cells or an inability of the stem cells to proliferate and/or differentiate (Okuda et al., 1996). Dysregulated CBF expression resulting from the chromosome rearrangements described above is likely to interfere with normal hematopoiesis so that rather than undergoing differentiation, the affected myeloid or lymphoid progenitor cells are arrested at a proliferative stage of development.

In order to determine whether the translocation-derived fusion proteins have a dominant-negative effect on CBF function in vivo, a knock-in experiment was performed in which homologous recombination in embryonic stem cells was utilized to generate a *Cbfb-MYH11* fusion gene at the mouse *Cbfb* locus (Castilla et al., 1996). When the recombinant ES cells were injected into a wild-type mouse blastocyst, the hematopoietic tissues of the resulting chimeric mice contained no ES cell derivatives. F_1 progeny of the chimeric mice that were germline-heterozygous for the *Cbfb-MYH11* fusion gene died at embryonic day 12.5 because of failure of definitive hematopoiesis, similar to mice homozygous for null alleles of *Cbfa2* or *Cbfb*. This experiment provides strong evidence that the AML1–MYH11 fusion protein has a dominant negative effect on CBF function and hematopoiesis in vivo. The severe effect of the presence of the *Cbfb-MYH11* fusion gene in all hematopoietic progenitor cells, rather than just a single clonal population as occurs during leukemogenesis, resulted in embryonic lethality and precluded the postnatal development of leukemia in the mice. These results thus confirm half of the pathophysiologic mechanism—that the fusion protein blocks differentiation of hematopoietic progenitor cells. It still remains to be formally demonstrated that these arrested cells retain the ability to proliferate, which may require additional mutations in other genes during the multistep process of leukemogenesis.

A similar knock-in strategy was utilized to generate mice heterozygous for an *Cbfa2-ETO* fusion gene (Yergeau et al., 1997). These mice died at midgestation with central nervous system hemorrhages and a block in fetal liver hematopoeisis, similar to the phenotype of the *Cbfa2*$^{-/-}$, *Cbfb*$^{-/-}$, and *Cbfb-MYH11*$^{+/-}$ mice described above. However, yolk sac cells from *Cbfa2-ETO*$^{+/-}$ embryos differentiated into macrophages ex vivo, whereas cells from *Cbfa2*$^{-/-}$ or *Cbfb*$^{-/-}$embryos formed no colonies, indicating that the AML1-ETO fusion protein may have other biological properties in addition to its dominant-negative effect on AML1 function. As in the case of the AML1-MYH11 fusion protein, there is good evidence that AML1-ETO prevents normal hematopoietic differentiation, but its role in promoting cellular proliferation remains to be determined. The AML1-ETO protein had a dominant-negative effect on AML1-mediated transcriptional activation of the genes encoding TCR-β and GM-CSF, but activated transcription of the gene encoding M-CSF synergistically with AML1 (Frank et al., 1995; Meyers et al., 1995), providing further evidence of the complex dysregulation of hematopoiesis caused by the fusion protein.

CBP and M4/M5 Acute Myeloid Leukemia

Acute myeloid leukemia associated with the translocation t(8;16)(p11; p13) is characterized by a block in differentiation at the myelomonocytic

(M4) or myelocytic (M5) stage of hematopoiesis and a poor clinical prognosis (reviewed by Borrow et al., 1996). Cloning of DNA across the translocation breakpoint on chromosome 16 revealed the presence of a fusion gene consisting of *CBP* coding sequences from chromosome 16p13 and chromosome 8p11 sequences encoding a novel protein designated MOZ (monocytic-leukemia zinc finger protein) (Borrow et al., 1996). As shown in Figure 15.8, the resulting fusion protein consists of amino acids 1–1547 of the 2004-residue MOZ protein fused to amino acids 266–2440 of CBP. As described in Chapters 3 and 13, CBP is a coactivator that is required for transcriptional activation mediated by a large number of DNA-binding factors, including glucocorticoid and retinoic acid receptors, cAMP response element binding protein, C-JUN, C-FOS, C-MYB, and E2F, and is likely to play an important role in the regulation of cellular proliferation. Although the function of MOZ is unknown, the protein contains two C2HC zinc fingers, also known as PHD fingers (Aasland et al., 1995), which have been found in several other proteins implicated in transcriptional regulation, including the putative coactivator protein XH2 (Gibbons et al., 1997; see Chapter 13).

What is most striking about this translocation is that it fuses genes that each encode proteins containing acetyltransferase domains, both of which are contained in the fusion protein (see Fig. 15.8). In addition to having intrinsic histone acetyltransferase activity, CBP interacts with

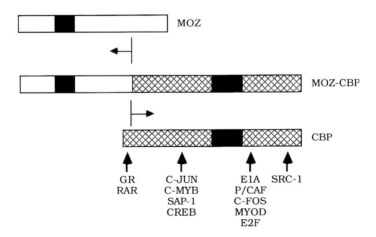

FIGURE 15-8. Structure of MOZ, CBP, and MOZ-CBP fusion protein expressed in M4–M5 subtype of acute myeloid leukemia cells carrying a t(8;16). The acetyltransferase domains of MOZ and CBP are indicated by solid boxes. The sites of CBP interaction with other transcription factors is indicated by arrows at bottom.

other proteins, including P/CAF (Yang et al., 1996) and SRC-1 (Spencer et al., 1997), which also have histone acetyltransferase activity. These results suggest that dysregulated chromatin acetylation may contribute to leukemogenesis. It is unclear whether the fusion protein exerts its pathophysiologic effects by interfering with normal expression of MOZ or CBP, or whether it acts via a gain-of-function mechanism. In this respect, it is of interest that patients with the Rubenstein-Taybi syndrome, who are heterozygous for a loss-of-function allele at the CBP locus (Petrij et al., 1995), have an increased incidence of tumors (Miller and Rubenstein, 1995).

PAX Genes in Cancer

Forced expression of PAX1, PAX2, PAX3, PAX6, or PAX8 was sufficient to induce cellular transformation in tissue culture and tumor formation in mice (Maulbecker and Gruss, 1993b). These data were consistent with the general principle that dysregulated expression of transcription factors that play key roles in embryogenesis can contribute to tumorigenesis, as previously described for HOX proteins (Maulbecker and Gruss, 1993a). Tumor-specific translocations involving *PAX* genes that result in the synthesis of fusion protein oncogenes have subsequently been described. Among the many translocations involving the *IGH* locus in lymphomas (see above), the characteristic t(9;14)(p13;q32) translocation found in small lymphocytic lymphomas contains a breakpoint in the 5'-flanking region of the *PAX5* gene, suggesting that dysregulated expression of PAX5 contributes to oncogenesis in these cells (Busslinger et al., 1996).

Translocations are less common in solid tumors. However, a t(2; 13)(q35;q14) or t(1;13)(p36;q14) translocation was identified in over 90% of alveolar rhabdomyosarcomas analyzed and contained breakpoints within *PAX3* or *PAX7*, respectively, and *FKHR*, which encodes a transcription factor of the forkhead DNA-binding domain class (Barr et al., 1993, 1995; Galili et al., 1993; Shapiro et al., 1993). In approximately 20% of tumors, the fusion gene is amplified (Barr et al., 1996). These results provide convincing evidence that PAX3-FKHR and PAX7-FKHR fusion proteins function as important oncogenes in the context of alveolar rhabdomyosarcoma. The PAX3-FKHR fusion protein, which contains the PAX3 DNA-binding domain and FKHR transcriptional activation domain, activated reporter gene transcription to a greater extent than did PAX3 (Fredericks et al., 1995). However, the targets for transcriptional activation by the fusion protein within tumors cells remain to be defined in future studies. The powerful oncogenic effect of these fusion proteins may explain why these tumors occur in the pediatric population—in contrast to most cancers, which do not develop until later in life.

References

Aas, T., A.-L. Borresen, S. Geisler, B. Smith-Sorensen, H. Johnsen, J. E. Vargaug, L. A. Akslen, and P. E. Lonning. Specific p53 mutations are associated with de novo resistance to doxorubicin in breast cancer patients. *Nat. Med.* 2:811–814, 1996.

Aasland, R., T. J. Gibson, and A. F. Stewart. The PHD finger: implications for chromatin-mediated transcriptional regulation. *Trends Biochem. Sci.* 20:56–59, 1995.

Adams, J. M., A. W. Harris, C. A. Pinkert, M. Corcoran, W. S. Alexander, S. Cory, R. D. Palmiter, and R. L. Brinster. The c-myc oncogene driven by immuno-globulin enhancers induces lymphoid malignancies in transgenic mice. *Nature* 318:533–538, 1985.

Aplan, P. D., D. P. Lombardi, G. H. Reaman, H. N. Sather, G. D. Hammond, and I. R. Kirsch. Involvement of the putative hematopoietic transcription factor SCL in T-cell acute lymphoblastic leukemia. *Blood* 79:1327–1333, 1992.

Bae, S. C., Y. Yamaguchi-Iwai, E. Ogawa, M. Maruyama, M. Inuzuka, H. Kago-shima, K. Shigesada, M. Satake, and Y. Ito. Isolation of PEBP2αB cDNA representing the mouse homolog of human acute myeloid leukemia gene, AML1. *Oncogene* 8:809–814, 1993.

Bae, S.-C., E. Takahashi, Y. W. Zhang, E. Ogawa, K. Shigesada, Y. Namba, M. Satake, and Y. Ito. Cloning, mapping, and expression of PEBP2αC, a third gene encoding the mammalian Runt domain. *Gene* 159:245–248, 1995.

Bain, G., E. C. Robanus Maandag, D. J. Izon, D. Amsen, A. M. Kruisbeek, B. C. Weintraub, I. Krop, M. S. Schlissel, A. J. Feeney, M. van Roon, M. van der Valk, H. P. J. te Riele, A. Berns, and C. Murre. E2A proteins are required for proper B cell development and initiation of immunoglobulin rearrange-ments. *Cell* 79:885–892, 1994.

Bargonetti, J., P. N. Friedman, S. E. Kern, B. Vogelstein, and C. Prives. Wild-type but not mutant p53 immunopurified proteins bind to sequences adjacent to the SV40 origin of replication. *Cell* 65:1083–1091, 1991.

Barr, F. G., J. Chatten, C. M. D'Cruz, A. E. Wilson, L. E. Nauta, L. M. Nycum, J. A. Biegel, and R. B. Womer. Molecular assays for chromosomal translo-cations in the diagnosis of pediatric soft tissue sarcomas. *JAMA* 27:553–557, 1995.

Barr, F. G., N. Galili, J. Holick, J. A. Biegel, G. Rovera, and B. S. Emanuel. Re-arrangement of the PAX3 paired box gene in the pediatric solid tumor al-veolar rhabdomyosarcoma. *Nat. Genet.* 3:113–117, 1993.

Barr, F. G., L. E. Nauta, R. J. Davis, B. W. Schafer, L. M. Nycum, and J. A. Biegel. In vivo amplification of the PAX3-FKHR and PAX7-FKHR fusion genes in alveolar rhabdomyosarcoma. *Hum. Mol. Genet.* 5:15–21, 1996.

Begley, C.G., P. D. Aplan, S. M. Denning, B. F. Haynes, T. A. Waldmann, and I. R. Kirsch. The gene SCL is expressed during early hematopoiesis and encodes a differentiation-related DNA-binding motif. *Proc. Natl. Acad. Sci. U.S.A.* 86:10128–10132, 1989.

Benezra, R. An intermolecular disulfide bond stabilizes E2A homodimers and is required for DNA binding at physiological temperatures. *Cell* 79:1057–1067, 1994.

Bernard, O., N. Lecointe, P. Jonveaux, M. Souyri, M. Mauchauffe, R. Berger, C. J. Larsen, and D. Mathieu-Mahul. Two site-specific deletions and t(1;14) translocation restricted to human T-cell acute leukemias disrupt the 5' part of the tal-1 gene. *Oncogene* 6:1477–1488, 1991.

Borrow, J., V. P. Stanton, Jr., J. M. Andresen, R. Becher, F. G. Behm, R. S. K. Chaganti, C. I. Civin, C. Disteche, I. Dube, A. M. Frischauf, D. Horsman, F. Mitelman, S. Volinia, A. E. Watmore, and D. E. Housman. The translocation t(8;16)(p11;p13) of acute myeloid leukemia fuses a putative acetyltransferase to the CREB-binding protein. *Nat. Genet.* 14:33–41, 1996.

Brockes, J. Reading the retinoid signals. *Nature* 345:766–768, 1990.

Brown, D., S. Kogan, E. Lagasse, I. Weissman, M. Alcalay, P. G. Pelicci, S. Atwater, and J M. Bishop. A PMLRARα transgene initiates murine acute promyelocytic leukemia. *Proc. Natl. Acad. Sci. U.S.A.* 94:2551–2556, 1997.

Brown, L., J. T. Cheng, Q. Chen, M. J. Siciliano, W. Crist, G. Buchanan, and R. Baer. Site-specific recombination of the tal-1 gene is a common occurrence in human T cell leukemia. *EMBO J.* 9:3343–3351, 1990.

Busslinger, M., N. Klix, P. Pfeffer, P. G. Graninger, and Z. Kozmik. Deregulation of PAX-5 by translocation of the Eμ enhancer of the IgH locus adjacent to two alternative PAX-5 promoters in a diffuse large-cell lymphoma. *Proc. Natl. Acad. Sci. U.S.A.* 93:6129–6134, 1996.

Cameron, S., D. S. Taylor, E. C. TePas, N. A. Speck, and B. Mathey-Prevot. Identification of a critical regulatory site in the human interleukin-3 promoter by in vivo footprinting. *Blood* 83:2851–2859, 1994.

Castaigne, S., C. Chommienne, M. T. Daniel, P. Ballerini, R. Berger, P. Fenaux, and L. Degos. All trans-retinoic acid as a differentiation therapy for acute promyelocytic leukemia. I. Clinical results. *Blood* 76:1704–1709, 1990.

Castilla, L. H., C. Wijmenga, Q. Wang, T. Stacy, N. A. Speck, M. Eckhaus, M. Marin-Padilla, F. S. Collins, A. Wynshaw-Boris, and P. P. Liu. Failure of embryonic hematopoiesis and lethal hemorrhages in mouse embryos heterozygous for a knocked-in leukemia gene CBFB-MYH11. *Cell* 87:687–697, 1996.

Chan, S.-K., L. Jaffe, M. Capovilla, J. Botas, and R. Mann. The DNA binding specificity of Ultrabithorax is modulated by cooperative interactions with extradenticle, another homeoprotein. *Cell* 78:603–615, 1994.

Chellappan, S. P., S. Hiebert, M. Mudryj, J. M. Horowitz, and J. R. Nevins. The E2F transcription factor is a cellular target for the RB protein. *Cell* 65:1053–1061, 1991.

Chen, P.-L., Y. Chen, R. Bookstein, and W.-H. Lee. Genetic mechanisms of tumor suppression by the human p53 gene. *Science* 250:1576–1580, 1990.

Cho, Y., S. Gorina, P. D. Jeffrey, and N. P. Pavletich. Crystal structure of a p53 tumor supressor-DNA complex: understanding tumorigenic mutations. *Science* 265:346–355, 1994.

Cleary, M. L. Oncogenic conversion of transcription factors by chromosomal translocations. *Cell* 66:619–622, 1991.

Cowell, I. G., A. Skinner, and H. C. Hurst. Transcriptional repression by a novel member of the bZIP family of transcription factors. *Mol. Cell. Biol.* 12:3070–3077, 1992.

Cross, S. M., C. A. Sanchez, C. A. Morgan, M. K. Schimke, S. Ramel, R. L. Idzerda, W. H. Rasking, and B. J. Reid. A p53-dependent mouse spindle checkpoint. *Science* 1353–1356, 1995.

de The, H., C. Lavau, A. Marchio, C. Chomienne, L. Degos, and A. Dejean. The PML-RARα fusion in RNA generated by the t(15;17) translocation in acute promyelocytic leukemia encodes a functionally altered RAR. *Cell* 66:675–684, 1991.

DeCaprio, J. A. , J. W. Ludlow, J. Figge, J. Y. Shew, C. M. Huang, W. H. Lee, E. Marsilio, E. Paucha, and D. M. Livingston. SV40 large tumor antigen forms a specific complex with the product of the retinoblastoma susceptibility gene. *Cell* 54:275–283, 1988.

Dedera, D. A., E. K. Waller, D. P. LeBrun, A. Sen-Majumbar, M. E. Stevens, G. S. Barsh, and M. L. Cleary. Chimeric homeobox gene E2a-Pbx1 induces proliferation, apoptosis, and malignant lymphomas in transgenic mice. *Cell* 74:833–843, 1993.

Diverio, D., F. LoCoco, F. D'Adamo, A. Biondi, M. Fagioli, A. Grignani, A. Rambaldi, V. Rossi, G. Avvisati, M. C. Petti, A. M. Testi, V. Liso, G. Specchia, G. Fioritoni, A. Recchia, S. Frassoni, S. Ciolli, and P. G. Pelicci. Identification of DNA rearrangements at the RAR-α locus in all patients with acute promyelocytic leukemia (APL) and mapping of APL breakpoints within the RARα second intron. *Blood* 79:1–5, 1992.

Donehower, L. A., M. Harvey, B. L. Slagle, M. J. McArthur, C. A. Montgomery Jr., J. S. Butel, and A. Bradley. Mice deficient for p53 are developmentally normal but susceptible to spontaneous tumors. *Nature* 356:215–221, 1992.

Duan, D. R., A. Pause, W. H. Burgess, T. Aso, D. Y. T. Chen, K. P. Garrett, R. C. Conaway, J. W. Conaway, W. M. Linehan, and R. D. Klausner. Inhibition of elongation by the VHL tumor suppressor protein. *Science* 269:1402–1406, 1995.

Dyson, N., P. M. Howley, K. Munger, and E. Harlow. The human papilloma virus-16 E7 oncoprotein is able to bind to the retinoblastoma gene product. *Science* 242:934–937, 1989.

El-Deiry, W. S., T. Tokino, V. E. Velculescu, D. B. Levy, R. Parsons, J. M. Trent, D. Lin, W. E. Mercer, K. W. Kinzler, and B. Vogelstein. WAF1, a potential mediator of p53 tumor suppression. *Cell* 75:817–825, 1993.

Erickson, P., J. Gao, K. S. Chang, A. T. Look, E. Whisenant, S. Raimondi, R. Lasher, J. Trujillo, J. Rowley, and H. Drabkin. Identification of breakpoints in t(8;21) acute myelogenous leukemia and isolation of a fusion transcript, AML1/ETO, with similarity to Drosophila segmentation gene, runt. *Blood* 80:1825–1831, 1992.

Field, S. J., F.-Y. Tsai, F. Kuo, A. M. Zubiaga, W. G. Kaelin, Jr., D. M. Livingston, S. H. Orkin, and M. E. Greenberg. E2F-1 functions in mice to promote apoptosis and suppress proliferation. *Cell* 85:549–561, 1996.

Finger, L. R., J. Kagan, G. Christopher, J. Kurtzberg, M. S. Hershfield, P. C. Nowell, and C. M. Croce. Involvement of the TCL5 gene on human chromosome 1 in T-cell leukemia and melanoma. *Proc. Natl. Acad. Sci. U.S.A.* 86:5039–5043, 1989.

Fitzgerald, T. J., G. A. Neale, S. C. Raimondi, and R. M. Goorha. c-tal, a helix-loop-helix protein, is juxtaposed to the T-cell receptor-beta chain gene by a reciprocal chromosomal translocation: t(1;7)(p32;q35). *Blood* 78:2686–2695, 1991.

Frank, R., J. Zhang, H. Uchida, S. Meyers, S. W. Hiebert, and S. D. Nimer. The AML1/ETO fusion protein blocks transactivation of the GM-CSF promoter by AML1B. *Oncogene* 11:2667–2674, 1995.

Fredericks, W. J., N. Galili, S. Mukhopadhyay, G. Rovera, J. Bennicelli, F. G. Barr, and F. J. Rauscher III. The PAX3-FKHR fusion protein created by the t(2;13) translocation in alveolar rhabdomyosarcoma is a more potent transcriptional activator than PAX3. *Mol. Cell. Biol.* 15:1522–1535, 1995.

Friend, S. H., J. M. Horowitz, M. R. Gerber, X. F. Wang, E. Bogenmann, F. P. Li, and R. A. Weinberg. Deletions of a DNA sequence in retinoblastomas and mesenchymal tumors: organization of the sequence and its encoded protein. *Proc. Natl. Acad. Sci. U.S.A.* 84:9059–9063, 1987.

Fukasawa, K., T. Choi, R. Kuriyama, S. Rulong, and G. F. Vande Woude. Abnormal centrosome amplification in the absence of p53. *Science* 271:1744–1747, 1996.

Galaktionov, K., X. Chen, and D. Beach. Cdc25 cell-cycle phosphatase as a target of c-myc. *Nature* 382:511–517, 1996.

Galili, N., R. J. Davis, W. J. Fredericks, S. Mukhopadhyay, F. J. Rauscher III, B. S. Emanuel, G. Rovera, and F. G. Barr. Fusion of a fork head domain gene to PAX3 in the solid tumor alveolar rhabdomyosarcoma. *Nat. Genet.* 5:230–235, 1993.

Gibbons, R. J., S. Bachoo, D. J. Picketts, S. Aftimos, B Asenbauer, J. Bergoffen, S. A. Berry, N. Dahl, A. Fryer, K. Keppler, K. Kurosawa, M. L. Levin, M. Masuno, G. Neri, M. E. Pierpont, S. S. Slaney, and D. R. Higgs. Mutations in a transcriptional regulator (hATRX) establish the functional significance of a PHD-like domain. *Nat. Genet.* 17:146–148, 1997.

Gnarra, J. R., S. Zhou, M. J. Merrill, J. R. Wagner, A. Krumm, E. Papavassiliou, E. H. Oldfield, R. D. Klausner, and W. M. Linehan. Post-transcriptional regulation of vascular endothelial growth factor mRNA by the product of the VHL tumor suppressor gene. *Proc. Natl. Acad. Sci. U.S.A.* 93:10589–10594, 1996.

Golub, T. R., G. F. Barker, S. K. Bohlander, S. Hiebert, D. C. Ward, P. Bray-Ward, E. Morgan, S. C. Raimondi, J. D. Rowley, and D. G. Gilliland. Fusion of the TEL gene on 12p13 to the AML1 gene on 21q22 in acute lymphoblastic leukemia. *Proc. Natl. Acad. Sci. U.S.A.* 92:4917–4921, 1995.

Gonzalez-Zulueta, M., C. M. Bender, A. S. Yang, T. Nguyen, R. W. Beart, J. W. Van Tornout, and P. A. Jones. Methylation of the 5' CpG island of the p16/CDKN2 tumor suppressor gene in normal and transformed human tissues correlates with gene silencing. *Cancer Res.* 55:4531–4535, 1995

Graeber, T. G., C. Osmanian, T. Jacks, D. E. Housman, C. J. Koch, S. W. Lowe, and A. J. Giaccia. Hypoxia-mediated selection of cells with diminished apoptotic potential in solid tumors. *Nature* 379:88–91, 1996.

Graeber, T. G., J. F. Peterson, M. Tsai, K. Monica, A. J. Fornace, Jr., and A. J. Giaccia. Hypoxia induces accumulation of p53 protein, but activation of a G_1-phase checkpoint by low-oxygen conditions is independent of p53 status. *Mol. Cell. Biol.* 14:6264–6277, 1994.

Greenblatt, M. S., W. P. Bennett, M. Hollstein, and C. C. Harris. Mutations in the

p53 tumor suppressor gene: clues to cancer etiology and molecular patho-
        genesis. *Cancer Res.* 54:4855–4878, 1994.

Greger, V., N. Debus, D. Lohmann, W. Hopping, E. Passarge, and B. Horsthemke.
        Frequency and parental origin of hypermethylated RB1 alleles in retinoblas-
        toma. *Hum Genet.* 94:491–496, 1994

Grignani, F., P. F. Ferrucci, U. Testa, G. Talamo, M. Fagioli, M. Alcalay, A. Men-
        carelli, F. Grignani, C. Peschle, I. Nicoletti, and P. G. Pelicci. The acute pro-
        myelocytic leukemia-specific PML-RAR fusion protein inhibits differentia-
        tion and promotes survival of myeloid precursor cells. *Cell* 74:423–431, 1993.

Gu, W., and R. G. Roeder. Activation of p53 sequence-specific DNA binding by
        acetylation of the p53 C-terminal domain. *Cell* 90:595–606, 1997.

Hainaut, P., T. Soussi, B. Shomer, M. Hollstein, M. Greenblatt, E. Hovig, C. C.
        Harris, and R. Montesano. Database of p53 gene somatic mutations in hu-
        man tumors and cell lines: updated compilation and future prospects. *Nu-
        cleic Acids Res.* 25:151–157, 1997.

Harper, J. W., G. Adami, N. Wei, K. Keyomarsi, and S. J. Elledge. The 21 kd Cdk
        interacting protein Cip1 is a potent inhibitor of G_1 cyclin-dependent kinases.
        Cell 75:805–816, 1993.

Hateboer, G., R. M. Kerkhoven, A. Shvarts, R. Bernards, and R. L. Beijersbergen.
        Degradation of E2F by the ubiquitin-proteasome pathway: regulation by re-
        tinoblastoma family proteins and adenovirus transforming proteins. *Genes
        Dev.* 10:2960–2970, 1996.

Haupt, Y., R. Maya, A. Kazaz, and M. Oren. Mdm2 promotes the rapid degra-
        dation of p53. *Nature* 387:296–299, 1997.

Herman, J. G., C. I. Civin, J. P. Issa, M. I. Collector, S. J. Sharkis, and S. B. Baylin.
        Distinct patterns of inactivation of p15INK4B and p16INK4A characterize
        the major types of hematological malignancies. *Cancer Res.* 57:837–841, 1997.

Herman, J. G., F. Latif, W. Yongkai, M. Lerman, B. Zbar, S. Liu, D. Samid, R.
        Dah-Shuhn, J. R. Gnarra, W. M. Linehan, and S. B. Baylin. Silencing of the
        VHL tumor-suppressor gene by DNA methylation in renal carcinoma. *Proc.
        Natl. Acad. Sci. U.S.A.* 91:9700–9704, 1994.

Hiebert, S. W., S. P. Chellappan, J. M. Horowitz, and J. R. Nevins. The interaction
        of RB with E2F coincides with an inhibition of the transcriptional activity of
        E2F. *Genes Dev.* 6:177–185, 1992.

Hofmann, F., F. Martelli, D. M. Livingston, and Z. Wang. The retinoblastoma
        gene product protects E2F-1 from degradation by the ubiquitin-proteasome
        pathway. *Genes Dev.* 10:2949–2959, 1996.

Hollstein, M., D. Sidransky, B. Vogelstein, and C. C. Harris. p53 mutations in
        human cancers. *Science* 253:49–53, 1991.

Hu, N., A. Gutsmann, D. C. Herbert, A. Bradley, W.-H. Lee, and E. H.-H. P. Lee.
        Heterozygous rb-1/+ mice are predisposed to tumors of the pituitary gland
        with a nearly complete penetrance. *Oncogene* 9:1021–1027, 1994.

Huang, M. E., Y. C. Ye, S. R. Chen, J. R. Chai, J. X. Lu, L. Zhoa, L. J. Gu, and
        Z. Y. Wang. Use of all-trans retinoic acid in the treatment of acute promye-
        locytic leukemia. *Blood* 72:567–572, 1988.

Hunger, S. P. Chromosomal translocations involving the E2A gene in acute lym-
        phoblastic leukemia: clinical features and molecular pathogenesis. *Blood* 87:
        1211–1224, 1996.

Hunger, S. P., R. Brown, and M. L. Cleary. DNA-binding and transcriptional regulatory properties of hepatic leukemia factor (HLF) and the t(17;19) acute lymphoblastic leukemia chimera E2A-HLF. *Mol. Cell. Biol.* 14:5986–5996, 1994a.

Hunger, S. P., P. E. Devaraj, L. Foroni, L. M. Secker-Walker, and M. L. Cleary. Two types of genomic rearrangements create alternative E2A-HLF fusion proteins in t(17;19)-ALL. *Blood* 83:2970–2977, 1994b.

Hunger, S. P., N. Galili, A. J. Carroll, W. M. Crist, M. P. Link, and M. L. Cleary. The t(1;19)(q23;p13) results in consistent fusion of E2A and PBX1 coding sequences in acute lymphoblastic leukemias. *Blood* 77:687–693, 1991.

Hunger, S. P., K. Ohyashiki, K. Toyama, and M. L. Cleary. HLF, a novel hepatic bZIP protein, shows altered DNA-binding properties following fusion to E2A in t(17;19) acute lymphoblastic leukemia. *Genes Dev.* 6:1608–1620, 1992.

Hupp, T. R., and D. P. Lane. Allosteric activation of latent p53 tetramers. *Curr. Biol.* 4:865–875, 1994.

Iliopoulos, O., A. P. Levy, C. Jiang, W. G. Kaelin, Jr., and M. A. Goldberg. Negative regulation of hypoxia-inducible genes by the von Hippel-Lindau protein. *Proc. Natl. Acad. Sci. U.S.A.* 93:10595–10599, 1996.

Inaba, T., T. Inukai, T. Yoshihara, H. Seyschab, R. A. Ashmun, C. E. Canman, S. J. Laken, M. B. Kastan, and A. T. Look. Reversal of apoptosis by the leukemia-associated E2A-HLF chimaeric transcription factor. *Nature* 382:541–544, 1996.

Inaba, T., W. M. Roberts, L. H. Shapiro, K. W. Jolly, S. C. Raimondi, S. D. Smith, and A. T. Look. Fusion of the leucine zipper gene HLF to the E2A gene in human acute B-lineage leukemia. *Science* 257:531–534, 1992.

Jacks, T., A. Fazeli, E. Schmitt, R. Bronson, M. Goodell, and R. Weinberg. Effects of an Rb mutation in the mouse. *Nature* 359:295–300, 1992.

Jayaraman, L., and C. Prives. Activation of p53 sequence-specific DNA binding by short single strands of DNA requires the p53 C-terminus. *Cell* 81:1021–1029, 1995.

Jeffrey, P. D., S. Gorina, and N. P. Pavletich. Crystal structure of the tetramerization domain of the p53 tumor suppressor at 1.7 angstroms. *Science* 267:1498–1502, 1995.

Kakizuka, A., W. H. Miller, Jr., K. Umesono, R. P. Warrell, Jr., and S. R. Frankel, V. V. V. S. Murtry, E. Dmitrovsky, and R. M. Evans. Chromosomal translocation t(15;17) in human acute promyelocytic leukemia fuses RARα with a novel putative transcription factor, PML. *Cell* 66:663–674, 1991.

Kamps, M. P., and D. Baltimore. E2A-Pbx1, the t(1;19) translocation protein of human pre-B-cell acute lymphocytic leukemia, causes acute myeloid leukemia in mice. *Mol. Cell. Biol.* 13:351–357, 1993.

Kamps, M. P., C. Murre, X. H. Sun, and D. Baltimore. A new homeobox gene contributes the DNA binding domain of the t(1;19) translocation protein in pre-B ALL. *Cell* 60:547–555, 1990.

Kern, S. E., K. W. Kinzler, A Bruskin, D. Jarosz, P. Friedman, C. Prives, and B. Vogelstein. Identification of p53 as a sequence-specific DNA-binding protein. *Science* 252:1708–1711, 1991.

Kern, S. E., J. A. Pietenpol, S. Thiagalingam, A. Seymour, K. W. Kinzler, and B. Vogelstein. Oncogenic forms of p53 inhibit p53-regulated gene expression. *Science* 256:827–830, 1992.

Kibel, A., O. Iliopoulos, J. A. DeCaprio, and W. G. Kaelin, Jr. Binding of the von

Hippel-Lindau tumor suppressor protein to elongin B and C. *Science* 269: 1444–1446, 1995.

Knudson, A. G., Jr. Mutation and cancer: statistical study of retinoblastoma. *Proc. Natl. Acad. Sci. U.S.A.* 68:820–823, 1971.

Knudson, A. G., Jr., H. W. Hethcote, and B .W. Brown. Mutation and childhood cancer: a probabilistic model for the incidence of retinoblastoma. *Proc. Natl. Acad. Sci. U.S.A.* 72:5116–5120, 1975.

Ko, L. J., and C. Prives. p53: puzzle and paradigm. *Genes Dev.* 10:1054–1072, 1996.

Krumm, A., and M. Groudine. Tumor suppression and transcription elongation: the dire consequences of changing partners. *Science* 269:1400–1401, 1995.

Kubbutat, M. H. G., S. N. Jones, and K. H. Vousden. Regulation of p53 stability by Mdm2. *Nature* 387:299–303, 1997.

Kussie, P. H., S. Gorina, V. Marechal, B. Elenbaas, J. Moreau, A. J. Levine, and N. P. Pavletich. Structure of the MDM2 oncoprotein bound to the p53 tumor suppressor transactivation domain. *Science* 274:948–953, 1996.

Laird, P. W., and R. Jaenisch. DNA methylation and cancer. *Hum. Mol. Genet.* 3: 1487–1495, 1994.

Lammer, E. J., D. T. Chen, R. M. Hoar, N. D. Agnish, P. J. Benke, J. T. Braun, C. J. Curry, P. M. Fernhoff, A. W. Grix, Jr., I. T. Lott, J. M. Richard, and S. C. Sun. Retinoic acid embryopathy. *N. Engl. J. Med.* 313:837–841, 1985.

Lee, S., B. Elenbaas, A. J. Levine, and J. Griffith. p53 and its 14 kDa C-terminal domain recognize primary DNA damage in the form of insertion/deletion mismatches. *Cell* 81:1013–1020, 1995.

Levanon, D., V. Negreanu, Y. Bernstein, I. Bar-Am, L. Avivi, and Y. Groneer. AML1, AML2, and AML3, the human members of the runt domain gene-family: cDNA structure, expression, and chromosomal localization. *Genomics* 23:425–432, 1994.

Levine, A. J. p53, the cellular gatekeeper for growth and division. *Cell* 88:323–331, 1997.

Levine, A. J., J. Momand, and C. A. Finlay. The p53 tumour suppressor gene. *Nature* 351:453–456, 1991.

Li, F. P., and J. F. Fraumeni, Jr. Soft-tissue sarcomas, breast cancer, and other neoplasms: a familial syndrome? *Ann. Intern. Med.* 71:747–752, 1969.

Lin, J., X. Wu, J. Chen, A. Chang, and A. J. Levine. Functions of the p53 protein in growth regulation and tumor suppression. *Cold Spring Harbor Symp. Quant. Biol.* 59:215–223, 1995.

Linke, S. P., K. C. Clarkin, A. DiLeonardo, A. Tsou, and G. M. Wahl. A reversible, p53-dependent G0/G1 cell cycle arrest induced by ribonucleotide depletion in the absence of detectable DNA damage. *Genes Dev.* 10:934–947, 1996.

Liu, P., N. Siedel, D. Bodine, N. Speck, S. Tarle, and F. S. Collins. Acute myeloid leukemia with inv(16) produces a chimeric transcription factor with a my-osin heavy chain tail. *Cold Spring Harbor Symp. Quant. Biol.* 59:547–553, 1994.

Liu, P., S. A. Tarle, A. Hajra, D. F. Claxton, P. Marlton, M. Freedman, M. J. Siciliano, and F. S. Collins. Fusion between transcription factor CBFα/ PEBP2β and a myosin heavy chain in acute myeloid leukemia. *Science* 261: 1041–1044, 1993.

Lowe, S. W., H. E. Ruley, T. Jacks, and D. E. Housman. p53-dependent apoptosis modulates the cytotoxicity of anticancer agents. *Cell* 74:957–968, 1993a.

Lowe, S. W., E. M. Schmitt, S. W. Smith, B. A. Osborne, and T. Jacks. p53 is required for radiation induced apoptosis in mouse thymocytes. *Nature* 362: 847–849, 1993b.

Lu, H., and A. J. Levine. Human TAF-31 is a transcriptional coactivator of the p53 protein. *Proc. Natl. Acad. Sci. U.S.A.* 92:5154–5158, 1995.

Lu, Q., P. S. Knoepfler, J. Scheele, D. D. Wright, and M. P. Kamps. Both Pbx1 and E2A-Pbx1 bind the DNA motif ATCAATCAA cooperatively with the products of multiple murine Hox genes, some of which are themselves oncogenes. *Mol. Cell. Biol.* 15:3786–3795, 1995.

Lu, X., and D. P. Lane. Differential induction of transcriptionally active p53 following UV or ionizing radiation: defects in chromosome instability syndromes? *Cell* 75:765–778, 1993.

Malkin, D. Germline p53 mutations and heritable cancer. *Annu. Rev. Genet.* 28: 443–465, 1994.

Malkin, D., F. P. Li, L. C. Strong, J. F. Fraumeni Jr., C. E. Nelson, D. H. Kim, J. H. Kassel, M. A. Gryka, F. Z. Bischoff, M. A. Tainsky, and S. H. Friend. Germ line p53 mutations in a familial syndrome of breast cancer, sarcomas, and other neoplasms. *Science* 250:1233–1238, 1990.

Maulbecker, C. C., and P. Gruss. The oncogenic potential of deregulated homeobox genes. *Cell Growth Differ.* 4:431–441, 1993a.

Maulbecker, C. C., and P. Gruss. The oncogenic potential of Pax genes. *EMBO J.* 12:2361–2367, 1993b.

Mellentin, J. D., C. M. Murre, T. Donlon, P. S. McCaw, S. D. Smith, A. J. Carroll, M. E. McDonald, D. Baltimore, and M. L. Cleary. The gene for enhancer binding proteins E12/E47 lies at the t(1;19) breakpoint in acute leukemias. *Science* 246:379–382, 1989a.

Mellentin, J. D., S. D. Smith, and M. L. Cleary. lyl-1, a novel gene altered by chromosomal translocation in T cell leukemia, codes for a protein with a helix-loop-helix DNA binding motif. *Cell* 58:77–83, 1989b.

Mellentin, J. D., J. Nourse, S. P. Hunger, S. D. Smith, and M. L. Cleary. Molecular analysis of the t(1;19) breakpoint cluster region in pre-B-cell ALL. *Genes Chrom.Cancer* 2:239–247, 1990.

Merlo, A., J. G. Herman, L. Mao, D. J. Lee, E. Gabrielson, P. C. Burger, S. B. Baylin, and D. Sidransky. 5' CpG island methylation is associated with transcriptional silencing of the tumor suppressor p16/CDKN2/MTS1 in human cancers. *Nat. Med.* 1:686–692, 1995.

Meyers, S., J. R. Downing, and S. W. Hiebert. Identification of AML-1 and the t(8;21) translocation protein (AML-1/ETO) as sequence-specific DNA-binding proteins: the runt homology domain is required for DNA binding and protein-protein interactions. *Mol. Cell. Biol.* 13:6336–6345, 1993.

Meyers, S., N. Lenny, and S. W. Hiebert. The t(8;21) fusion protein interferes with AML-1B-dependent transcriptional activation. *Mol. Cell. Biol.* 15:1974–1982, 1995.

Mietz, J. A., T. Unger, J. M. Huibregtse, and P. M. Howley. The transcriptional transactivation function of wild-type p53 is inhibited by SV40 large T-antigen and by HPV-16 E6 oncoprotein. *EMBO J.* 11:5013–5020, 1992.

Miller, R. W., and J. H. Rubenstein. Tumors in Rubenstein-Taybi syndrome. *Am. J. Med. Genet.* 56:112–115, 1995.

Milner, J., and E. A. Medcalf. Cotranslation of activated mutant p53 with wild type drives the wild-type p53 protein into the mutant conformation. *Cell* 65: 765–774, 1991.

Mitani, K., S. Ogawa, T. Tanaka, H. Miyoshi, M. Kurokawa, H. Mano, Y. Yazaki, M. Ohki, and H. Hirai. Generation of the AML-1-EVI-1 fusion gene in the t(3;21)(q26;q22) causes blastic crisis in chronic myeloid leukemia. *EMBO J.* 13:504–510, 1994.

Mitelman, F. *Catalog of Chromosome Aberrations in Cancer*, 3rd ed. New York: Alan R. Liss, Inc., 1988.

Miyamoto, A., X. Cui, L. Naumovski, and M. L. Cleary. Helix-loop-helix proteins LYL1 and E2a form heterodimeric complexes with distinctive DNA-binding properties in hematolymphoid cells. *Mol. Cell. Biol.* 16:2394–2401, 1996.

Miyoshi, H., T. Kozu, K. Shimizu, K. Mitani, H. Hirai, T. Imai, K. Yokoyama, E. Soeda, and M. Ohki. The t(8;21) translocation in acute myeloid leukemia results in production of an AML1-MTG8 fusion transcript. *EMBO J.* 12:2715–2721, 1993.

Miyoshi, H., K. Shimizu, T. Kozu, N. Maseki, Y. Kaneko, and M. Ohki. t(8:21) breakpoints on chromosome 21 in acute myeloid leukemia are clustered within a limited region of a single gene, AML1. *Proc. Natl. Acad. Sci. U.S.A.* 88:10431–10434, 1991.

Moll, U. M., M. LaQuaglia, J. Benard, and G. Riou. Wild-type P53 protein undergoes cytoplasmic sequestration in undifferentiated neuroblastomas but not in differentiated tumors. *Proc. Natl. Acad. Sci. U.S.A.* 92:4407–4411, 1995.

Moll, U. M., G. Riou, and A. J. Levine. Two distinct mechanisms alter p53 in breast cancer: mutation and nuclear exclusion. *Proc. Natl. Acad. Sci. U.S.A.* 89:7262–7266, 1992.

Momand, J., G. P. Zambetti, D. C. Olson, D. George, and A. J. Levine. The mdm-2 oncogene product forms a complex with the p53 protein and inhibits p53-mediated transactivation. *Cell* 69:1237–1245, 1992.

Monica, K., N. Galili, J. Nourse, D. Saltman, and M. L. Cleary. PBX2 and PBX3, new homeobox genes with extensive homology to the human proto-oncogene PBX1. *Mol. Cell. Biol.* 11:6149–6157, 1991.

Monica, K., D. P. LeBrun, D. A. Dedera, R. Brown, and M. L. Cleary. Transformation properties of the E2A-Pbx1 chimeric oncoprotein: fusion with E2A is essential but the Pbx1 homeodomain is dispensable. *Mol. Cell. Biol.* 14: 8304–8314, 1994.

Nelson, W. G., and M. B. Kastan. DNA strand breaks: the DNA template alterations that trigger p53-dependent DNA damage response pathways. *Mol. Cell. Biol.* 14:1815–1823, 1994.

Nervi, C., C. E. Poindexter, F. Grignani, P. P. Pandolfi, F. Lo Coco, G. Avvisati, P. G. Pelicci, and A. M. Jetten. Characterization of the PML/RARα chimeric product of the acute promyelocytic leukemia-specific t(15;17) translocation. *Cancer. Res.* 52:3687–3692, 1992.

Nisson, P. E., P. C. Watkins, and N. Sacchi. Transcriptionally active chimeric gene derived from the fusion of the AML1 gene and a novel gene on chromosome 8 in t(8;21) leukemic cells. *Cancer Genet. Cytogenet.* 63:81–88, 1992.

Nourse, J., J. D. Mellentin, N. Galili, J. Walkinson, E. Stanbridge, S. D. Smith, and M. L. Cleary. Chromosomal translocation t(1;19) results in synthesis of a homeobox fusion mRNA that codes for a potential chimeric transcription factor. *Cell* 60:535–545, 1990.

Nuchprayoon, I., S. Meyers, L. M. Scott, J. Suzow, S. Hiebert, and A. D. Friedman. PEBP2/CBF, the murine homolog of the human myeloid AML1 and PEBP2β/CBFβ proto-oncoproteins, regulates the murine myeloperoxidase and neutrophil elastase genes in immature myeloid cells. *Mol. Cell. Biol.* 14: 5558–5568, 1994.

Ogawa, E., M. Inuzuka, M. Maruyama, M. Satake, M. M. Naito-Fujimoto, Y. Ito, and K. Shigesada. Molecular cloning and characterization of PEBP2β, the heterodimeric partner of a novel Drosophila runt-related DNA binding protein PEPB2α. *Virology* 194:314–331, 1993.

Okuda, T., J. van Deursen, S. W. Hiebert, G. Grosveld, and J. R. Downing. AML1, the target of multiple chromosomal translocations in human leukemia, is essential for normal fetal liver hematopoiesis. *Cell* 84:321–330, 1996.

Oliner, J. D., K. W. Kinzler, P. S. Meltzer, D. George, and B. Vogelstein. Amplification of a gene encoding a p53-associated protein in human sarcomas. *Nature* 358:80–83, 1992.

Oliner, J. D., J. A. Pietenpol, S. Thiagalingam, J. Gyuris, K. W. Kinzler, and B. Vogelstein. Oncoprotein MDM2 conceals the activation domain of tumour suppressor p53. *Nature* 362:857–860, 1993.

Pandolfi, P. P., F. Grignani, M. Alcalay, A. Mencarelli, A. Biondi, F. Lo Coco, F. Grignani, and P. G. Pelicci. Structure and origin of the acute promyelocytic leukemia myl/RARα cDNA and characterization of its retinoid-binding and transactivation properties. *Oncogene* 6:1285–1292, 1991.

Pause, A., S. Lee, R. A. Worrell, D. Y. T. Chen, W. H. Burgess, W. M. Linehan, and R. D. Klausner. The von Hippel-Lindau tumor-suppressor gene product forms a stable complex with human CUL-2, a member of the Cdc53 family of proteins. *Proc. Natl. Acad. Sci. U.S.A.* 94:2156–2161, 1997.

Perkins, A., and S. Cory. Conditional immortalization of mouse myelomonocytic, megakaryocytic and mast cell progenitors by the Hox-2.4 homeobox gene. *EMBO J.* 12:3835–3846, 1993.

Petrij, F., R. H. Giles, H. G. Dauwerse, J. J. Saris, R. C. M. Hennekam, M. Masuno, N. Tommerup, G.-J. van Ommen, R. H. Goodman, D. J. M. Peters, and M. H. Breuning. Rubinstein-Taybi syndrome caused by mutations in the transcriptional coactivator CBP. *Nature* 376:348–351, 1995.

Pietenpol, J. A., T. Tokino, S. Thiagalingam, W. S. el-Deiry, K. W. Kinzler, and B. Vogelstein. Sequence-specific transcriptional activation is essential for growth suppression by p53. *Proc. Natl. Acad. Sci. U.S.A.* 91:1998–2002, 1994.

Prosser, H. M., D. Wotton, A. Gegonne, J. Ghysdael, S. Wang, N. A. Speck, and M. J. Owen. A novel phorbol ester response element within the human T cell receptor β enhancer. *Proc. Natl. Acad. Sci. U.S.A.* 89:9934–9938, 1992.

Prowse, A. H., A. R. Webster, F. M. Richards, S. Richard, S. Olschwang, F. Resche, N. A. Affara, and E. R. Maher. Somatic inactivation of the VHL gene in von Hippel-Lindau disease tumors. *Am. J. Hum. Genet.* 60:765–771, 1997.

Rabbitts, T. H. Chromosomal translocations in human cancer. *Nature* 372:143–149, 1994.

Raimondi, S. C., E. Privatera, D. L. Williams, A. T. Look, F. Behm, G. K. Rivera, W. M. Crist, and C.-H. Pui. New recurring chromosomal translocations in childhood acute lymphoblastic leukemia. *Blood* 77:2016–2022, 1991.

Romana, S. P., M. Mauchauffe, M. Le Coniat, I. Chumakow, D. Le Paslier, R.

Berger, and O. A. Bernard. The t(12;21) of acute lymphoblastic leukemia results in a tel-AML1 gene fusion. *Blood* 85:3662–3670, 1995.

Sakai, T., N. Ohtani, T. L. McGee, P. D. Robbins, and T. P. Dryja. Oncogenic germ-line mutations in Sp1 and ATF sites in the human retinoblastoma gene. *Nature* 353:83–86, 1991.

Scheffner, M., B. A. Werness, H. Huibregtse, A. J. Levine, and P. M. Howley. The E6 oncoprotein encoded by human papillomavirus types 16 and 18 promotes the degradation of p53. *Cell* 63:1129–1136, 1990.

Shapiro, D. N., J. E. Sublett, B. Li, J. R. Downing, and C. W. Naeve. Fusion of PAX3 to a member of the forkhead family of transcription factors in human alveolar rhabdomyosarcoma. *Cancer Res.* 53:5108–5112, 1993.

Shaulian, E., A. Zauberman, D. Ginsberg, and M. Oren. Identification of a minimal transforming domain of p53: negative dominance through abrogation of sequence-specific DNA binding. *Mol. Cell. Biol.* 12:5581–5592, 1992.

Sherr, C. J. Cancer cell cycles. *Science* 274:1672–1677, 1996.

Shivdasani, R. A., E. L. Mayer, and S. H. Orkin. Absence of blood formation in mice lacking the T-cell leukaemia oncoprotein tal-1/SCL. *Nature* 373:432–434, 1995.

Shurtleff, S. A., S. Meyers, S. W. Hiebert, S. C. Raimondi, D. R. Head, C. L. Wilman, S. Wolman, M. L. Slovak, A. J. Carroll, F. Behm, et al. Heterogeneity in CBFB/MYH11 fusion messages encoded by the inv(16)(p13;q22) and the t(16;16)(p13;q22) in acute myeologenous leukemia. *Blood* 85:3695–3703, 1995.

Slansky, J. E., and P. J. Farnham. Introduction to the E2F family: protein structure and gene regulation. *Curr. Top. Microbiol. Immunol.* 208:1–30, 1996.

Spencer, C. A., and M. Groudine. Control of c-myc regulation in normal and neoplastic cells. *Adv. Cancer Res.* 56:1–47, 1991.

Spencer, T. E., G. Jenster, M. M. Burcin, C. D. Allis, J. Zhou, C. A. Mizzen, N. J. McKenna, S. A. Onate, S. Y. Tsai, M. J. Tsai, and B. W. O'Malley. Steroid receptor coactivator-1 is a histone acetyltransferase. *Nature* 389:194–198, 1997.

Strong, L. C., M. Stine, and T. L. Norsted. Cancer in survivors of childhood soft tissue sarcoma and their relatives. *J. Natl. Cancer Inst.* 79:1213–1220, 1987.

Swafford, D. S., S. K. Middleton, W. A. Palmisano, K. J. Nikula, J. Tesfaigzi, S. B. Baylin, J. G. Herman, and S. A. Belinsky. Frequent aberrant methylation of p16^{INK4a} in primary rat lung tumors. *Mol. Cell. Biol.* 17:1366–1374, 1997.

Takahashi, A., M. Satake, Y. Yamaguchi-Iwai, S.-C. Bae, J. Lu, M. Maruyama, Y. W. Zhang, H. Oka, N. Arai, K. Arai, and Y. Ito. Positive and negative regulation of granulocyte-macrophage colony-stimulating factor (GM-CSF) promoter activity by AML1-related transcription factor, PEBP2. *Blood* 86:607–616, 1995.

Thut, C. J., J. L. Chen, R. Klemin, and R. Tjian. p53 transcriptional activation mediated by coactivators TAF$_{II}$40 and TAF$_{II}$60. *Science* 267:100–104, 1995.

Trouche, D., C. Le Chalony, C. Muchardt, M. Yaniv, and T. Kouzarides. RB and hbrm cooperate to repress the activation functions of E2F1. *Proc. Natl. Acad. Sci. U.S.A.* 94:11268–11273, 1997.

Ueda, H., S. J. Ullrich, J. D. Gangemi, C. A. Kappel, L. Ngo, M. A. Feitelson, and G. Jay. Functional inactivation but not structural mutation of p53 causes liver cancer. *Nat. Genet.* 9:41–44, 1995.

Van Dijk, M. A., and C. Murre. Extradenticle raises the DNA-binding specificity of homeotic selector gene products. *Cell* 78:617–624, 1994.

Vaupel, P., F. Kallinowski, and P. Okunieff. Blood flow, oxygen and nutrient supply, and metabolic microenvironment of human tumors: a review. *Cancer Res.* 49:6449–6465, 1989.

Versteeg, R. Aberrant methylation in cancer. *Am. J. Hum. Genet.* 60:751–754, 1997.

Vogelstein, B., and K. W. Kinzler. p53 function and dysfunction. *Cell* 70:523–526, 1992.

Wang, Q., T. Stacy, M. Binder, M. Marin-Padilla, A. H. Sharpe, and N. A. Speck. Disruption of the Cbfa2 gene causes necrosis and hemorrhaging in the central nervous system and blocks definitive hematopoiesis. *Proc. Natl. Acad. Sci. U.S.A.* 93:3444–3449, 1996a.

Wang, Q., T. Stacy, J. D. Miller, A. F. Lewis, T.-L. Gu, X. Huang, J. H. Bushweller, J.-C. Bories, F. W. Alt, G. Ryan, P. P. Liu, A. Wynshaw-Boris, M. Binder, M. Marin-Padilla, A. H. Sharpe, and N. A. Speck. The CBFβ subunit is essential for CBFα2 (AML1) function in vivo. *Cell* 87:697–708, 1996b.

Wang, S., Q. Wang, B. E. Crute, I. N. Melnikova, S. R. Keller, and N. A. Speck. Cloning and characterization of subunits of the T-cell receptor and murine leukemia virus enhancer core-binding factor. *Mol. Cell. Biol.* 13:3324–3339, 1993.

Wang, X. W., K. Forrester, H. Yeh, M. A. Feitelson, J.-R Gu, and C. C. Harris. Hepatitis B virus X protein inhibits p53 sequence-specific DNA binding, transcriptional activity and association with transcription factor ERCC 3. *Proc. Natl. Acad. Sci. U.S.A.* 91:2230–2234, 1994.

Weinberg, R. A. The retinoblastoma protein and cell cycle control. *Cell* 81:323–330, 1995.

Weintraub, S. J., K. N. B. Chow, R. X. Luo, S. H. Zhang, S. He, and D. C. Dean. Mechanism of active transcriptional repression by the retinoblastoma protein. *Nature* 375:812–815, 1995.

Weintraub, S. J., C. A. Prater, and D. C. Dean. Retinoblastoma protein switches the E2F site from positive to negative element. *Nature* 358:259–261, 1992.

Whyte, P., K. J. Buchkovich, J. M. Horowitz, S. H. Friend, M. Raybuck, R. A. Weinberg, and E. Harlow. Association between an oncogene and an anti-oncogene: the adenovirus E1A proteins bind to the retinoblastoma gene product. *Nature* 334:124–129, 1988.

Wijmenga, C., P. E. Gregory, A. Hajra, E. Schrock, T. Ried, R. Eils, P. P. Liu, and F. S. Collins. Core binding factor β-smooth muscle myosin heavy chain chimeric protein involved in acute myeloid leukemia forms unusual nuclear rod-like structures in transformed NIH 3T3 cells. *Proc. Natl. Acad. Sci. U.S.A.* 93:1630–1635, 1996.

Williams, B. O., L. Remington, D. M. Albert, S. Mukai, R. T. Bronson, and T. Jacks. Cooperative tumorigenic effects of germline mutations in Rb and p53. *Nat. Genet.* 7:480–484, 1994.

Xia, Y., L. Brown, C. Y. Yang, J. T. Tsan, M. J. Siciliano, R. Espinosa III, M. M. Le Beau, and R. J. Baer. TAL2, a helix-loop-helix gene activated by the (7; 9)(q34;q32) translocation in human T-cell leukemia. *Proc. Natl. Acad. Sci. U.S.A.* 88:11416–11420, 1991.

Xiong, Y., G. J. Hannon, G. J. Zhang, D. Casso, R. Kobayashi, and D. Beach. p21 is a universal inhibitor of cyclin kinases. *Nature* 366:701–704, 1993.

Yamasaki, L., T. Jacks, R. Bronson, E. Goillot, E. Harlow, and N. J. Dyson. Tumor induction and tissue atrophy in mice lacking E2F-1. *Cell* 85:537–548, 1996.

Yang, X.-J., V. V. Ogryzko, J.-i. Nishikawa, B. H. Howard, and Y. Nakatani. A p300/CBP-associated factor that competes with the adenoviral oncoprotein E1A. *Nature* 382:319–324, 1996.

Yergeau, D. A., C. J. Hetherington, Q. Wang, P. Zhang, A. H. Sharpe, M. Binder, M. Marin-Padilla, D. G. Tenen, N. A. Speck, and D.-E. Zhang. Embryonic lethality and impairment of hematopoiesis in mice heterozygous for an AML1-ETO fusion gene. *Nat. Genet.* 5:303–306, 1997.

Yew, P. R., and A. J. Berk. Inhibition of p53 transactivation required for transformation by adenovirus early 1B protein. *Nature* 357:82–85, 1992.

Yoshihara, T., T. Inaba, L. H. Shapiro, J.-Y. Kato, and A. T. Look. E2A-HLF-mediated cell transformation requires both the trans-activation domains of E2A and the leucine zipper dimerization domain of HLF. *Mol. Cell. Biol.* 15: 3247–3255, 1995.

Zhang, D. E., C. J. Heterington, S. Meyers, K. L. Rhoades, C. J. Larson, H. M. Chen, S. W. Hiebert, and D. G. Tenen. CCAAT enhancer-binding protein (C/EBP) and AML1 (CBFa2) synergistically activate the macrophage colony-stimulating factor receptor promoter. *Mol. Cell. Biol.* 16:1231–1240, 1996.

Zhuang, Y., P. Soriano, and H. Weintraub. The helix-loop-helix gene E2A is required for B cell formation. *Cell* 79:875–884, 1994.

Epigenetic Disease: **16**
Teratogenesis

In contrast to germline mutations, which are hereditable and result in malformation syndromes, and somatic mutations, which are nonhereditable and contribute to oncogenesis, teratogenesis can be viewed as resulting from changes in gene expression that are induced by *in utero* exposure of the developing embryo to an exogenous compound or to increased amounts of an endogenous compound. This differs from the traditional view of teratogenesis as representing the effect of toxins that cause cell death. Although teratogens undoubtedly cause cell death, they may do so not by nonspecific toxic effects on cellular metabolism but by activating specific genetic pathways that lead to an active form of cell death, termed apoptosis, which is an essential process of normal development. Teratogenic exposure of mouse embryos to ethanol or retinoic acid (RA) results in an increased area and density of dying cells at sites of developmentally programmed cell death (Kotch and Sulik, 1992a, b; Sulik et al., 1988). In this chapter, evidence will be presented indicating that the effects of two well-studied teratogens, retinoic acid and ethanol, may be mediated by specific changes in gene expression.

Retinoic Acid Embryopathy

Retinoic Acid as a Developmental Morphogen and Teratogen

An extensive body of research spanning over half of a century indicates a key role for retinoic acid in a wide variety of developmental processes. Either excess or inadequate retinoic acid levels have profound effects on developing tissues (Kochar et al., 1973; Warkany and Nelson, 1940). For example, placement of a retinoic acid–soaked bead in the anterior aspect of the developing chick limb bud resulted in a dramatic mirror-image duplication of the distal limb (Tickle et al., 1982). These results and subsequent studies have indicated that retinoic acid plays a key role in establishing the anterior-posterior axis of the developing limb bud via its endogenous expression within the zone of polarizing activity in the posterior limb bud (reviewed by Tabin, 1995). However, when retinoic acid is present at high levels throughout the limb bud, deficiencies rather than duplications of structures result (Tickle et al., 1985). In addition to dosage-dependence, the teratogen effects of retinoic acid are also temporally defined. Limb malformations are observed only when mouse embryos are exposed to retinoic acid between embryonic day (E)10.5 and E11.5, the stage at which the limb bud is developing (Kochar et al., 1973).

Human Retinoic Acid Embryopathy

In 1982, isotretinoin (13-*cis* retinoic acid) was introduced for the treatment of cystic acne under the brand name Accutane. Because of the known teratogenicity of retinoids, Accutane was labeled as a Category X medication contraindicated for use during pregnancy. This contraindication implies a knowledge of the pregnancy status of each patient to whom drug administration is under consideration and such was not the case at its introduction and for several years thereafter. As a result, a significant proportion of children born after *in utero* exposure to 13-*cis* retinoic acid were found to have major developmental malformations. In a landmark study of 154 pregnancies at risk due to maternal isotretinoin intake of 0.5 to 1.0 mg/kg/d, the outcomes were 95 elective abortions, 12 spontaneous abortions, 21 infants with major malformations (12 of whom were stillborn or died in the perinatal period), and 26 infants without major malformations (Lammer et al., 1985). Malformations involved craniofacial (microtia/anotia, micrognathia, and cleft palate), cardiac (conotruncal heart defects and aortic arch anomalies), thymic, and central nervous system defects that were similar to those previously described in animal models of retinoid embryopathy. Embryonic exposure to isotretinoin was associated with a 25-fold increased risk of developing one of the major malformations described above (Lammer et al., 1985). Craniofacial, cardiac, thymic and CNS structures all require the contribution of cephalic neural crest cells for normal development. Exposure of chick, hamster, and mouse embryos to high levels of vitamin A or retinoic acid resulted in deficiencies of cephalic neural crest cells within the hindbrain and branchial arches (Hassell et al., 1977; Keith, 1977; Poswillo, 1975; Sulik et al., 1988; Wiley et al., 1983).

Influence of Retinoic Acid on Hox *Gene Expression in Mouse Embryos*

Exposure of mouse teratocarcinoma cells to retinoic acid was shown to induce expression of *Hox* genes and the concentration of retinoic acid required for induction of a particular gene depended on its position within the gene cluster (Breier et al., 1986). Treatment of *Xenopus* embryos with retinoic acid and growth factors led to the induction of *Hox* gene expression (Cho and De Robertis, 1991). Because both retinoic acid and *Hox* genes are known to play key roles in establishing the body plan, it was reasonable to hypothesize that retinoic acid might exert teratogenic effects by altering *Hox* gene expression.

To test this hypothesis, pregnant female mice were administered all-*trans* retinoic acid at a dose of 10 mg per kilogram of body weight or 13-*cis* retinoic acid at a dose of 450 mg/kg on E8.5 (Kessel and Gruss, 1991). These represent very high doses compared to the 0.5 to 1.0 mg/kg/d intake of pregnant women that caused human retinoic acid embryopathy. In this study, the effect of retinoid exposure on the development of the vertebral column was analyzed. The *Hox* genes are expressed in an overlapping pattern in the vertebral column. As described in Chapter 9, genes at the 5' end of the *Hox* clusters are expressed posteriorly whereas genes at the 3' end are expressed more anteriorly (Fig. 16.1).

Mouse embryos exposed to retinoic acid on E7 were found to have abnormalities in the specification of the vertebral column. In wild-type embryos, 7 cervical, 13 thoracic, and 6 lumbar vertebrae were found, whereas some retinoic acid–exposed embryos contained only 6 cervical or 5 lumbar vertebrae. Analysis of the vertebrae suggested that some vertebrae had taken on the identities of more anteriorly placed structures (a so-called anterior transformation). In addition, *in situ* hybridization revealed that in retinoic acid–treated embryos the expression of individual *Hox* genes was shifted anteriorly (Kessel and Gruss, 1991). These results suggest that (1) the pattern of *Hox* gene expression ("Hox code") determines the identity of individual vertebrae and (2) retinoic acid exposure alters the pattern of *Hox* gene expression and thus vertebral identity. At E8.5, a different pattern of malformations was seen, as retinoic acid–exposed embryos contained 14 or 15 thoracic vertebrae and in some cases only 5 lumbar vertebrae. In these embryos, analysis of the vertebral columns suggested that RA exposure had resulted in posterior transformations. Thus, the precise teratogenic effect of RA appeared to be time-dependent, although a difference due to the administration of 13-*cis* retinoic acid as opposed to all-*trans* retinoic acid was not excluded, nor was the rationale for using two different drugs provided. Since all-*trans* and

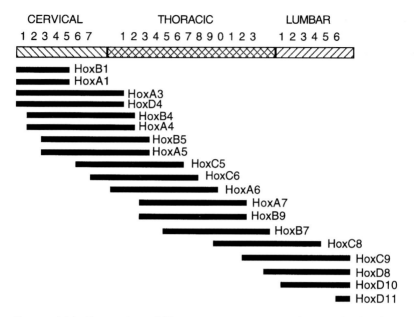

FIGURE 16-1. Expression of *Hox* gene expression in the vertebral column. The approximate location of expression of selected *Hox* genes in the developing cervical, thoracic, and lumbar vertebrae is shown. (Based on data summarized by Kessel and Gruss, 1991.)

9-*cis* retinoic have subsequently been shown to have different biological properties by serving as ligands for the retinoic acid receptors (RARα, RARβ, and RARγ) and retinoid X receptors (RXRα, RXRβ, and RXRγ), respectively (reviewed by Linney, 1992), it would also be important to know whether 13-*cis* retinoic acid is metabolized to all-*trans* or 9-*cis* retinoic acid. It is also interesting to note that the interpretation of the teratogenic effects of retinoic acid presented in this landmark paper was based exclusively on changes in gene expression affecting cellular identity and that the role, if any, of apoptosis in this process was not discussed.

Role of RARγ in Retinoic Acid Embryopathy

The biological effects of retinoids are believed to be mediated by binding to RAR/RXR heterodimers that function as ligand-activated transcription factors (see Chapter 6). Analysis of mice homozygous for a null mutation in the gene encoding RARγ manifested minor skeletal malformations (Lohnes et al., 1993). The relative minor degree of malformation associated with loss of RARγ function suggested functional overlap with RARα and RARβ, a hypothesis that was confirmed by the more severe phenotypes of RAR double-mutant mice (Lohnes et al., 1994; Mendelsohn et al., 1994). The most remarkable aspect of the phenotype of RARγ$^{-/-}$ mice was the effect of retinoic acid on vertebral column development. When wild-type embryos were exposed to a maternal retinoic acid dose of 100 mg/kg at E8.5, a striking caudal regression syndrome was noted in which the vertebral column was truncated near the thoracolumbar junction with complete aplasia of the lumbar, sacral, and caudal segments. This loss of segments cannot be easily explained by a Hox code model and obviously involves increased cell death associated with the much higher dose of retinoic acid used compared to the previous study.

In contrast to wild-type mice, RARγ$^{-/-}$ embryos were resistant to the teratogenic effects of retinoic acid, and RARγ$^{+/-}$ mice manifested a phenotype that was intermediate between RARγ$^{-/-}$ and RARγ$^{+/+}$ mice (Lohnes et al., 1993). These results demonstrate that the teratogenic effects of retinoic acid on vertebral development are mediated by RARγ. In contrast, the teratogenic effects of retinoic acid on craniofacial and limb development were not affected by the RARγ genotype, suggesting that either RARα or RARβ mediated these effects. There also appears to be specificity with respect to the RXR partner because mice lacking expression of RXRα were resistant to the teratogenic effects of retinoic acid on limb development (Sucov et al., 1995). The gene-dosage sensitivity of the resistance phenomenon suggests that the risk for, and severity of, retinoic acid embryopathy is determined by both the amount, timing, and duration of retinoic acid exposure as well as the expression level of each RAR and RXR in different developing tissues, which invokes another level of genetic control and of genetic predisposition to teratogen-induced malformations. These studies thus provide important insights into the mechanisms by which a teratogen can disrupt normal development. Whether this model will also apply to teratogens such as ethanol that have no known endogenous role in development remains to be determined. However, the basic principle that teratogens affect development through changes in gene expression is an appealing hypothesis to guide further investigation in this area.

Ethanol Embryopathy

Human Fetal Alcohol Syndrome

The adverse effects of ethanol on human development have been appreciated since Biblical times, as evidenced by the following passage from

Judges 13:7: "Behold thou shalt conceive, and bear a son; and now drink no wine or strong drink." Ethanol can pass freely across the placenta from the maternal to fetal circulation and exert its teratogenic effects, resulting in retarded somatic and central nervous system growth, abnormalities of craniofacial development, and increased risk of cardiac, genitourinary, and skeletal malformations (reviewed by Clarren and Smith, 1978; Streissguth et al., 1980). The phenotype of the fetal alcohol syndrome (Table 16.1) is extremely variable, presumably reflecting differences in the timing, duration, and intensity of the teratogenic exposure as well as other environmental and/or genetic factors. Chronic ingestion of at least 89 ml of ethanol per day (approximately six drinks) has been established as constituting a major risk for teratogenesis (National Institute of Alcohol Abuse and Alcoholism, 1977). It remains controversial whether there is a threshold effect or whether in fact ethanol exposure represents a graded risk to the developing fetus. It is clear, however, that maternal ethanol abuse is the most common teratogenic cause of mental retardation in the Western world (Clarren and Smith, 1978), given that an estimated 1 in 750 live-born infants in the United States are affected by the fetal alcohol syndrome (Streissguth et al., 1980).

Investigation of Teratogenic Mechanisms in Mouse Models of Fetal Alcohol Syndrome

Exposure of mouse embryos to ethanol results in malformations similar to those observed in humans (reviewed by Sulik et al., 1988). The teratogenic effects of ethanol vary with the timing of the exposure. When

TABLE 16.1. Cardinal features of the fetal alcohol syndrome

Affected Process	>80% of Patients	>50% of Patients
Central nervous system development	Mild to moderate retardation Microcephaly Irritability in infancy	Poor coordination Hypotonia Hyperactivity in childhood
Body growth (prenatal/postnatal)	Length and weight >2 SD below mean for age	Decreased adipose tissue
Craniofacial development	Short palpebral fissures Hypoplastic philtrum Thin upper vermillion Hypoplastic mandible	Short, upturned nose Hypoplastic maxilla

Data from Clarren and Smith, 1978.

pregnant female mice were given two intraperitoneal injections of ethanol at a dose of 4 mL/kg body weight on day 8 of gestation (E8), increased cell death was observed in specific regions of the developing
embryos (Kotch and Sulik, 1992b). Two aspects of this cell death were
particularly interesting. First, the cell death occurred in those areas of
the embryo in which malformations would ultimately occur, including
exencephaly, bilateral or unilateral cleft lip, maxillary hypoplasia, and
median facial cleft. Second, in ethanol-exposed embryos, the areas of cell
death specifically coincided with areas of normally occurring developmentally programmed cell death. These results suggest that the teratogenic effects of ethanol are due to the dysregulation of a normal developmental program.

As described in Chapter 9, the malformations observed in ethanol-
exposed embryos are very similar to those observed in mice transgenic
for the human *MSX2* gene (Winograd et al., 1997). Furthermore, in chick
embryos, *msx2* expression is associated with programmed cell death of
cranial neural crest cells (progenitors of all craniofacial structures) in the
hindbrain rhombomeres (Graham et al., 1994). These results led to the
hypothesis that ethanol and retinoic acid may exert their teratogenic effects by increasing expression of MSX2 in cranial neural crest cells. Increased MSX2 would cause increased cell death and craniofacial malformations would then result from a deficiency of cranial neural crest cells
(Winograd et al., 1997).

Mouse embryos were exposed to ethanol on E8 and then analyzed
on E11–11.5 for the presence of malformations and expression of *Msx2*
(Rifas et al., 1997). The ethanol-exposed mice exhibited multiple craniofacial malformations as previously described. In contrast to control embryos, which demonstrated *Msx2* expression in a wide variety of developing craniofacial structures, *Msx2* expression could not be detected at
all in the ethanol-exposed embryos. The investigators concluded that ethanol inhibited *Msx2* expression (Rifas et al., 1997). However, the opposite
conclusion, that ethanol exposure was associated with increased *Msx2*
expression, is not excluded by the data presented, because increased
Msx2 expression may have resulted in the death of *Msx2*-expressing cells
so that, 3 days later, no *Msx2* expression would be detected. Because
increased cell death was detected within 12 hours after ethanol administration (Kotch and Sulik, 1992b), it will be essential to analyze *Msx2*
expression during this early time period. Regardless of the outcome of
such studies, the reported data are consistent with the hypothesis that
ethanol exerts its teratogenic effects through the dysregulation of a transcription factor that plays a key role in craniofacial development by controlling the number of progenitor neural crest cells.

Neural Tube Defects and Folic Acid

Whereas excessive intake of certain bioactive molecules such as ethanol or retinoic acid can lead to developmental defects, deficient intake of essential compounds can also have a deleterious effect on embryogenesis. For example, maternal vitamin A deficiency results in a variety of malformations (Warkany and Nelson, 1940; Wilson and Barch, 1949; Wilson et al., 1953). Recently, a deficiency of folic acid was implicated as a contributing factor in the pathogenesis of the neural tube defects myelomeningocele (spinal bifida), encephalocele, and anencephaly. Administration of folic acid to women before and during pregnancy significantly reduced the incidence of offspring with neural tube defects compared to an untreated control population in multiple studies (Czeizel and Dudas, 1992; MRC Vitamin Study Research Group, 1991; Smithells et al., 1989). As a result, the Food and Drug Administration will require the fortification of enriched grain foods with folic acid beginning in 1998, and specific recommendations regarding folate intake have been published (American College of Medical Genetics, 1997). A study of 440 pairs of monozygotic twins and 331 pairs of dizygotic twins indicated that 46% of the variance in red blood cell folate levels in these adult females was caused by genetic factors, whereas less than 20% of the variance was considered to be the result of environmental factors, including diet (Mitchell et al., 1997). From these results it is reasonable to conclude that different females may require different levels of folate intake in order to prevent neural tube defects.

Neural tube defects occur with an incidence of approximately 1 per 1000 live births (Edmonds and James, 1990) and represent a category of malformations consisting of multiple specific subtypes (as described above), each of which is likely to have multiple contributing genetic and environmental factors. The mouse *Cart1* gene was shown to encode a homeodomain protein that is expressed in the developing head beginning on embryonic day 9.5. In knockout mice lacking *Cart1* expression, forebrain mesenchymal cells undergo apoptosis and the deficiency of these cells results in abnormal neural tube formation and anencephaly, the most severe neural tube defect (Zhao et al., 1996). Whereas all homozygous mutant mice exhibited anencephaly on a strain 129/SvEv inbred genetic background, only 65% of homozygotes on a C57BL/6 X 129 hybrid background were anencephalic, demonstrating effects of modifier loci elsewhere in the genome. Because of the striking similarity between the phenotype of *Cart1*-mutant mice and human anencephaly, the homozygotes (on the strain 129 inbred genetic background) were treated with folic acid during the first half of gestation. Remarkably, only 3 of

16 (19%) treated homozygotes developed anencephaly compared to 100% in the absence of folate supplementation (Zhao et al., 1996). The *Cart1*-mutant mice thus provide an interesting model for studying neural tube defects, as they demonstrate the effects of both multiple genes and environmental factors on disease incidence, and may provide a means to understand the protective effects of folic acid—which will, it is hoped, result in a dramatic reduction in the incidence of neural tube defects. The new recommendations may bring even greater joy: some, but not all, studies suggest that multivitamin supplementation may increase the incidence of multiple births (Werler et al., 1997).

Closing Thoughts

Transcriptional regulation represents a fundamental mechanism underlying development and homeostasis. Disruption of transcription factor functioning by germline mutation, somatic mutation, or by the epigenetic effects of environmental agents provides the pathophysiological basis for a significant proportion of human congenital malformation syndromes ("birth defects") and cancer, major causes of infant and adult mortality, respectively. Mutations in *cis*-acting transcription factor binding sites, as well as *trans*-acting factors, are also likely to contribute to more subtle alterations in gene expression that nevertheless play an important role in determining the development of birth defects as well as susceptibility to common multifactorial diseases of adulthood, including asthma, cancer, cardiovascular disease, diabetes, osteoporosis, and neuropsychiatric disorders. In these multifactorial disorders, environmental factors are likely to interact with genetic factors to further influence disease susceptibility. A more complete understanding of these complex processes will hopefully lead to a greater integration of molecular biology and clinical medicine and will provide a foundation for developing more effective approaches to disease prevention and treatment. The power and promise associated with the ever-accelerating accumulation of scientific knowledge provide great excitement and hope for the future.

References

American College of Medical Genetics. *Statement on Folic Acid: Fortification and Supplementation.* American College of Medical Genetics, Bethesda, Maryland, 1997.

Breier, G., M. Bucan, U. Francke, A. M. Colberg-Poley, and P. Gruss. Sequential expression of murine homeobox genes during F9 EC cell differentiation. EMBO J. 5:2209–2215, 1986.

Cho, K W. Y., and E. M. De Robertis. Differential activation of Xenopus homeobox genes by mesoderm-inducing growth factors and retinoic acid. *Genes Dev.* 4:1910–1916, 1991.

Clarren, S. K., and D. W. Smith. The fetal alcohol syndrome. *N. Engl. J. Med.* 298: 1063–1067, 1978.

Czeizel, A. E., and I. Dudas. Prevention of the first occurrence of neural-tube defects by periconceptional vitamin supplementation. *N. Engl. J. Med.* 327: 1832–1835, 1992.

Edmonds, L. D., and L. M. James. Temporal trends in the prevalence of congenital malformations at birth based on the birth defects monitoring program, United States, 1979–1987. *MMWR CDC Surveill. Summ.* 39:19–23, 1990.

Graham, A., P. Francis-West, P. Brickell, and A. Lumsden. The signaling molecule BMP4 mediates apoptosis in the rhombencephalic neural crest. *Nature* 372: 684–686, 1994.

Hassell, J. R., J. H. Greenberg, and M. C. Johnston. Inhibition of cranial neural crest cell development by vitamin A in the cultured chick embryo. *J. Embryol. Exp. Morphol.* 39:267–271, 1977.

Keith, J. Effects of excess vitamin A on the cranial neural crest in the chick embryo. *Ann. R. Coll. Surg.* 59:479–483, 1977.

Kessel, M., and P. Gruss. Homeotic transformations of murine vertebrae and concomitant alteration of Hox codes induced by retinoic acid. *Cell* 67:89–104, 1991.

Kochar, D. M. Limb development in mouse embryos: I. Analysis of teratogenic effects of retinoic acid. *Teratology* 7:289–299, 1973.

Kotch, L. E., and K. K. Sulik. Experimental fetal alcohol syndrome: proposed pathogenic basis for a variety of associated fetal and brain anomalies. *Am. J. Med. Genet.* 44:168–176, 1992a.

Kotch, L. E., and K. K. Sulik. Patterns of ethanol-induced cell death in the developing nervous system of mice: neural fold states through the time of anterior neural tube closure. *Int. J. Dev. Neuroscience* 10:273–279, 1992b.

Lammer, E. J., D. T. Chen, R. H. Hoar, N. D. Agnish, P. J. Benke, J. T. Braun, C. J. Curry, P. M. Fernhoff, A. W. Grix, Jr., I. T. Lott, J. M. Richard, and S. C. Sun. Retinoic acid embryopathy. *N. Engl. J. Med.* 313:837–841, 1985.

Linney, E. Retinoic acid receptors: transcription factors modulating gene regulation, development, and differentiation. *Curr. Topics Dev. Biol.* 27:305–350, 1992.

Lohnes, D., P. Kastner, A. Dierich, M. Mark, M. LeMeur, and P. Chambon. Function of the retinoic acid receptor γ in the mouse. *Cell* 73:643–658, 1993.

Lohnes, D., M. Mark, C. Mendelsohn, P. Dolle, A. Dierich, P. Gorry, A. Gansmuller, and P. Chambon. Function of the retinoic acid receptors (RARs) during development: (I) Craniofacial and skeletal abnormalities in RAR double mutants. *Development* 120:2723–2748, 1994.

Mendelsohn, C., D. Lohnes, D. Decimo, T. Lufkin, M. LeMeur, P. Chambon, and M. Mark. Function of the retinoic acid receptors (RARs) during development: (II) Multiple abnormalities at various stages of organogenesis in RAR double mutants. *Development* 120:2749–2771, 1994.

Mitchell, L. E., D. L. Duffy, P. Duffy, G. Bellingham, and N. G. Martin. Genetic effects on variation in red-blood-cell folate in adults: implications for the familial aggregation of neural tube defects. *Am. J. Hum. Genet.* 60:433–438, 1997.

MRC Vitamin Study Research Group. Prevention of neural tube defects: results of the Medical Research Council Vitamin Study. *Lancet* 338:131–137, 1991.

National Institute of Alcohol Abuse and Alcoholism. *Critical Review of the Fetal Alcohol Syndrome.* Alcohol, Drug Abuse, and Mental Health Administration, Rockville, Maryland, 1977.

Poswillo, D. The pathogenesis of the Treacher Collins syndrome (mandibulofacial dysostosis). *Br. J. Oral Surg.* 13:1–26, 1975.

Rifas, L., D. A. Towler, and L. V. Avioli. Gestational exposure to ethanol suppresses msx2 expression in developing mouse embryos. *Proc. Natl. Acad. Sci. U.S.A.* 94:7549–7554, 1997.

Smithells, R. W., S. Sheppard, J. Wild, and C. J. Schorah. Prevention of neural tube defect recurrences in Yorkshire: final report. *Lancet* 2:498–499, 1989.

Streissguth, A. P., S. Landesman-Dwyer, J. C. Martin, and D. W. Smith. Teratogenic effects of alcohol in humans and laboratory animals. *Science* 209:353–361, 1980.

Sucov, H. M., J.-C. Izpixua-Belmonte, Y. Ganan, and R. M. Evans. Mouse embryos lacking RXRα are resistant to retinoic-acid-induced limb defects. *Development* 121:3997–4003, 1995.

Sulik, K. K., C. S. Cook, and W. S. Webster. Teratogens and craniofacial malformations: relationships to cell death. *Development* 103 (Suppl.):213–232, 1988.

Tabin, C. The initiation of the limb bud: growth factors, Hox genes, and retinoids. *Cell* 80:671–674, 1995.

Tickle, C., B. Alberts, L. Wolpert, and J. Lee. Local application of retinoic acid to the limb bud mimics the action of the polarizing region. *Nature* 296:564–566, 1982.

Tickle, C., J. Lee, and G. Eichele. A quantitative analysis of the effect of all-transretinoic acid on the pattern of chick wing development. *Dev. Biol.* 109:82–95, 1985.

Warkany, J., and R. C. Nelson. Appearance of skeletal abnormalities in the offspring of rats reared on a deficient diet. *Science* 92:383–384, 1940.

Werler, M. M., J. D. Cragan, C. R. Wasserman, G. M. Shaw, J. D. Erickson, and A. A. Mitchell. Multivitamin supplementation and multiple births. *Am. J. Med. Genet.* 71:93–96, 1997.

Wiley, M. J., P. Cauwenbergs, and I. M. Taylor. Effects of retinoic acid on the development of the facial skeleton in hamsters: early changes involving cranial neural crest cells. *Acta Anat* (Basel) 116:180–192, 1983.

Wilson, J. G., and S. Barch. Fetal death and maldevelopment resulting from maternal vitamin A deficiency in the rat. *Proc. Soc. Exp. Biol. Med.* 72:687–693, 1949.

Wilson, J. G., C. B. Roth, and J. Warkany. An analysis of the syndrome of malformations induced by maternal vitamin A deficiency: Effects of restoration of vitamin A at various times during gestation. *Am. J. Anat.* 92:189–217, 1953.

Winograd, J., M. P. Reilly, R. Roe, J. Lutz, E. Laughner, X. Xu, L. Hu, T. Asakura, C. vander Kolk, J. D. Strandberg, and G. L. Semenza. Perinatal lethality and multiple craniofacial malformations in *MSX2* transgenic mice. *Hum. Mol. Genet.* 6:369–379, 1997.

Zhao, Q., R. R. Behringer, and B. de Crombrugghe. Prenatal folic acid treatment suppresses acrania and meroanencephaly in mice mutant for the Cart1 homeobox gene. *Nat. Genet.* 13:275–283, 1996.

Index

ABD-A, ABD-B, 57, 324
Accutane, 348
Acetyltransferase activity. *See* Histone
Activators. *See* Trans-acting factors
ADA genes, 74
Adenovirus, 64
Adrenal hypoplasia congenita, 144–146
Adrenocorticotropic hormone (ACTH), 263
Agouti, 179
AHR, 52, 68–69
AIDS, 54
Albumin gene, 34–35, 283
Alcohol dehydrogenase genes, 30
Alternative splicing, 70, 158, 200
Alternative translation initiation, 70
Amino acid codes, 128 *table*
AML1, 329–331
Androgen receptor (AR), 118, 129–130, 132–138, 234
Aniridia, 155, 156, 171 *table*, 183–185
Anophthalmia, 171 *table*, 184
anterior digit deformity, 161
Anti-mullerian hormone (AMH), 249. *See also* Mullerian inhibiting substance
ANTP, 57
AP-1, 48–49, 51, 54, 55, 84–87, 202. *See also* C-FOS, C-JUN
APC, 67
Apert syndrome, 208
Apoptosis, 215–216, 220–221, 313, 315, 327, 347, 350, 354
Architectural transcription factors, 66–67, 249
ARNT, 51–52, 68
ARNT-2, 52

ATF family, 49–50, 66
Atherogenesis, 54
ATPase activity, 75–76
    DNA-dependent, 15, 291, 302–304
ATR-X syndrome, 290–293

B lymphocytes, 62, 64–65, 277–278, 323–325
BAFs. *See* BRG-1
Bare lymphocyte syndrome, 277–279
BEAF-32, 39
bHLH. *See* Helix-loop-helix
bHLH-ZIP, 51, 70–72, 199–205
BICOID, 60–62
BOB-1, 65
Bone morphogenetic protein 4 (BMP4), 216
Boundary elements, 38–39
Brachyury, 272
Branchial arches, 215, 221
BRG-1, 75–76
    associated factors, 76
BRN4, 261
Bromodomain, 64
Burkitt's lymphoma, 321–322
bZIP. *See* Leucine zipper

C/EBP, 30, 117–118
C-FOS, 35, 48, 54, 63, 69–70, 77, 84, 202
C-JUN, 48, 54, 63, 69–70, 77, 84
C-MYB, 63
C-MYC, 35, 51, 70–71, 73, 82, 312, 321–322, 325
C-RAF, 83–84
CIIA, 278
Calcineurin, 56